D0839483

Hearts of Wisdom

Hearts of Wisdom:

American Women Caring for Kin, 1850–1940

EMILY K. ABEL

HARVARD UNIVERSITY PRESS

Cambridge, Massachusetts
London, England   2000

To Rick, Laura, Sarah, and Heather

Library of Congress Cataloging-in-Publication Data

Abel, Emily K.
   Hearts of wisdom : American women caring for kin, 1850–1940 /
Emily K. Abel.
      p. cm.
   Includes bibliographical references and index.
   ISBN 0-674-00314-4
   1. Caregivers—United States—History—19th century.   2. Caregivers—
United States—History—20th century.   3. Medical personnel-caregiver
relationships—United States—History—19th century.   4. Medical
personnel-caregiver relationships—United States—History—20th century.
5. Women—United States—Social conditions—19th century.   6. Women—
United States—Social conditions—20th century.   7. Home nursing—United
States—History—19th century.   8. Home nursing—United States—
History—20th century.   I. Title.

R727.47 .A24 2000
362.1′082′0973—dc21   00-033596

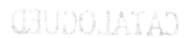

Contents

Acknowledgments

The best part of writing a book is thanking the many people who contributed to it. I first wrote about caregiving with my sister, Margaret K. Nelson. Since then, I have watched her continually translate theory into practice.

Important themes in this book also arose from discussions with Carole H. Browner and Andrea Sankar during joint writing projects. Other people with whom I frequently discussed this book include Richard L. Abel, Karen Brodkin, Mary Felstiner, Dorein Grunbaum, Sondra Hale, Sandra Harding, Sybil Houlding, Joanne Leslie, Ruth Milkman, Mary Rothschild, Vivian Rothstein, and Ann Shalleck.

The many scholars who helped me locate relevant sources include Karen Anderson, Barbara Bates, Eileen Boris, Janice Brockley, Karen Buhler-Wilkerson, Suzanne L. Bunkers, Ellen Dwyer, Sharla Fett, Joanne L. Goodwin, Dawn Greeley, Molly Ladd-Taylor, Judith Walzer Leavitt, Joan Nolte Lensink, Joan E. Lynaugh, Howard Markel, Regina Morantz-Sanchez, René Obrecht, Leigh Pruneau, Susan M. Reverby, David Rosner, Sheila M. Rothman, Mary Rothschild, Susan L. Smith, Marlene Springer, and Brenda Stevenson.

I owe a large debt of gratitude to Nancy Reifel, who conducted interviews with elderly American Indians and coauthored the article on which the second section of Chapter 7 is based. Susan Markens provided excellent research assistance on slavery.

The staffs of various archives provided invaluable help, including those at Arizona State Historical Society, Tucson; Special Collections and Archives, Cline Library, Northern Arizona University, Flagstaff; Huntington Library, San Marino; Archives of the Catholic University of America, Washington, D.C.; Rare Book and Manuscript Library, Columbia University, New York; Special Collections, New York Academy of Medicine, New York; New York State Archives, Albany; New York City Municipal Archives, New York; YIVO Institute for Jewish Research, New York; Kansas State Historical Society, Topeka; State Historical Society of Iowa, Iowa City; Library of Congress, Washington, D.C.; National Archives, Washington, D.C.; National Archives, Pacific-Southwest Region, Laguna Niguel; and Special Collections, Young Research Library, University of California, Los Angeles.

I received funding to conduct research for this book from the UCLA American Indian Studies Center and the UCLA Center for the Study of Women.

My husband, Richard L. Abel, was, as always, my first and best editor. At Harvard University Press, Ann Downer-Hazell and Lee Simmons made important improvements. The manuscript also benefited enormously from the comments of other people who read all or parts of it, including Douglas C. Baynton, Carole H. Browner, Mary Felstiner, Sharla Fett, Evelynn M. Hammonds, Barbara Melosh, Regina Morantz-Sanchez, Penny Richards, Vivian Rothstein, and Deborah Stone. All errors, of course, are my own.

⁓ PORTIONS OF Chapters 1, 4, 6, and 7 and the conclusion appeared in a different form as "Parental Dependence and Filial Responsibility in the Nineteenth Century: Hial Hawley and Emily Hawley Gillespie, 1884–1885," *Gerontologist* 32, no. 4 (1992): 519–526; "Family Caregiving in the Nineteenth Century: Emily Hawley Gillespie and Sarah Gillespie, 1858–1888," *Bulletin of the History of Medicine* 68, no. 4 (Winter 1994): 573–599; "A 'Terrible and Exhausting' Struggle: Family Caregiving During the Transformation of Medicine," *Journal of the History of Medicine and Allied Sciences* 50, no. 4 (October 1995): 474–502; "Interactions between Public Health Nurses and Clients on American Indian Reservations during the 1930s," *Social History of Medicine* 9, no. 1 (1996): 89–108 (with Nancy Reifel); "Appealing for Children's Health Care: Conflicts between Mothers and Officials in the 1930s," *Social Service Review* 70, no. 2 (June 1996): 282–304; "Taking the Cure to the Poor: Patients' Responses to New York City's Tuberculosis Program, 1894–1918," *American Journal of Public Health* 87, no. 11 (November 1997): 1808–1815; "Hospitalizing Maria Germani," in *"Bad" Mothers: The Politics of Blame in Twentieth-Century America*, ed. Molly Ladd-Taylor and Lauri Umansky (New York: New York University Press, 1998), pp. 58–66; and "A Historical Perspective on Care," in *Care Work: Gender, Labor, and Welfare States*, ed. Madonna Harrington Meyer (New York: Routledge, 2000).

⌐Introduction

$\mathcal{D}$URING THE TIME I have been studying family caregiving, the model of the self-reflexive scholar increasingly has challenged that of the detached observer. Simultaneously, a set of personal experiences has enriched my understanding of the meaning of care. Shortly after I began this book, my mother was diagnosed with lymphoma and turned to her five children for emotional, practical, and occasional nursing assistance during the five months she battled the disease. Her death left me and my siblings responsible for my father, who had suffered from a series of disabling strokes for over a decade. He experienced a number of major medical crises until his death six years later. A year after my mother died, I was diagnosed with cancer and added to my siblings' burden by relying on them, as well as on my husband, children, and friends, during my six-month treatment. As both a provider and receiver of care, I have seen firsthand how caregiving can reignite family conflicts, impose financial stress, and encroach on both work and leisure. But I also have gained a deeper appreciation of caregiving as a transformative experience, introducing us to new forms of human connectedness. One goal of this study is to identify both the conditions that make this essential endeavor rewarding and meaningful and those that increase its burdens.

My immersion in the world of care is hardly unusual. Although many of us take health for granted, illness and disability are omnipres-

1

ent. As the population ages, increasing numbers of people devote substantial periods of time to caring for frail, elderly spouses, parents, and grandparents. Despite the rise of a vast health care system in the United States since 1900, care for sick and disabled people remains a predominantly private responsibility. And recent policy changes have reimposed caregiving obligations on households. Between the mid-1950s and the mid-1970s, state mental hospitals discharged the majority of their patients, some onto the streets but many others into the care of their families. Subsequent state measures attempted to reduce the size of the nursing home population and thus increase family responsibilities for the frail elderly. The establishment in 1983 of a Medicare prospective payment system for acute hospital care resulted in a drop in the average length of stay, again shifting care back to the home. The dramatic growth of health maintenance organizations also has led to shorter hospital stays and, thus, more work for family members.

Despite its central place in all of our lives, caregiving receives little social recognition. The dominant culture extols the virtues of independence, seeks distance from such basic life experiences as birth, illness, and death, and trivializes most unpaid work done by women in the home. The history of this activity remains almost completely hidden. Although studies of nineteenth-century doctors and nurses have proliferated in recent decades, few scholars investigate the care provided by family and friends. Most historians pass quickly over informal care, noting only those domestic healing practices that were later incorporated into the formal system of health care delivery. Studies of women healers still concentrate on the exceptional few who can be considered forerunners of contemporary female health professionals. Although it is commonplace to note that most care was delivered by women at home, we know little about women's lifelong work as caregivers. Laurel Thatcher Ulrich, in *A Midwife's Tale*, explores "social medicine" in the late eighteenth and early nineteenth centuries. She demonstrates that caregiving was a "universal female role" and that midwives worked closely with a broad network of neighborhood women.[1] Yet even Ulrich focuses on a woman who had earned public recognition as a healer.

We know still less about how informal care has changed over time. Because caregivers deal with fundamental aspects of human existence—birth, pain, infirmity, disability, and death—we might expect their experiences to remain constant. A complex series of historical changes, however, has profoundly altered both the content and the cultural meaning of care. This book examines the impact of various forces between 1890 and 1940, including the bacteriological revolution, new concepts of disease, the transformation of the formal health care system, and the spread of domestic technologies.

This history addresses several major issues. One is the relationship between power and knowledge. Throughout the nineteenth century, women could consider themselves skilled medical providers. Although physicians sought the rewards and privileges of professional status by touting the superiority of their formal knowledge, they did not hold a monopoly of competence. Female caregivers employed many of the same diagnostic and therapeutic practices. Then, at the turn of the century, dramatic bacteriological discoveries bolstered physicians' claims of special expertise and helped them construct a powerful profession. Although many medical practices remained unchanged, physicians had new grounds for dismissing women's healing knowledge as folk belief. What factors encouraged caregivers to defer to medical authority, and what enabled them to retain control of medical decisions? Were some groups of caregivers especially likely to rely on physicians' judgment? Following Foucault, many scholars emphasize the subtle ways in which medical knowledge and power were diffused throughout society. The medical authority encountered by many caregivers, however, was indistinguishable from state systems of control. Public health programs established in the early twentieth century sought to regulate poor people's lives, emphasized surveillance, and relied on powerful sanctions to compel compliance. How did caregivers experience and respond to such programs?

This book also illuminates the value placed on the emotional and spiritual aspects of caregiving. Throughout the nineteenth century, caregivers were encouraged to draw on their own experiences of suffering in order to establish close bonds with sick and disabled people and respond to their emotional needs. Widespread belief in the importance of personal ties lent prestige to the private world of caring. Assuming a close connection between mind and body, physicians declared that psychic distress contributed to ill health. Female kin were considered especially qualified to offer the attention, sympathy, and reassurance that alleviated emotional stress and facilitated healing. Close association with others can provide the basis for what I call *empathic knowledge*. Evelyn Fox Keller describes empathy as "a form of knowledge of other persons that draws explicitly on the commonality of feelings and experiences in order to enrich one's understanding of another in his or her own right."[2] With the growing emphasis on scientific rationality at the end of the nineteenth century, however, professionals encouraged caregivers to suppress their emotions, distance themselves from care recipients, and monitor their behavior. To what extent were different groups of caregivers able to rely on their own understandings of patients to challenge the new advice of various professionals?

Although scholars of caregiving today do direct attention to the emotional work involved in care, they tend to slight its spiritual dimension. Religious beliefs suffused the caregiving practices of enslaved women in the antebellum South. Caregivers viewed their healing knowledge and skills as divine gifts and assumed that their medicines had spiritual powers. With death often the inevitable outcome of disease, white caregivers routinely prayed with sick relatives, urged them to accept death with equanimity, and relied on their own faith to quell despair. During the late nineteenth and early twentieth centuries, however, caregivers increasingly were exhorted to use their time and energy fighting for recovery rather than preparing for death. How did that advice affect different groups of caregivers?

This history also explores the extent to which caregiving undermines autonomy. A principal theme in much feminist writing today is that women are compelled to provide care by oppressive ideological and material forces. Have women caregivers simply been responding to external pressures? Did caregiving obligations conflict with women's own self-determination? Or, in fact, did caregiving contribute to women's autonomy and maturity? How have poor women, especially women of color, struggled to be able to care for intimates? In what contexts have caregivers asserted the dignity and human worth of lives that others disparaged? How did impoverished and disenfranchised caregivers contend with the professionals and bureaucrats who sought to wield authority over them?

While exploring the effect of caregiving on autonomy, I will also aim to expose the limitations of that quintessentially American ideal. Dependence is an inescapable feature of human existence. As Willard Gaylin has written, "All of us . . . inevitably spend our lives evolving from an initial to a final stage of dependency. If we are fortunate enough to achieve power and relative independence along the way it is a transient and passing glory."[3] What did caregivers gain from providing an essential human service? What groups of caregivers were most likely to receive respect? Caregivers themselves often depended on others for economic resources and emotional sustenance. In what circumstances were caregivers most likely to be able to rely on community networks of support?

The breadth of this topic has made it especially challenging methodologically. I not only trace changes across ninety years and examine a wide range of diseases and disabilities but also discuss women in diverse social positions, with very different relationships to the care recipients. Although caregiving today is concentrated on the elderly population, nineteenth- and early-twentieth-century women cared for people of all ages. In an attempt to avoid overgeneralizing, I have selected specific topics that illuminate broader themes. I concentrate on chronic, rather than acute, illnesses because "persistent, debilitating sickness," as Sue E. Estroff writes, "may be more readily observed and more reliably documented than a brief illness or injury."[4] Although a growing literature examines men's caregiving responsibilities,[5] I focus on women because historically they provided most of the care and because I came to see that caregiving was intertwined with prevailing notions of femininity. Although I discuss care for people with mental handicaps, I omit care for those with mental illness, another enormous topic deserving separate examination. Likewise, I write little about laying out the dead, despite the centrality of this task to nineteenth-century caregivers.

My research on caregiving adds to a growing historical literature based on "illness narratives," in Arthur Kleinman's phrase.[6] Sheila M. Rothman extended our understanding of tuberculosis by moving from the "medical archives" to what she calls the "general archives" in order to understand patients' experiences with that disease.[7] In this study I draw heavily on general archives to elucidate the meaning of caregiving in women's lives. Two chapters are based entirely on the diaries of individual women, reminding us that caregiving is embedded in intimate relationships and cannot be understood apart from them.

General archives, of course, have limitations as well as advantages. Female diarists and letter writers during the nineteenth and early twentieth centuries tended to be overwhelmingly white, eastern, affluent, and relatively leisured. I tried, therefore, to oversample the personal writings of less privileged women. To elucidate the caregiving responsibilities of enslaved women, I draw on published slave narratives, as well as the extensive secondary literature on slavery. I base my examination of poor women, immigrant women, and women of color between 1890 and 1940 primarily on the reports of charity workers, public health nurses, and government officials. Although these "texts of the dominant" must be read with caution, they provide glimpses into the experiences of women too frequently ignored.

The first part of this book examines caregiving between 1850 and 1890. It opens with an examination of the caregiving responsibilities of Emily Hawley Gillespie, a white Iowa farm woman, and her daughter Sarah. Although neither Emily nor Sarah had unusual knowledge or skills, both regularly cared for their neighbors and kin. When Emily's health deteriorated in 1886, Sarah abandoned the teaching career she loved in order to nurse her mother. Because both Emily and Sarah kept diaries, their experience can be examined from the perspectives of the recipient as well as the giver of care.

Chapter 2 provides an overview of caregiving between 1850 and 1890. I first discuss the forces that compelled white women to provide care, the impact of caregiving responsibilities on their lives, the availability of community support, and their relationships to formal health providers. Some women derived enormous satisfaction from honing and using healing skills, which partially compensated for the labor and exhaustion caregiving entailed. The emotional and spiritual components of care also offered gratification. The chapter concludes with a brief examination of enslaved African American women, whose caregiving experiences contrasted sharply with those of whites. This section highlights the theme of power and conflict, which is central to subsequent chapters.

The bedsides of sick patients were contested sites in the nineteenth century. Chapter 3 examines the struggles for power between doctors and white women. Doctors disparaged women's healing skills, belittled the emotional care they rendered, and sought to restrict the medical knowledge available to them. Lacking any way to demonstrate a monopoly of expertise, however, doctors failed to usurp women's authority as healers.

Chapter 4 focuses on Martha Shaw Farnsworth, a white woman

from Kansas, between 1890 and 1924. This chapter introduces many of
the themes examined throughout the second part of the book: conflict
between paid employment and informal care, changing conceptions of
disease, the extent to which women surrendered control over medical
decision-making, and the effect on family caregivers of the communi-
cations revolution, the greater availability of consumer goods and services, and the growth of the formal sector of health care. The story of
Martha Farnsworth, who cared for two husbands, an infant daughter,
and a niece, challenges the persistent assumption that family members
lost responsibility for health care after the late nineteenth century.

The relationships between diverse groups of caregivers and various
forms of medical authority underwent a profound transformation between 1890 and 1940. Chapter 5 first discusses mothers who solicited
advice from the Children's Bureau and then analyzes correspondence
between family members of tuberculosis sufferers and a prominent
tuberculosis specialist. Chapter 6 examines how indigent caregivers
around the beginning of the twentieth century responded to New York
City's pioneering program of tuberculosis control, which sought to impose medical authority from the top down.

Chapter 7 focuses on two groups of caregivers during the Great Depression. Relying on mothers' letters to Eleanor and Franklin D. Roosevelt, I begin by describing the fury, resentment, and sense of helplessness of women seeking health care for their children. The public
officials who investigated the women's appeals delegitimized their empathic knowledge, denied the children's medical problems, and refused
treatment. I then describe interactions between public health nurses
and American Indian caregivers on reservations. Although the nurses
assumed that American Indian people would follow a linear progression from understanding the benefits of white medicine to accepting
the entire public health program, the caregivers made selective use of
the nurses' services.

Extreme hostility was directed toward children labeled "feebleminded" or epileptic during the late nineteenth and early twentieth
centuries. Chapter 8 examines the ways various groups of mothers responded to pressures to place such children in institutions and how
some mothers were able to sustain contact with their offspring after admission.

Chapter 9 describes the experiences of mothers who struggled to conform to the tenets of "oralism" in rearing deaf children. In order to enable their children to "pass" in a hearing world, mothers were expected to display enormous determination and optimism while devoting themselves to an intensive training regime.

The conclusion briefly chronicles the medical, political, and social developments that have transformed caregiving since 1940, explores several reasons why caregiving commands little social respect, and suggests how the legacy of the past should influence current policy decisions.

Although virtually none of the family members, friends, and neighbors I discuss labeled their endeavor as "caregiving" or themselves as "caregivers," I use those terms as shorthand.

The title comes from the Bible: "Teach us to number our days, That we may attain a heart of wisdom." In this book I wish to show how caregivers acquire a kind of knowledge that comes from personal connection. At its best, caregiving promotes insight and personal integrity by heightening our awareness of the fragility of all human life.

⌒Part One
1850–1890

~1

"Hot Flannels, Hot Teas, and a Great Deal of Care": Emily Hawley Gillespie and Sarah Gillespie, 1858–1888

*O*N OCTOBER 14, 1871, Emily Hawley Gillespie, an Iowa farm woman, wrote in her diary, "Mrs. Houghton and I sat up all last night with old Mrs. Stephens, 74 yrs, she died 10 minutes past 9 this morning. We lay her out in black dress—I came home this afternoon." Although Emily had no exceptional medical knowledge or skills, she routinely incorporated care for birthing women, the sick, and the dying into her daily life. In turn, various neighbors, friends, and relatives cared for her whenever she was in need. Emily taught her daughter Sarah to nurse the sick along with other household and farm chores. When Emily's health began to fail in the mid-1880s, Sarah became her primary caregiver. The story of Emily and Sarah Gillespie between 1858, when Emily's diary begins, and 1888, the year she died, helps to illuminate the nineteenth-century world of caregiving.[1]

Emily Hawley Gillespie

Emily Gillespie was born in 1838, the oldest of four children of Hial Newton Hawley and Sarah Baker Hawley, Michigan farmers. From an early age she participated in household and farm labor. Because her parents' farm was less prosperous than the average, she also was compelled to take advantage of the few opportunities for young women to

11

make money. In addition to teaching school, sewing for neighbors, and peddling books, she nursed invalids.

While in her early twenties, Emily wrote frequently of her fear of death. At least one of her nursing experiences may well have sharpened her sense of vulnerability. On May 20, 1860, she spent the night with a neighbor suffering from consumption. "Am at Mrs. Wiley's this evening," she wrote. "Poor woman, I do pity her, she took my hand and said 'your hand will be like mine sometime; mine was once like yours.'" The absence of other people in the house appears to have added to Emily's terror. "I alone with one almost dying," she complained. At other times Emily could draw comfort from the presence of the women around her. On July 1 she wrote, "Called at Mrs. Wileys. She is no better. I with Mrs. Converse, Mrs. Evans and Mrs. Culver sit up with her to night, how sick she is." And on July 5 she wrote, "Edna and I, Harriet Sutherland, Adison and Augusta Stone and Maria Dawes sit up to night with the corpse. Mrs. Wiley died this morning about 4." The following day Emily wrote, "The Dr's. came this morning to dissect Mrs. Wiley, her heart and lungs were grown *fast*. Right *lung all gone* and left one except a part about the size of a hickory nut."[2] It is possible that Emily's graphic description of physical deterioration helped her cope with her anxieties. As Elizabeth Hampsten notes, working-class women in the nineteenth century frequently wrote about death and decay with a frankness that startles late-twentieth-century readers.[3]

Emily left home in June 1861 at the age of twenty-three to work as a housekeeper for her uncle, an innkeeper in a small town in Iowa. Fourteen months later she married James Gillespie, a twenty-five-year-old farmer. The marriage was not happy. James was subject to deep depressions and uncontrollable rages, and he occasionally threatened suicide. By the early 1880s, Emily feared for her own safety. After James had one of his "bad spells" on October 4, 1883, she wrote, "It makes my blood run cold and I shake like a leaf." Driving with him in a carriage on April 19, 1884, she felt "perfectly terror struck." On December 19, 1884, she wrote that the children "dare not leave me alone with him." Emily also worried that James would expel her from the farm, depriving her of livelihood as well as home.

In addition, marriage confined Emily to a life she had hoped to avoid. From an early age she had aspired to become a lady.[4] "I had wanted to be married in silk and was real sorry," she confessed in a letter to her parents soon after the wedding.[5] As a farm woman, she engaged in a constant round of grueling labor. James plowed and planted the fields, chopped wood, churned the butter, cared for the horses, and repaired the farm equipment. Emily kept a vegetable garden and did all the housework. Although James built their house, she cleaned it, painted the walls, laid flooring and carpeting, and constructed closets. During the last decades of her life, a variety of store-bought goods lightened her burdens. She no longer had to spin and weave cloth or make soap and candles. In addition, she benefited from technological advances: she bought a wringer for washing in 1878, a new coal stove in 1882, and a sewing machine in 1883. She continued, however, to sew overalls and shirts for her husband and son, bake bread, and can vegetables and fruit. On September 19, 1883, she reported that she had just filled 108 cans. "It is a sight of work to put up so much fruit," she commented. Moreover, in order to pay for the manufactured goods and appliances that were available, she had to increase her workload. She sold butter, eggs, honey, vegetables, and poultry for cash. On July 26, 1883, she noted that she had 118 turkeys, 78 chickens, and 20 other fowl. In addition to feeding them regularly, she built and cleaned their cages, chased them when they escaped onto neighbors' land, and protected them from skunks, gophers, and cats.

James and Emily had two children, a son, Henry, born in 1863 and a daughter, Sarah, in 1865. Although both worked on the farm from an early age, Emily devoted considerable time and energy to their care and socialization.

Despite the burdens Emily shouldered as both a farm woman and a mother, she assumed that she would render care whenever it was needed. In addition to nursing her husband and children through assorted illnesses, she tended many of her kin and neighbors. "Oh! Oh!! Oh!!! what awful news again," Emily wrote on August 21, 1868. "Uncle got hurt in the reaper—we went to see him, he is in dreadful pain." Once again, she described bodily affliction in detail, writing that "about 3 inches flesh, bones, arteries, cords and all" had to be removed from her uncle's arm. She continued to visit him regularly during the succeeding three weeks.

On July 22, 1869, Emily commented that "they sent for me" to attend the childbirth of Nell Thomas, a neighbor. On September 7 Emily wrote, "stay at Mr. Thomas' most all day, their Baby is *sick*." She returned to the Thomas house the following day to attend the baby's burial. Two months later, Emily again had responsibility for nursing a critically ill patient. On November 5 she noted that James's brother "come and tell us Ma is worse, we go and stay most all day, come home and do chores, then go back. I stay all night, James went home." The following day she wrote, "Ma *died* just 23 minutes of 2 o'clock this morning—died without a struggle." On October 14, 1871, she noted that she had "sat up" all night with Mrs. Stephens, an elderly woman, and then helped to lay her out. On September 22, 1872, Emily recorded that she had assisted Mrs. McMillen when she gave birth to a boy, and six months later she spent a night watching Mr. Stephens, who had been sick for several months. "He died this morning half past three," she reported on March 21, 1873.

Some observers argue that the chores and household responsibilities of nineteenth-century farm women gave them the satisfaction of honing skills and demonstrating competence.[6] Caregiving offered similar opportunities. In 1858, when Emily was still living at her parents' house, she described her prowess in dispensing medicine: "Aunt Mary came here," she wrote on November 25. "She has not spoken loud in fourteen weeks. I gave her a teaspoon of 'Chamberlains Relief' and in about half an hour she talked aloud; she was so pleased that she cried." Emily exhibited similar self-confidence whenever James became ill. "I have made up my mind its a 'nervous fever,'" she pronounced on August 18, 1863. Two days later she noted, "I wash him and make him some catnip tea, rub his stomach with liniment he said he felt better." On January 6, 1868, she again made her own diagnosis and decided what treatment to administer. "I think he has symptoms of infection of the bowels," she wrote. "Have kept hot cloths wet with vinegar across him all day." Emily also felt competent to act on her own when Henry hit his thumb with an axe and "cut it nearly off" in 1884. "Deara-me it is too bad," she wrote on May 13. "He held it on while I done it up. I hope it will grow on again without leaving too bad a scar."

In providing Emily with a sense of mastery, caregiving resembled much of her other work. But in one important respect, Emily's responsibilities for care were unique. Most household and farm labor isolated her from the community around her; she often complained that the constant demands of work left little time for socializing. Moreover, although she received some help with her chores, first from her sister

Harriet and later from her daughter, Sarah, she rarely, if ever, shared tasks with neighborhood women. Emily's success as a farm woman also separated her from the broader community. Partly as a result of her efforts, she and James prospered. Although they lived with James's parents at the time of their marriage, they were able to move to their own land in 1864 and built a new house in 1872. Their farm thrived during the agricultural depression of the 1870s, a time when many others failed.

As Emily's fortunes rose, she spurned those she left behind. She attributed the plight of others to their personal failings. Jealously guarding her possessions, she responded with rage when neighbors sought to borrow farm implements. One of her sharpest grievances against James was that he was too generous toward his extended family and neighbors, helping anyone in need. Believing that "charity begins at home first," Emily wanted him to focus on bettering his immediate family (September 23, 1879).

Nor did Emily view the farm as a joint enterprise with her husband. The two fought bitterly about the amount of work each did. Emily complained that James imposed an excessive workload on her and belittled her economic contributions to the family. Moreover, instead of sharing the money she earned with James, she spent it herself.[7] Although James had no interest in acquiring the trappings of the genteel life, she improved their home—for example, spending $50.40 for new carpets in 1880; James, she scornfully wrote, considered them "too nice" (June 22, December 16, 1880). She adorned herself and her children as well, buying silk, cashmere, and velvet to make clothes. On February 17, 1886, Emily noted that the cost of Sarah's new dresses was $43.84. Emily's most prized possession was a carriage, which she had wanted for years and finally bought for $65 in 1885. "It is splendid," she wrote on September 27, after riding in it for the first time, "but James is *too harsh* for anything *so fine*."

If farmwork ruptured social bonds, caregiving helped to restore them. The sufferings of others elicited Emily's sympathy. Whenever James fell ill, she expressed a tenderness and solicitude toward him that was absent from her diary at other times. On August 16, 1863, she wrote, "'Tis sad when he is sick . . . I read him the letter I wrote to my folks. I had said in it a few words about his being sick; the tears came trickling from his eyes." And she expressed admiration for his courage:

"O. how good he is; he said he did not know but he was as ready to go now, as ever, if his time had come, and if he found out he must die, he would settle up his business and die in peace with all. O. with what composure of mind he talks, O. God I pray that when I die I may be as well prepared to go as James is" (January 20, 1863). James's second major illness, in 1868, prompted equally loving comments. "O my prayer is that he may get well, for O. Lord . . . wilt Thou spare him to me a while longer for I feel I have no other friend on Earth . . . Ah me all seems bad when dear ones are sick. James groans so mournfully" (January 6).

Caregiving also enabled Emily to exhibit concern for her sister Harriet, who came to Iowa to visit in September 1869 and remained with the Gillespies for two years. Although Harriet taught school, she also helped with the housework. Emily's two children were young, and she was grateful for her sister's assistance. After Harriet married John McGee in November 1871 and moved to his farm, the two women continued to exchange gifts and favors. Emily attended Harriet in October 1872 when Harriet had a stillbirth and again in August 1873 when her first daughter was born.

The relationship cooled considerably as Harriet's fortunes declined. When Harriet and John owed "debts to the amount of twenty-six hundred dollars" in 1876, Emily noted on October 1 that they had been "advised to do different." But Emily continued to assist at Harriet's confinements. On May 16, 1878, she wrote, "Harriet has another Boy it was born to day tween four and five o'clock. I have been there all day." The agony Emily witnessed troubled her. "Ah what suffering one can endure," she wrote. The relationship between the sisters continued to deteriorate after Harriet and her husband lost their farm. When Harriet failed to return a garden tool promptly, on May 9, 1881, Emily wrote, "I wanted to dig some roots in the garden this afternoon. Our potatoe-fork was down to Harriets. I *was* provoked that I had to go after it when I was so tired . . . When I work and get things to use I do not like to have them gone when I want them . . . I hope . . . it may learn them a lesson that they can not always expect some one of their relatives to help them. They must work to a better advantage for themselves."

When Emily helped Harriet after an "abortion" in 1882, she again expressed sympathy for her sister.[8] "She looks very bad indeed. I am really sorry for her," Emily wrote on March 19. "Ah me! such is the life of most women." Although conflicts continued to erupt between the sisters, Emily did not doubt that she would offer assistance to Harriet in any crisis. On August 26, 1883, Emily vowed never to visit Harriet again "except that she sends for me or any of them are sick."

Caring activities also bound Emily to a large female network. Despite the contempt Emily displayed for many of her neighbors, she routinely attended their childbirths, nursed their sick, and sat up with their dying. When she went to neighbors' homes to dispense such services, other women occasionally did the housework she left behind.

Births, illnesses, and deaths frequently were communal events. Although Emily performed most farm chores by herself, she typically shared caregiving tasks with others. On October 11, 1873, she wrote, "Go with Harriet to see Isabelle, she is sick, her baby 1 week old." When Emma Brook's husband died in January 1886, Emily spent the day at her house with three other women. One was Mrs. Chapman, with whom Emily had previously enjoyed a close bond, but from whom she had recently become estranged. On May 23, 1884, Emily had complained that Mrs. Chapman appeared "unfriendly toward me." When she had invited Mrs. Chapman to visit her the following September, her friend had declined, pleading an excess of work. As Emily cleaned the Brook house and cooked the dinner, however, she healed the breach in the relationship. "Mrs. Chapman and I had a good visit," Emily reported on January 14, 1886. "I asked her to come and see me. She invited me to come and see her. I mean to go too."

Emily's experiences as a recipient, as well as a giver, of care tied her to a community of women. Her diary entry for September 4, 1863, reads,

> Ah me, what I have to write for this day; was real sick all night (last night), did not sleep a minute . . . about daylight James sent for some help to take care of me. Pa went, got Mrs. Lewis, Mrs. Coats, Mrs. Parliman and Margaret, Ma [James's mother] *was* here. Mrs. Lewis was the Dr. (paid her $2.00) she is a real good woman. Baby [her son Henry] was born about half past ten A.M. . . . About three o'clock I felt that all was well; was lying com-

fortably in bed; the boy beside me, the Ladies, all but Margaret
went home. Mrs. Lewis kissed me, O. she seemed like one kind
deliverer, and they were all kind.

It is likely that, despite Emily's use of the term "Dr.," Mrs. Lewis was
the midwife.[9] Although male physicians officiated at some of the deliveries Emily attended, for her own childbirth she marshaled the help of
women alone. The presence of James's mother also is noteworthy. By
this time, Emily and James had been living at the home of his parents
for almost a year, and the relationship between Emily and her in-laws
had grown increasingly conflictual. Emily accused them of compelling
James to work too hard and paying him too little. Nevertheless, to Emily's evident surprise, Ma attended the birth. It was customary for one
woman to remain at the home of the birthing woman for several days
to provide practical assistance; in this case the helper was James's married sister, Margaret Doolittle.[10]

The women who attended Emily's second confinement confronted
death as well as birth. "Ah. ah," Emily wrote on July 7, 1865, "can it be
possible that we have a little daughter born this morning that weighs 5
lbs. 7 oz. Her twin brother did not live to even breathe." Once again,
Mrs. Lewis delivered the baby and James's mother provided assistance,
despite growing tensions between her and Emily.

When Emily, then in her late forties, became seriously ill in 1886,
even more neighbors and kin offered their services. Sarah reported that
during the first two weeks, six women sat with Emily through the
night, one woman as many as four times. Many others came during the
day to provide both nursing and practical assistance. After listing various women who visited her in the late spring and summer of 1886, Emily wrote on June 3, "All the neighbors all round every where they all
seem every one like real true friends far different than ever before."
The visits of Mrs. Chapman were especially precious. The two women
had reestablished their friendship the previous January, and Mrs.
Chapman's care in June cemented their bond. "She was here yesterday," Emily wrote on June 3. "She was talking about how Her and I
used to visit together and she cried about it . . . and as soon as I can ride
am going up there."

Nevertheless, caregiving could not overcome all conflicts. We have
seen that tensions between Emily and Harriet continued after Emily

provided assistance at Harriet's childbirth. Harriet visited Emily daily and "sat up" with her on at least two occasions in May and June 1886, but Emily did not welcome her sister's ministrations. On June 3 she wrote, "That Harriet comes up every day but most everytime she comes has something to say about the past that makes it unpleasant Im fraid all the time when [she] comes here that when I get well that there will be something." After seeing Harriet on October 20, Emily exclaimed, "No! I did *not* have a *good* Visit with her." James's sister, Margaret Doolittle, had stayed with Emily and had helped with the housework after Henry's birth in 1863, but whatever closeness may have developed between the women at that time vanished when Margaret sided with James in his battles with Emily. Like many other relatives and friends, Margaret visited Emily when her health failed in the spring of 1886. However, that summer James left home, and when Margaret appeared at the Gillespie door in October, Emily threatened to have her arrested.

Elder Care

Emily Gillespie's truncated experience caring for her father, Hial Newton Hawley, further cautions us against romanticizing nineteenth-century caregiving. In 1884 he was seventy-seven years old and suffered from a number of physical problems. His most serious disability was lameness. Although he still tried to do farm labor, he experienced great difficulty and had to lie down much of the day.

After leaving home at the age of twenty-three, Emily corresponded with her parents and visited them twice in Michigan, but she considered herself outside the circle of her natal family. The only sibling to whom she remained close was her sister Harriet; by 1884, however, that tie had also frayed. The death of her mother in 1882 increased Emily's sense of alienation from her family. Their attachment had been especially strong, and her grief engulfed her diary for several months. The death also precipitated a major clash between Emily and her siblings. In July 1882 she had responded angrily to a suggestion from her brother Henry that Harriet receive the bulk of their mother's clothes and other personal items. When their mother's effects arrived in Iowa in October, Emily was shocked to discover that Harriet's box contained five times as much as her own. The sale of the family farm, which occurred nine months later, added insult to injury. Emily had considered herself entitled to receive a portion of her parents' property, and she felt aggrieved when her brother kept the proceeds of the sale himself.

Emily had first expressed a desire to assist her father when she entered a lottery in 1884. "Should I be so fortunate as to draw a prize I shall try to take care of Father the rest of his life," she promised in her diary entry of January 23. When she failed to win, she wrote nothing further about caring for him. She visited her father in March, assuring him that he always "would have a place" with her (April 2); she was confident, however, that he would not take up her offer.

She was stunned, therefore, when he appeared on her doorstep six weeks later. On May 15 Emily's daughter, Sarah, described the shock of his arrival: "Last night just as we had retired, and were about to enter in the sweet slumber of 10 o'clock: we were quickly awakened by a loud knock, and who should appear but Grandpa Hawley." Emily recorded her own dismay in her diary the same day: "I feel it an imposition upon us all."

If Emily viewed her father's presence as an "imposition," she also realized that her sister Harriet was jealous that Hial had chosen Emily's home rather than her own. Responsibility for Hial was an honor as well as a burden, and Emily tried to behave like a good daughter. When Hial seemed "despondent," she comforted him, promising to "make it as pleasant for him as I can" (May 18). She also welcomed him by making up "a nice bed" for him in the sewing room and carefully putting away his clothes. When he tried to work around the farm, she encouraged him to rest. She refused payment for making him a coat.

Emily, in turn, received Hial's support. He gave her a $1,000 note he held against his son Henry and expressed the hope that she "would collect every cent interest and all" (May 28). He also took her side against Harriet. After he paid his first visit to Harriet's house on May 18, Emily reported, "He does not approve of Harriet talking as she does about me and the children." On May 24 Emily wrote that her father found Harriet's family "too noisy for him." On August 31, according to Emily, he declared himself "perfectly disgusted with the way Harriet talked."

Hial's support of Emily's claim to her mother's bureau was especially gratifying. This bureau arrived at the Gillespie house along with Hial's possessions on May 26. Although Harriet argued that their mother had left the bureau to her, Emily found an inscription on the bottom, proving her ownership. On May 27 she wrote, "When I was washing the last drawer (the small one that I kept my trinkets in when I lived at home) I beheld on the underside of it where Mother had written on two different times that she wanted me to have her beauro when she was dead and gone. It seems to me as from the dead." Because Emily cherished material possessions and demonstrated affection through gifts, this bequest symbolized her mother's love. "I have always felt that Mother loved me above all others, but could not know it until to day," she continued. "It seemed almost when I read her gift to me that she came to tell me." Emily was even more delighted when her father expressed his pleasure at the resolution of the dispute. "Now Father loves me, too—best of his children," she proclaimed two days later.

It is not clear why the relationship between Emily and her father soon soured. She claimed that both James and Harriet turned him against her, portraying her as lazy and deceitful. Because we have no access to Hial's version of events, we can only speculate about how he perceived their relationship. We do know, however, that by the time he came to Emily's house, he had suffered several major blows, including the death of his wife, his departure from Michigan, and his failing health. The sale of his farm meant that instead of being able to wield power over his children, he now was dependent on them.[11] The evidence indicates that Hial hated his dependency. As we have seen, he sought to pay his own way insofar as possible and tried to contribute to the work of the farm.

Although we cannot know how Emily treated her father, her diary suggests that she did little to bolster his dignity and self-esteem. His labor, she repeatedly claimed, was primarily therapeutic; he worked only because "he wants something to do." And he had difficulty accomplishing the chores he undertook. She wrote that he hoed "too close" to the strawberry vines (May 22). When he sawed wood, "his cane went into a hole—he fell against a post and hurt his face" (June 6). Two months later he "fell down three times" while pulling weeds in the garden (August 12).

Hial did not passively accept the subservient status his daughter assigned him. If she belittled him because of his age and infirmities, he expressed contempt for all women. According to Sarah, he argued that women should be denied the vote, and he expressed disapproval of Sarah's driving a carriage. "Grandpa can't bear to see a woman be anybody," she complained in her diary on September 6, 1884. Hial also asserted his independence by allying himself with James. The two men spent their days together, and Hial increasingly took James's side in the conflicts that raged within the household. On July 31, according to Sarah, both men "laughed" at Emily's account of her attempts to make money. As Emily displayed less and less sympathy for her father, he withdrew into silence. On the rare occasions when he spoke, Emily noted, he was "sarcastic and cross" (October 22). On November 1 she wrote, "It is sometimes as much as I can endure . . . continually being obliged to be on my guard to be able to be calm at all times."

By the end of October, Hial was spending more and more time at Harriet's house. On November 2 Emily lamented, "When he first came he said . . . that Harriet tried to set him up against me and make trouble between him and me but she could not. And now he has sided with her."

On November 7, six months after his arrival, Hial announced that he would move permanently to Harriet's house. Although stung by his defection, Emily agreed to pack his possessions. But conflicts continued to erupt after his departure. He asked for the $2.00 he had given her to buy a present; she responded that the amount was just $1.75. When he demanded the return of Henry's $1,000 note, she asked for compensation for the sheep she had lent him twenty-five years earlier. Their worst fight concerned the bureau. He insisted on taking this heirloom to Harriet's house, but Emily refused, reminding him that it had been passed down through the female line. She had received it from her mother, who had bought it with money she received from her own mother. When he threatened to sue, she finally admitted defeat. "Dear-a-me," Emily wrote on December 16, after he came to collect the bureau, "I felt as if he stole it from me and from the dead and that I believed it would haunt him every night of his life." As she later commented, the loss of this cherished possession demonstrated the legal power of men. "Father took it just because he could," she wrote on January 8, 1885.

Hial's departure may have damaged Emily's reputation in the community. According to James, a rumor circulated that she had expelled her father after making him work at her house all summer. James also charged that her treatment of her father provided evidence of her difficult personality.

Hial's situation remained difficult. Although Harriet had been jealous that her father initially chose to live with Emily, Harriet now found him a trial. On February 13, 1885, Emily wrote that Harriet was having a "terrible time with Father." In June, having exhausted his children's goodwill, he was compelled to apply to the local authorities for assistance.[12]

Operating within hierarchies of gender and generation, Emily and Hial were both losers in their struggle for control. Both women and the elderly had low status in the second half of the nineteenth century. Emily and Hial could undermine each other's limited power, but neither could escape nineteenth-century structures of subordination.

Henry and Sarah

Although Emily never wavered in her love for her children, her feelings toward them were complex. The texture of her relationships with Henry and Sarah shaped the nature of the care they rendered when she became ill. On August 29, 1877, Emily wrote that the "only happiness" of farm women "lies in their children. With fond hopes that *they* may rise higher, that *they* perhaps may be an ornament to society." Emily taught Henry and Sarah to disdain the drudgery of farmwork and encouraged them to seek upward mobility through education.[13] She paid their tuition at a private academy where they could associate with "young Ladies and gentlemen," carefully supervised their schoolwork, and urged them to enter such "noble" professions as teaching and medicine.[14] On August 28, 1886, she declared that Henry and Sarah were her "reward" for "all the sorrows" of her marriage; "pure and noble minds with high aims. No more could be asked."

Looking to her children for the affirmation and companionship she missed from others, Emily was devastated when they began to leave home. In September 1882 Henry was the first to go, traveling to Nebraska County, 120 miles from the farm, to work as a peddler for six months. In 1883 he spent a term at Adrian College in Michigan, and in January 1886 he sought work in Missouri. At other times he found employment reasonably close to the farm but still had to live away from home at least part of the time. When Sarah began to teach in 1883, she boarded at the homes of her students during the school term. Although both Henry and Sarah returned home often, Emily experienced each departure as a fresh blow. On January 20, 1886, she wrote, "Grief at parting with my children is almost unbearable."

Viewing herself as a self-denying mother, Emily wanted to take pleasure in her children's growing independence and encourage them to leave home. Because she lacked any other satisfaction in her life, however, she felt bereft and abandoned when they did. Her diary entry for July 11, 1883, reveals her struggle. She hoped Sarah would pass her exam for a teaching certificate "because she would be disappointed if not, I would so like for her to stay at home with me, yet if she wants to teach I am willing and wish her the best success. No no I would not keep my children at home away from doing what is right and best for them to do. Though I am so lonely without them. Yes I will help them all I can." At other times Emily reminded herself that "it is *happiness* to know they are doing *so well*" (January 30, 1884), that "we cannot expect to keep our children always at home" (June 28, 1884), and that she "must try to not be so lonesome for they must be gone" (November 8, 1885). Nevertheless, she remained convinced that it was best when everyone was at home.

In her desire to reconcile herself to this loss, Emily may well have sent her children a double message, drawing them to her while pushing them away. She often vowed not to upset Henry and Sarah by letting them know how deeply she mourned them, but she poured out her grief in letters to them as well as in the pages of her diary. Although she wanted them to see her as strong and self-sufficient, she was very grateful whenever they responded to her problems and appears to have been aware that her neediness kept them tied to her. We will see that Emily's illness enabled her to have her daughter at her side without violating her image of herself as a self-abnegating mother.

Mother and Daughter

Although Emily was devoted to both children, her tie to Sarah seems to have been especially intense. Emily frequently claimed to see herself in her daughter. As she wrote on February 13, 1886, *"she is myself living over again."* Emily rarely made any distinction between her emotional and physical responses to events and those of Sarah. After they spent a day working, Emily commented that both were tired. When Henry left home, they both "missed" him; when he published an article in the paper, they were united in their pride. A typical refrain in Emily's diary was "Sarah too feels just the same." Ironically, the differences between Emily and Sarah may have helped to cement their bond. Both Emily and Henry were quick to take offense, and misunderstandings arose frequently between them; Sarah appears to have enjoyed an easier relationship with her mother partly because she was less sensitive to slights.

Emily watched especially closely over Sarah's teaching career, preparing arithmetic problems Sarah could use in the classroom, consoling her during periods of discouragement, giving her hints about enforcing discipline, and offering her rest at the farm on weekends. Emily also hoped Sarah would marry well and was delighted when Sarah appeared to win the admiration of Joseph Hutchinson, a local banker whose father was "supposed to be worth several hundred thousand dollars" (November 15, 1885). Emily took vicarious pleasure in Sarah's other conquests as well. Although relieved when Sarah declined proposals that had little promise of elevating her from farm life, Emily proudly noted each new suitor Sarah attracted. "Sarah is much like myself when I was her age," Emily wrote on November 15, 1885. "It seemed as if young boys, young and old men, bachelors and married men admired."

But Emily's attitude toward Sarah was not all of a piece. We have seen that Emily urged her children to pursue individual achievement while simultaneously seeking to keep them home. Although welcoming Sarah's career and social success, Emily also expressed jealousy and resentment of her daughter's many advantages. Sarah was enjoying youth just when Emily, then forty-five, was newly conscious of aging. "Care and hard work," she wrote, had harmed her "once youthful looks" (September 18, 1882). Her hands were "like a faded rose," and her hair had turned gray (November 25, 1883). While Sarah was attracting men, Emily was losing her sexual powers. And Emily was keenly aware that Sarah had opportunities she had been denied. When Sarah attended a preparatory course for a teaching certificate in the summer of 1882, Emily enthusiastically followed her daughter's progress but also noted that such programs had not been available to her. Similarly, although Emily was proud of the salary Sarah earned as a teacher, she commented that the sum far exceeded what she herself had received for teaching. Above all, Sarah had the maternal support that Emily felt she had lacked. "O that I could have had the sympathy and encouragement when I was young and trying to rise above poverty, trying to gain a high place in society," she wrote on February 17, 1885. Although Emily wanted Sarah to lead a better life than she had, Sarah's opportunities often served as a painful reminder of her own deprivations.

The close relationship between Emily and Sarah had a material, as well as an emotional, base. Until Sarah left home in 1883, the two women shared the rhythms of daily life. Sarah helped her mother can tomatoes, plant strawberries, sell eggs, honey, and butter in town, prepare supper, cut carpet rags, and sew clothes.

Sarah also shared her first major nursing experience with her mother. On October 3, 1884, Sarah's brother, Henry, was helping to rebuild a church in a nearby town when he suffered an accident. "O dear I can hardly write in my journal," Emily wrote three days later. "Last Friday noon Mr. Morse came for me to go to Manchester that Henry was hurt. O. O. he had fallen from the church spire I could not be thankful enough that he was not killed . . . The first place he hit anything was 9 ft. then 20 ft. to the roof and from there it was 45 ft. *Oh, terrible.* I have been with him all the time . . . It is too bad, terrible to think of—to fall 74 feet, not a bone broken . . . he is seriously hurt it seems as if he is bruised in every place . . . It is indeed the hardest time in my life." According to Sarah, for the first four days and nights, "he was fanned and rubbed every second by myself and Ma. He was taken to Mrs. Nell Smiths where he boarded . . . He was literally covered with black and blue spots and had to be bathed in hot water—and cold clothes kept on his head. O such pain and suffering as he endured. He was light headed a couple of times at night and we had to work so hard to keep him alive" (October 19).

The two women were attentive to each other, not just to Henry. Sarah described Emily's response as well as her own: "Ma did not cry but was as white as a corpse, She is almost sick at best" (October 19). Emily noted that "it is very hard" for Sarah too (October 12). While Emily stayed with Henry during the day, Sarah returned to the farm each morning to do the household and farm chores. On October 19 she described her workload this way: "I can't tell how many washings and ironings I have done. But a doz. pillow slips had to be changed each day besides sheets and clothes and I [remember] washing and ironing 23 slips one day when I came home and then baking a doz. pumpkin pies

and making cake and washing all the dishes making the beds and to see
to every thing else." She also complained about the toll caring took on
her own health: "I wrenched my back lifting and turning Henry and
now my left wrist is 'gun' out. He can not turn over or get on or off the
bed without lifting."

But there were compensations. After recounting all the housework
she did, Sarah commented, "Why I am stronger than I thot I was." She
also believed that she was uniquely equipped to minister to Henry's
needs. Although many friends offered to sit up with Henry, she noted
that she "couldn't trust such a care to anyone." And it is likely that Sarah knew that Emily considered her indispensable. "O what would I do
without her," Emily wrote three days after the accident. Henry was
able to return to the farm on October 11 and to walk with the aid of
crutches by October 19. Nevertheless, he continued to need substantial
care from both his mother and Sarah for several more weeks.

Emily's Illness

Sarah's sense of responsibility for Emily began even before Henry's accident. Although Emily prided herself on offering protection to her
children, she appeared much weaker in Sarah's diary than in her own.
Sarah was well aware that Emily suffered intensely from James's out-
bursts and threats of violence. "Poor Ma," she wrote often, or, "I feel so
sorry for her." Although we lack Henry's account, both Emily's and Sarah's diaries suggest that he too viewed his mother as an object of pity.
Emily frequently expressed her determination to appear strong and in
control before her daughter. Whenever Sarah witnessed an attack of
"nerves," Emily vowed to act "pleasant" in the future.

During the spring and summer of 1884, when Emily was forty-six,
Sarah first began to notice her mother's physical ailments. She wrote
that Emily appeared "sickly" and that her hands were "numb." On September 9 Emily wrote, "My fingers and hands have had a queer feeling
for some time. I will be glad if they get their natural feeling and thankful, too, they feel as if the cuticle was about worn out." Two weeks later
she noted that a local doctor had corroborated her self-diagnosis: "Dr.
Sherman said I must bathe my hands in alcohol, that the cuticle was so
thin. Just as I thought."

Emily attributed her physical problems to the burdens she shouldered and especially to the stresses engendered by James's violent and erratic behavior. "Ah! James," she wrote in her journal on May 11, 1886. "Had you have treated me as half human I do believe I should have been in better health now, but instead of being a protector, you have hundreds of times almost broke my heart."

Because Sarah's caregiving responsibilities were intertwined with her teaching career, they must be described together. Although teaching was one of the few respectable occupations open to nineteenth-century women, it had numerous disadvantages. It paid poorly, conferred little security, and was physically and emotionally demanding. Teachers often had large and unruly classes with students of vastly disparate ages. Many teachers viewed their work solely as a way of making money before marriage and happily abandoned it on their wedding days.[15]

But Sarah invested great hopes in her career. She enjoyed making an independent income and had a strong sense of mission about the work. After her first day at a new school on November 16, 1885, she wrote that her students "had been used to do about as they pleased, whispering, chewing gum, and a general shuffling noise." She vowed to "work diligently to overcome these formed habits." She took equal pride in the attention she devoted to teaching the fundamentals of spelling and arithmetic. Sarah also found happiness in her life away from the farm. Most of the homes in which she boarded had a son or daughter her age. One taught her to play the organ, another to sew a lace pattern. Together they went sleigh riding, visited friends, and held impromptu parties. She was always pleased to see her mother again, but she occasionally found days at home dreary and was glad to return to her hosts.

Nevertheless, Sarah did not enjoy undiluted success. Especially in the beginning, she confronted several major setbacks. She failed her first teaching certification examination and had to remain home as her friends departed for jobs. She did receive a certificate the following year but could not immediately find a post. In her first term as a teacher, she found it difficult to exercise discipline and was not rehired for the following term.

Sarah first felt secure as a teacher during her second term, from November 1884 to March 1885. Her growing professional confidence, however, coincided with increased anxiety about her mother. When Sarah left for school, she confessed on November 30 that she did not like "to leave Ma so miserable." And, indeed, as soon as Sarah departed,

Emily's health grew worse. On December 3 Emily wrote, "My hands feel real bad and in fact I have a singular feeling all over; when I rub my flesh it gives a peculiar sensation a shudder almost hurts. My nerves must be in a bad condition. I hope I may be better sometime." During the next few months she complained that the problems had spread to her feet and head.

Soon after Sarah returned to the farm for a vacation in the spring of 1885, Emily described her condition thus: "I have a nervous chill and fever every day. When I move around it seems as if my head would almost burst and every time my heart beats I can hear and feel the flow of blood on the top of my head so much that the sound is some of the time unendurable" (April 6). Sarah reported on April 8 that she "kept cold water" on Emily's head. Emily also found relief in a remedy she prescribed for herself. "I feel better when I eat dandelion greens," she noted on April 30. Before leaving, Sarah recruited a "hired girl" to do some of the housework she left behind.[16]

Sarah's worries intensified during her third term, which began on May 3, 1885. Although she was "glad" to see the family with whom she boarded, she wondered how her mother was faring in her absence. "Ma was sick abed and had a burning fever when we came away I do hope and pray she may get better soon," she wrote that day. Returning home for a visit three weeks later, she commented, "I tell you I've cried more than once since Fri. evening when I first saw her this time. Something must be done for her." She found that her mother had increased difficulty walking and could feed the turkeys only by lying down. Back at school on June 4, Sarah recorded her concerns about leaving Emily with only the hired girl to help: "Ma has the dropsy to her body—Im so afraid it will get all over her—and wish I knew what could be done to help her. She did not sleep she said her feet and legs pain her so badly— Now if I was there Id rub them for her—But there is nothing done for her at all."[17] Emily also compared the hired girl invidiously with Sarah. When Sarah returned from school in July, Emily wrote, "Sarah wash, mop and do up the work before eleven A.M. O so much nicer than it has been done for three months" (July 27).

During Sarah's fourth term as a teacher, from November 1885 to March 1886, Emily's condition continued to deteriorate. On February 5 she wrote that when she tried to move a chair she "fell flat upon the floor. I could have cried for its very discouraging to be so weak." Re-

turning to the farm that weekend, Sarah reported that she found Emily
"ever so much weaker." Sarah also had to contend with the intense hostility between her parents. Emily complained that James purposely aggravated her condition. He drove the carriage too fast when they were
together, refused to supply her with the proper food, and made her
faint by cleaning a kerosene lantern too close to her room. During her
vacation in the spring of 1886, Sarah chastised her father for his behavior, watched over Emily, rubbed her swollen legs, and brought the
food she desired. On April 17, the day before Sarah left, Emily again
stressed her dependence on Sarah: "She *is* such a *blessed good* girl. If it
were not for her it seems as if I would almost starve. And no one else to
do the slightest errand."

When Sarah began a new term in April 1886, she increasingly was
torn between her responsibilities as a daughter and as a teacher. Her
last day at home she wondered if she "ought to go and leave" her
mother. When she arrived at her boarding place later that day, she described herself as "very homesick" because she had left her mother
"failing so badly." Her spirits rose when she entered the classroom.
"Seems like home again," she wrote on April 19. "Think we will have
a good school." But the following day she noted that her students
thought she was "crosser" than she had been the previous term. "I
guess I am worrying about Ma," she explained. "Wish I might see her."
On April 30 Emily wrote that she could "hardly walk" and that she
felt "entirely broken down. Both nerve and muscle and courage." The
same day, Sarah commented in her diary, "Ma is just dying for want of
care I'm almost a mind to give up my school." When Sarah returned
for a short visit, Emily noted on May 2 that Sarah "dreads to leave me
feeling so bad." On May 3 Sarah wrote, "Don't believe I'll try to teach
any more for I have to worry so much. I'm thinking of Ma every minute." Two days later, however, she again dwelt on the joys of her job:
"We had a splendid school to-day. Seems as though I could take them
in my arms and kiss them all."

Sarah returned to the farm for the weekend ten days later. She slept
with her mother on the night of Saturday, May 15. When she awoke
the following morning, she discovered that her mother "did not realize
anything." Although Emily soon regained consciousness, she continued to require around-the-clock care for several weeks. Sarah resigned
her job and stayed home to nurse her mother. Emily reported on May

21 that Sarah "comes every minute to see how I feel." Sarah also described her care. On May 20 she wrote that Emily "had been to weak to sit up much for 2 or 3 days. But has to be rubbed and hot flannels Kept on and hot teas and a great deal of care." Whenever death seemed imminent, Sarah "sat up" in order to forestall "sinking spells." Although neighbors and a hired girl provided some assistance, Sarah frequently was alone at night. She often noted that she slept just one or two hours. On June 2 she slept from 11:30 P.M. to 12:30 A.M. and from 2:15 to 3:45 A.M. On June 22 she reported that her eyes ached and that she was sick herself as a result of "irregular sleep." Six days later, she wrote that she undressed and went to bed for the first time in six weeks. The following week, however, she cared for her mother between two and six times each night.

Sarah accepted without question that her primary duty as a daughter and a woman was to provide this nursing care. Because she felt strongly attached to her mother, caregiving was a labor of love. Nevertheless, she also longed to be back at school. Four days after this crisis began, she wrote, "It makes me cry to think of them (My pupils)." Two weeks later, a rumor that she would be rehired the following term "much pleased" her (June 6). She also was glad to learn that the students preferred her to the replacement and that the director thought the school was not functioning well in her absence.

Henry Gillespie had been working in Kansas City when the crisis began and returned on May 19; however, he immediately found another job in the vicinity. Although he lived at the farm and cared for his mother when he could, he was away most days. Sarah complained that her father added to, rather than alleviated, her burdens. According to her account, James was indifferent to her difficulties. "Pa does not seem to think but that I can work all night and all day," she commented bitterly on May 26. She was "provoked" when he would not relieve her even "1 hr. of the night" (June 10). When James asked Sarah to not bother him and to allow him to sleep, she remarked indignantly, "I thot I needed rest if any one" (June 17). James left home a few weeks later, and he and Emily never again lived together.

Sarah also received relatively little assistance from formal health providers. During May and June 1886, physicians from town occasionally stopped by the house, left medicine, discussed Emily's prognosis, and offered advice. On June 28, Sarah noted, "Dr. Fuller said for me to get asparagus root and steep it and put in a drop or two of alcohol to keep it and let Ma smell of it." It seems likely that Sarah took this recommendation seriously and attempted to follow it. Most of the time, however, she administered remedies without a doctor's direction.

Emily loathed the enforced dependency of an invalid. On August 7, 1886, she wrote, "I pray I may walk again and be so that I can get around and wait upon myself . . . To be helpless is *so bad* I can not tell *how* bad." The following month she explained why she had neglected her diary: "Each time when I felt like writing no one was near to ask for pen and ink and Book, or were busy. It seems to me a *deep, sorrowful and bad affliction* that I *can not* wait upon myself" (September 5). On October 2 she complained, "I could sew some but can not get at any of my things to get any thing to do and to ask for every thing I want is *surely* the hardest work I ever done."

But her children's attentiveness also gave her enormous pleasure. Shortly after becoming seriously ill, she wrote, "I have lived for them and now they have sacrificed time and money, and they can not do too much for me" (May 21). She expressed her gratitude again on August 4: "The Children have been so kind and faithful to care for me. Doing and watching . . . *I thank Henry and Sarah* for their watchful care."

Nevertheless, Emily also worried that the work was a strain on her son and daughter. As she commented on June 3, "Sarah sits up most nights and does a good deal of cooking and it is too much for her." It is likely that she also had concerns about Sarah's teaching career. Emily had wanted Sarah to achieve the upward mobility that had been denied to her, but Sarah was now marooned on the farm, engulfed in domestic obligations. Rather than pursuing professional success, she seemed to be repeating the narrow pattern of her mother's life.

Emily slowly regained her health throughout the summer and early fall of 1886, and Sarah was able to return to school in November. She wrote only sporadically in her journal during the next few months. Emily's diary, however, indicates that she continued to experience new health problems. As a result of lying down so much, her hip joints became sore, and at the end of December, she burned her foot. Although Henry and a hired girl tended to her regularly, she was convinced that Sarah alone could meet her needs. When Sarah returned for spring vacation in 1887, she recorded on March 11 that she "put on a poultice of potato, changing it often during the day." At night she applied "bread and milk and sugar." The following day, Emily noted that her sore foot had greatly improved. "I verily believe," she asserted, "my foot might not have ever healed and got well had not Sarah have come home to take care of it."

During this vacation Sarah also sent for a "magnetic doctor."[18] "I believe he can cure Ma," she wrote on March 19. She was not immediately disappointed. Two days after his arrival, she wrote, "Ma is constantly better. It is wonderful what the simplicity of rubbing will do. And it is not so simple either, for there is the will and the magnetism which develops and enshrouds the healer and is passed from him to the patient" (April 10). Emily expressed even greater faith in his powers, writing on April 12 that her hair was not as white as before and that she felt he could almost bring "the dead back to earthly life." He stayed at the house for five weeks, administering a total of thirty-three treatments.

His presence added to Sarah's burdens. She had to cook his meals, and when he expressed distaste for her food, she had to help him find other places to eat. Because James refused to pay his fee, the responsibility fell on Henry and Sarah. Worst of all, because Sarah often lacked the protection of her father and brother, she was vulnerable to unwanted sexual advances. "Dr. Munson is a free-lover," she complained on April 20. "I do not believe in his doctrine . . . The idea of an old man wanting to kiss and hug me Its surely unreasonable and below my dignity."

Sarah accepted another job for the term beginning in April 1887 but deferred opening the school to stay home an extra week. Instead of boarding in the community, she traveled the nine miles between the farm and school each morning and evening to tend her mother. While she was away, Henry and the hired girl shared responsibility for Emily's care. When the hired girl left abruptly, Sarah had to find a replacement. This, too, was an onerous job. On April 25 she wrote, "Saturday morning at 9 o'clock I drove to town for the mail as I heard nothing from Mrs. McFarland the woman who wished to work for us I concluded to drive to Dorsetville for her . . . A Scotchman led [the horse] past a brush fire . . . The place where they said Mrs Mc. was, she was not for she had gone 7 mi. farther to Lamont. I engineered the way and drove there . . . I saw Jas. Grey and he found out for me where Mrs Mc. was." They did not reach the Gillespie farm until eight o'clock in the evening. As Emily commented in her diary that night, it was "a real hard jaunt for Sarah."

When the school term ended, Sarah returned home and devoted herself to her mother's care. She later wrote, "School closed the 25th of June . . . I was very tired that Saturday night and thankful too, for I felt as though my school days were ended, not thankful for my own sake as much as Ma's and Henry's. Ma was so glad to have me with her again" (November 6). Emily was aware of Sarah's mixed emotions, noting on June 29 that Sarah would "so much rather teach than to stay." Sarah did not return to the classroom until several years after her mother's death the following spring.

Although Sarah's departure from school freed her from the burden of reconciling the competing demands of work and home, it also deprived her of her primary way of limiting her caregiving responsibilities. As Emily worsened, Sarah spent her days bathing her mother, lifting her from bed, turning her over, dressing her, and helping her use the bedpan. In addition, Sarah gave Emily catnip tea, bathed her hip in smartweed water, and cleaned her bedsores. On March 15, 1888, two weeks before Emily died, Sarah wrote, "Her bedsores are very painful—one which is a trifle better now is 3 in. deep and 2½ in. in diameter. I have to cut out the 'puss' and cleanse them often and it fairly makes my veins refuse to carry the blood sometimes." Even when Sarah did not provide direct care, she could not escape the sight of her mother's deteriorating body. On February 3, she suddenly lost her appetite when she saw her mother lying in an unusually convoluted position. "She was in a terrible shape . . . Well—it spoiled my meal. I was choked and had to leave the table. I was so hungry and had some nice mashed potatoes on my plate; but somehow I was not the least hungry in less than a minute." It is possible that Emily's infirmities affected Sarah so intensely because she identified closely with her mother. Watching Emily, Sarah may have imagined her own future.

Sarah's concern for her mother's emotional well-being also meant that Sarah had to conceal the toll that caregiving inflicted on her. Emily hated being a burden, and she wanted to believe that her children rendered care with "willing hearts." Six weeks before Emily's death, Sarah complained, "My side and back are very lame and, though I very much dislike to own it I feel very tired; a kind of tired sick. And if I make visible complaint, such as to lie down or go without a meal why,

Ma will look so much worse and worry so" (February 2). Just as Emily took pride in being "pleasant" despite her troubles, so Sarah had to mask her own feelings. Although various friends and relatives called and offered their services, the bulk of the work fell on Sarah. Once again she complained about her exhaustion. Because she had little time to eat, she lost weight. She also wrote about painful back problems, which she attributed to the strain of lifting her mother.

Emily continued to express both concern about the burdens imposed on Henry and Sarah and gratitude for their help. On February 19 she wrote, "Sarah is lying down to rest. She is tired it grieves my heart that she has had to get up to care for me every night." Because Henry and Sarah frequently wrote Emily's diary for her during the months before her death, her comments served as a way of conveying sentiments to them. An entry in Sarah's handwriting on December 28 reads, "Sarah takes the best care of me she can." On February 12, 1888, Emily was able to write for herself. In an entry clearly intended for Sarah to read, she stated, "Sarah is here and cares for me . . . Dear Daughter it is to Ma more than words or pen can tell." Emily died the following month, on March 24, 1888.

〜 ARTHUR KLEINMAN WRITES, "Acting like a sponge, illness soaks up personal and social significance from the world of the sick person."[19] The deterioration of Emily's marriage, coupled with the tensions in her female friendships, made her especially dependent on her daughter. Although Emily encouraged Sarah to pursue individual achievement and furthered her career in many ways, Emily also expected Sarah to respond to her emotional and physical crises. Because Sarah had long been solicitous of her mother's well-being, caregiving represented an extension of previously established patterns in their relationship, not an abrupt change. Sarah's strong attachment to her mother had advantages as well as disadvantages. Because Sarah experienced Emily's pain as if it were her own, the process of rendering care frequently was overwhelming. But Sarah also was able to give her mother extremely sensitive care, and she had the gratification of knowing that she alone could satisfy her mother's conflicting needs.

The accidents of personal history also help us understand how Emily Gillespie's filial caregiving experience unfolded. Hial Hawley's attempts to receive assistance from his daughter Emily quickly became entangled in the ongoing conflicts in her life. His seven-month stay intensified her battle with her sister Harriet. The women competed for their father's affection and contested his one valuable possession. Hial's presence also exacerbated Emily's marital conflict. She accused James of slandering her to her father; James used her poor filial relationship as evidence of her personal failings. This chapter thus reminds us that family caregiving is an intensely personal experience that can be fully understood only in the context of the relationships that nest it.

But Emily and Sarah Gillespie's "world" also included the broader social and cultural context that helped to shape their personal lives and relationships. Both Emily and Sarah became caregivers partly to fulfill the prevailing definition of female virtue. Neither could transfer care to formal providers. The following chapter will demonstrate that many other white women of their era similarly assumed very expansive caregiving responsibilities, made medical decisions on their own, relinquished paid jobs whenever kin fell ill, relied on female support networks, and struggled to make sense of their encounters with sickness, dependency, and death.

~2
An Overview of
Nineteenth-Century Caregiving

$\mathcal{C}$AREGIVING DOMINATED women's lives throughout the nineteenth century. Women from diverse social strata administered medications, applied poultices, watched for dangerous symptoms, changed dressings, and cleaned up vomit, excrement, and pus. Beginning as early as girlhood and extending into middle and old age, caregiving simultaneously exacted a terrible toll and conferred significant benefits. This chapter focuses first on white women, who left the most extensive records. Because caregiving varied little across geographic regions, I discuss white women living in many parts of the country. Although I focus on the period between 1850 and 1890, I occasionally use earlier or later examples that illustrate themes central to that period. The chapter then briefly examines enslaved African American women in the antebellum South; that discussion, of course, stops in 1865. The caregiving experiences of enslaved women provide a counterpoint to those of whites and introduce the theme of power and conflict, which recurs repeatedly in later chapters.

"Supplying All Her Needs and Fancies": White Women, 1850–1890

We can explain white women's preoccupation with caregiving in various ways. Because mutual aid was often a requirement of participating in social life as well as a form of insurance, responsibilities extended very broadly.[1] Women in isolated rural areas sometimes cared for strangers who needed assistance far from home. When George Cutter was wounded in a battle in Kansas in 1856, he was taken to the home of John and Sarah Everett, who nursed him for more than six months.[2] Women moving west from the East Coast stopped to assist strangers they passed along the way. Charlotte Stearns Pengra, a traveler on the Overland Trail, rode with women from other parties to help a woman afflicted with "camp colic": "I thought her case almost helpless, but after applying numerous remedies we succeeded in relieving her."[3] Frances Sawyer, another woman who made the trip west, wrote in her diary, "Tonight we visited an adjoining camp to see a lady and her little daughter who had been turned over in a carriage today with coming down a steep mountain-side."[4]

Many women also cared for an extensive network of kin and neighbors. In 1867 Laura Stebbens explained why she could not join her friend in reform work: "My eldest Aunt, almost eighty, is so very frail and feeble, that I ques[tion] very seriously the propriety of my leaving—for both [aunts] are very helpless and in case of sudden illness—or of accident, they might suffer much; and then I should reflect upon myself exceedingly."[5] As we have seen, despite Emily Gillespie's strained relationships with many members of her community, she responded immediately to their calls for help.

A diary written by Nannie Stillwell Jackson in 1890 and 1891 portrays women's neighborhood obligations in unusually rich detail.[6] The wife of a small farmer in Arkansas, Nannie saw her close friend Fannie Morgan as often as four times a day. In addition, Nannie frequently exchanged goods and services with at least twenty other women, both white and African American. Care for sick and dying people was embedded in this collective female life. When Mrs. Dyer "was terribly afflicted with boils," Nannie visited her, along with several other women.[7] Both Nannie and Fannie spent time at the home of Mrs. Caulk when her baby was ill.[8] When Nannie herself fell ill, Fannie cooked breakfast for her; Mrs. Gifford and Bettie Newby came by in the evening.[9] After Mrs. Hornbuckle's son died, Nannie and her husband stayed with her at night. The following day, Nannie returned to the Hornbuckle house, got material for the coffin lining, and went to the home of Fannie, who helped her "make the pillow and face cover."[10]

Sickness at the Archdale home required a range of services from several women. On March 22 Nannie "set a while" with Mrs. Archdale's sons Bill and Lee, both of whom had pneumonia. She continued to visit the house regularly over the next few days, reporting on March 28 that the sons were better but that the daughter had contracted the disease. On April 8 Mrs. Archdale became ill and sent for Nannie; Nannie, in turn, summoned Fannie, and together they gave Mrs. Archdale "a dose of oil and turpentine and some gum camphor." Various other women spent the next few nights with the patient. Mrs. Archdale's son Lee came to the Jacksons' house for dinner and then took food to Fannie, who also was not well. On April 11 all members of the Archdale family appeared to be recovering. Nannie "cleaned up the dishes and stratened things about there some"; she also gave Lee Archdale two of his meals. The following day, Nannie had time to visit three ailing women in addition to Mrs. Archdale. Then, on April 13, Mrs. Archdale took a turn for the worse. Nannie visited her "5 or 6 times," and she and Fannie spent the night. On April 14 Mrs. Archdale died. "Mrs. Morgan [Fannie], Mrs. Newby and I Mr. Jackson Kate McNiel and Fannie Totten all set up . . . and we dressed her and laid her out." Although a flood prevented the women from attending the burial, Nannie "fixed things about in Mrs. Archdale's house."[11]

When Nannie was too busy to engage in caregiving activities herself, she relied on her daughters—Lizzie (twelve) and Sue (nine)—to fulfill her responsibilities. In this way, she was able to extend the range of her neighborly services and socialize her daughters into a major female role. Nannie sent both girls to stay with Fannie when the latter was sick and the two women who might have been expected to tend her had gone to spend the night at the home of a boy who had just died. The following day, Fannie took Lizzie with her to visit the bereaved mother.[12]

Two obligations of neighborliness were especially onerous. Because infectious diseases were rampant, infants and children frequently required nursing care. Common killers included pneumonia, typhus, typhoid fever, diphtheria, scarlet fever, measles, whooping cough, dysentery, and tuberculosis. During epidemics, women moved continually from house to house in the community, exposing themselves and their own families to disease. Women also received frequent calls to lend assistance at deliveries. Although the fertility rate of white women dropped throughout the century, it remained high by present standards; moreover, each confinement involved several female attendants. Birth was a hazardous event in the nineteenth century, and attendants often had to assume responsibility for critically ill newborns and women. Some birth attendants completed their work by laying out the infants they had helped to deliver. On January 9, 1890, Emily French recounted the events of the previous night: "Mrs. Sloans sick all the night, I up with her, the child a girl still born at 8 this morning . . . Her Annie, 16 months old, is her baby yet. I put all away as best I could, got a place for the child, a nice smooth box."[13] Common maternal complications included hemorrhage, convulsions, and puerperal fever. When anesthesia was absent, as it often was, many women suffered severe pain.

Few formal services were available to relieve women of these responsibilities. According to Charles E. Rosenberg, "Most Americans in 1800 had probably heard that such things as hospitals existed, but only a minority would have ever had occasion to see one."[14] The situation had not changed greatly seventy years later. When the first government survey was conducted in 1873, the nation had only 120 hospitals, most of which were custodial institutions serving the "deserving poor."[15] Middle-class patients rarely entered hospitals. Although low-income people had fewer options, most families were reluctant to entrust sick relatives to such facilities. After hearing that her husband had been wounded in battle, Harriet Jane Thompson wrote to him, "Dear William, do take care of yourself and not go into the hospital if you can possibly avoid it for there you are apt to get disease and not be taken care of."[16] Other medical institutions also were sparse. Although tuberculosis was a common scourge throughout the century, the sanatorium movement was not launched until the 1880s, and in the absence of nursing homes, the sole facilities for the elderly were poorhouses; only the most desperate sought refuge within their walls.

Caregivers also received little help from health professionals. Many families could not afford the fees physicians charged. Without telephones or automobiles, summoning physicians involved considerable time and effort. When a young woman had a miscarriage in Oregon in 1890, one of her relatives reported that the doctor "arrived in a wonderfully short time, about hours."[17] A man volunteered to call for the doctor when Anne Ellis's mother was dying in a Colorado mining camp. Anne later described his journey: "It is seventeen miles over Ute Pass—the snow in dreadful drifts, but he makes it, sometime riding, other times leading his horse and breaking trail. He is all night, then starts the doctor, who has a horse and buggy, on his forty-mile trip."[18] Some doctors were visiting other patients when travelers reached their destinations. A few refused to come.[19]

Transportation difficulties not only delayed doctors' arrivals but also prevented them from providing continuing care. Emma Reid sent a messenger eleven miles to summon a doctor when her baby was "terribly burned" in Idaho in 1879. "The doctor came and dressed the burns once," Emma wrote to her father a few weeks later. "Since then I have taken care of them myself."[20] Dr. Francis A. Long recounted the following incident in the life of a "railroad surgeon":

> A physician a hundred miles up the line telegraphed him to come on the evening train prepared to amputate. Reaching the [other] physician's home he was told the patient lived in the Dakota Indian country two days' pony drive away. They started early in the morning, drove all that day and all the next before reaching the ranch home of the patient who had gangrene of the leg . . . [T]hey amputated above the knee and remained with the patient the rest of that day and the following night. Necessary dressings were left with the family.[21]

Skepticism about physicians further deterred many people from relying on them. According to Nannie T. Alderson, a Montana woman, "Some of those who practiced out west in the early days spent much of their time in the clutches of the demon rum, having come here because they couldn't keep a practice back east."[22] Although physician assistance at childbirth became increasingly common during the nineteenth century, horror stories abounded. Alderson wrote that the doctor attending a neighbor's confinement "boasted of having nine diplomas, and was considered first rate, but when she had been in labor for a night and a day, uselessly, and they saw she would die like this, he confessed that he had never had a baby case before, and he fell on his knees and begged for forgiveness."[23]

Children's illnesses also revealed the limits of doctors' knowledge. Many nineteenth-century doctors did not bother to learn about children's health, assuming that mothers were competent to treat their own offspring.[24] In 1840 Rachel Simmons, an Ohio woman, wrote to her mother, "We are all well but my little babe. It has been sick for two weeks and last Wednesday she was taken with hard fits . . . We sent for Dr. Thompson. He came and gave her calomel. In a day or two he came back. Did not think he could do much for a child so young." Rachel beseeched her mother to come and help.[25] In another case, Maria D. Brown resolved to avoid physicians whenever possible after her daughter died of diphtheria in Iowa in 1862. She later told her daughter-in-law,

> With any fair treatment, she would have pulled through. But old Dr. Farnsworth gave her terrible doses of quinine and cayenne pepper . . . [A]fter she was gone, I said to myself: "Never again! When the next trouble comes, it will be between me and my God. I won't have any doctor." . . . I had a pretty hard test. Three of my children, Charlie, Lizzie, and Gus, came down at the same time with scarlet fever. All but Will were ill, and I was expecting another baby. Nevertheless, I nursed them through without the help of doctor or nurse.[26]

Women who did trust doctors typically resorted to them only after exhausting home remedies. According to a history of nursing in nineteenth-century Kansas, when epidemics of diphtheria, scarlet fever, smallpox, whooping cough, and typhoid fever swept through the state, families sought "professional advice so rarely that when a physician was called it was understood that death was probably imminent."[27]

Moreover, medical aid did not replace neighborhood assistance. When the daughter of Mary Ann Owen Sims "was taken with a sevier attact of the croup," the mother "sent for Mrs. garrett and Dr. galispe a Physi[ci]an."[28] Isaac Neff Ebey described the events occurring at the beginning of his wife's labor: "In the afternoon to Coveland for Dr. Lansdale in the evening went for Mrs. Alexander"; Ebey's brother-in-law "went for Mrs. Ann Crockette and Mrs. Ivans."[29] When Samuella Curd gave birth, she called for "Mrs. McKinney and cousin Mary," and only "later for Dr. Abbott."[30] As we will see in the next chapter, during both sickness and childbirth, female friends and kin continued to make major treatment decisions and exercise medical skills after doctors arrived.

Most caregivers had even less contact with nurses. Although nursing did not begin to organize into a profession until late in the century, many women worked as "professed" nurses.[31] Ralph Waldo Emerson's daughter Ellen wrote that a nurse had eased her burdens during her mother's final illness: "It was not hard to take care of Mother this last year, at least all the hardness came on Miss Leavitt, not on me, and I am not in the least tired."[32] Although Emerson may have underestimated her own contributions, she escaped the overwhelming exhaustion experienced by many women caring for seriously ill family members.

But the cost of hiring nurses was prohibitive for many families, and those who could afford to pay for nursing care often chose not to. Some were unaccustomed to depending on strangers for care and fearful of allowing them into their homes. Class prejudices may have heightened such anxieties. Whereas most families employing nurses were of the middle or upper class, nurses came overwhelmingly from less privileged backgrounds.[33] Louisa May Alcott claimed that she intended to hire a nurse during her mother's long illness but could find none who met her standards. She later employed a nurse to care for her father, but only because her own poor health prevented her from caring for him herself.[34]

Still another reason caregiving consumed women's attention is that the reigning ideology assigned that endeavor to women alone. The domestic manuals, religious tracts, etiquette guides, and women's magazines flooding the market in the mid-nineteenth century expounded a new doctrine exalting women's sphere. At the heart of the domestic code lay the belief that women were calmer, purer, more loving, and more sensitive than men. The traits that are considered essential to caregiving—responsiveness to the needs of others, patience, and an ability to adapt to change—became part of the cultural definition of womanhood. In addition, prescriptive literature exhorted women to strive to please others and subordinate their own needs.[35]

Some women explained their motives in providing care in terms of duty. In her autobiography, Lucy Sprague Mitchell, a famous educator, recalled that she had not questioned her family's expectation that she would nurse her parents and cousin. "As a dutiful daughter, I simply did my job . . . I accepted the standards of the times that daughters belonged to their families."[36] Women who resented caregiving obligations occasionally tried to conform their emotions to the prevailing ideology. Judith C. Breault notes that after Emily Howland began caring for her father, her letters to friends were filled with phrases such as "'I try to do right,' 'I must,' 'I should,' . . . 'I should feel,' 'I strain with all my might.'"[37]

To be sure, caregiving was not exclusively women's work. Men escorted neighborhood women to and from their homes and fetched doctors, an exceedingly onerous task in some cases. Although the primary responsibility for family nursing rested with women, the gender division of labor frequently dissolved in the midst of medical emergencies. During Emily Gillespie's long illness, her son, Henry, filled in when Sarah was unavailable, rubbing his mother's legs, making her special teas, and watching her throughout the night. Some men spooned soup and broth into the mouths of sick children, wiped their fevered brows, and administered medications. In remote areas many men cared for sick and dying wives without any assistance. "My husband has been my only nurse, and he has done all he could for me," wrote Almira Raymond from Oregon to her sister in 1852. "It has been as hard for him as for me."[38] It is commonly assumed that husbands in the nineteenth century were exiled from the birthing room, but some fathers did attend their wives' deliveries.[39]

Outside the household, however, gender lines remained more firmly entrenched. Men kept vigil at the bedsides of other men, watching for signs of danger or impending death. But women alone assumed the two major community obligations—caring for children and parturient women.

The Burdens of Care

Caregiving was a powerful force restricting women to the home. Although increasing numbers of single women went out to work during the nineteenth century, female workers at all levels of the occupational hierarchy quit their jobs when family members fell ill. After Malenda M. Edwards left her employment in the mills of New Hampshire to care for her parents in 1845, she wrote to a friend that she was serving as "physician and nurse too" and that she would travel west were it not for the need to provide care.[40] Velma Leadbetter had learned dressmaking in hopes of achieving economic independence. Her work separated her from her family in Nanticoke Valley in New York, but she was recalled periodically to assist during sickness. Her daughter later wrote,

"The maiden woman in a country family belongs to everybody in case of illness . . . [C]all on her and she'd come home and take care of the mother or the father who was ill. So Mother would have to hang a sign out, saying 'I'm sorry but I've gone up to my father's . . .' They thought *nothing* of calling her out like that."[41]

Even entry into a profession did not excuse single women from the duty to provide care. Mary Holywell Everett was a successful New York physician when her sister became ill in 1876. A male colleague to whom she had written counseled her thus: "Even at the risk of losing your practice entirely, duty commands you to remain by the side of your old mother and help her to carry the burden."[42] At least one of Everett's female patients concurred with this advice. Writing to Everett about her absence from practice, the patient commented, "Being that you have no husband, your dear mother has the first claim to you."[43]

The history of nineteenth-century women teachers is filled with stories of women who left their posts to nurse family members. Lettie Teeple had just begun her first teaching job in Michigan in 1848 when she "was hurried away from school by [family] sickness."[44] Sarah Gillespie withdrew from the work force twice when her mother was ill and once postponed the opening of school. Preoccupation with her mother's well-being also prevented her from adhering to the high standards she set herself. When her students found her "crosser" than usual, she feared she was violating her own code of professional behavior. Even when Emily lay dying in March 1888, the offer of a new teaching job sorely tempted Sarah, much as she tried to convince herself otherwise. "No—I can not teach—no use to think of it now," she wrote nine days before her mother's death.[45]

Caregiving obligations not only brought teachers back home but also followed them to work. On May 12, 1886, Sarah Gillespie described the various misfortunes that had befallen three of her students: "Rena Allen went to town this forenoon and had Dr. Trim cut out a tumor which was as large as a hazlenut above her eye. She came this afternoon. Alice Traver has a poisoned foot—She hobbles around on the other—I had her home with me to stay till Amos McNeil came past with the milk. Charley Mead had the sick-head-ache so I have been a Homeopathic to day."[46] Pamela Brown, a teacher in Plymouth, Vermont, noted in her journal on January 25, 1837, that she was boarding at the home of a Mrs. Taylor, whose "babe had a fit."[47] Two days later

Pamela reported that she "sat up with Mrs. Taylor's babe until three o'clock."[48] On February 10 Pamela dismissed school because the baby "died in a fit," and the family needed help.[49] Pamela also visited students who were too ill to attend school. "Called to Philinda Hall's," Pamela wrote on January 18. "She was taken sick in school Monday. Is not quite sick."[50] Pamela "called again (at noon) to see Philinda" on January 20, this time pronouncing the girl "a very sick child."[51]

During most of the nineteenth century, however, caregiving was more likely to conflict with domestic chores than with paid employment. Household labor for most women was extremely arduous. The making of textiles, soap, and candles had moved from the home to the factory by the early years of the century, but indoor plumbing did not reach most households until 1900 or later.[52] Laundry alone was a day-long ordeal, demanding that women carry and heat gallons of water, lug pails of wet clothes, scrub and rinse each item and hang it on the line, exposing their hands to lye and other caustic soaps.[53] "To-day Oh! horrors how shall I express it; is the dreded washing day," wrote America Butler in her diary in 1853.[54]

I have noted that women routinely cared for an extensive network of kin, friends, and neighbors, as well as immediate family. Sickness among members of this broad community pulled women away from home, often for extended periods. Mary Wilder Foote wrote that when her baby was very ill, "My kind friend, Mrs. Pierson, sat with me *four* days, leaving all her family cares. Nobody ever tended a child so exquisitely, and in her lap I could place my darling, and feel at ease."[55] Other women performed the same tasks in their neighbors' homes that they left undone in their own. Abbie Bright was a young woman living with her brother on a Kansas claim in 1871 when she learned that her neighbors were ill. Arriving at their house, she "fixed to bake bread next day, then commenced at the dishes which sat around in confusion." The following morning she "washed dishes, pots and pans, I had not found the evening before, dressed a chicken, [roasted] coffee, and what not. Had chicken and sweet potatoes for dinner. It was long after noon when the bread was baked, and house tidied up."[56]

In some cases, women who responded to pleas for help were able to draw on a large structure of labor exchange to get their own work done. When Emily Gillespie was summoned to attend her sister Harriet in childbirth, Harriet's sister-in-law Lilly went to Emily's house to bake her bread and cook James Gillespie's dinner.[57] A friend's daughter churned for Fannie Morgan when she spent the night with her sick mother.[58]

But more often, the caregiver's housework simply accumulated in her absence. Nannie Jackson and her husband watched a sick woman throughout most of one night. When they returned home, Nannie's husband "laid down and took a nap." Her work, however, could not wait. "I churned and cooked breakfast and had it ready before daylight," she wrote in her diary.[59] A week later, Nannie noted that she had spent most of the day caring for another sick friend and, as a result, had "done no work."[60] A mission of mercy had more serious economic consequences for Effie Hanson, a North Dakota farm woman. Writing to a friend about the assistance she and her husband rendered when her mother-in-law was dying, Effie noted, "We lost some chickens [during] those cold spells as we wasn't home to take care of them as we should."[61]

Caregiving intruded on Effie's household responsibilities even when she remained at home. In another letter she explained that she hadn't washed any clothes for two weeks in the one-room house she shared with her husband and three children because "the children were all sick and I didn't like to have wet clothes hanging in here."[62] Some of the tasks women performed when family members fell ill were indistinguishable from their routine household labor. But sickness also imposed extra burdens, such as cooking custards, gruels, and broths, preparing special tonics, and washing blood-and sweat-stained sheets and clothes. Marian Louise Moore, an Ohio homesteader, remembered her experience nursing her mother: "In the Spring of the year 1872 . . . she was sick three months, part of the time helpless [with] typhoid inflammatory rheumatism . . . This sickness of hers brought more work upon me, washing and other work, when I had more work of my own than I could possibly do well."[63]

When husbands or older children were ill, caregivers had to add the patients' chores to their own. Mary Ann Webber was in her early sixties when her husband's health began to decline. In January 1865 she wrote to her children, "Your Father and myself, or rather, I perform our daily round of chores. I am able to cope, but he feels it a great burden many times. His health is not very good."[64] A few months later, he injured his ankle in a fall on the cellar steps and was unable to walk without crutches. "This has been a great disadvantage," she wrote. "It has also made it very hard on me, as I have to be now Man, woman, and chore boy."[65] Emily Gillespie's illness meant that Sarah assumed responsibility for her mother's household and family labor. Even when caring for her mother "night and day," Sarah rose at half past five in the morning to prepare her brother's breakfast, fed more than two hundred turkeys, baked bread and pies, mopped the kitchen, washed the family's clothes, and took berries to the market. "Dear me," she wrote in March 1887, "the clock strikes 8 and now I've my dishes to wash and Ma's foot to dress. Beds to make, etc, etc."[66]

When illness struck men who were wage earners, their wives often were thrust into the job market. Emily Conine Dorsey of Indiana wrote to her sister in March 1854, "John's health is poor and I fear likely to remain so. This is the evil wind which blew me again into the school room." Because the school was close by and she could earn a decent salary, "it would not have been bad at all" had she been able to afford a hired girl to help with the household chores.[67] But the combination of teaching, housework, and caregiving overwhelmed her.

Because hospitalization was rarely an option, women had to provide personal care and skilled nursing services, even for critically ill patients. "It is hard to have the care of a poor sick man day after day, week after week," wrote Mary Ann Webber to her son when her husband lay dying in 1871.[68] Dressing him, getting him in and out of bed, helping him walk, and bathing him consumed time and energy she previously had devoted to her daily chores. As he grew progressively weaker, her burdens multiplied. She was used to heavy farm work, but lifting a bedridden man several times a day taxed her strength.[69]

Although the members of Nannie Jackson's close-knit Arkansas community could draw on a ready source of support in times of trouble, women in more remote areas often delivered care alone.[70] Some caregivers had to tend several patients at once. And some were either pregnant or ill themselves. Emma Reid wrote to her father from Idaho territory in 1881, "For three weeks preceding my confinement, we had six children down at once, five of ours and one of the Warrens who had come to help us. Twenty nights I took my turn sitting up half the night, then when I knew that I, too, must soon be a care, I finished the night. And the next day, just across the hall from my little boys moaning in their delirium, I gave birth to twin girls."[71]

Not surprisingly, women often attributed their own ill health to the stresses of caregiving. We saw that when Emily Gillespie lay dying, Sarah complained constantly about exhaustion, weight loss, and back problems. Louisa May Alcott wrote five months after her mother's death, "I too have been ill and still am ordered to keep still for some months. Too much nursing last summer was bad for me."[72]

Caregiving had other consequences as well. When snow or mud made rural roads impassable, trips to the sick could be slow and arduous. Abigail Baldwin, a Vermont woman, wrote on December 23, 1853, "Snowed, started with wagon to go and see Mother, snow increased, stopped at Moses', stayed all night, wind blowed hard through the night, in the morning cold. Husband went with the horse . . . for the sleigh, drifted very badly at the hill but they broke through with the oxen so we got along very well. Found mother feeble and wasting away."[73] When Samuella Curd went by foot to visit a neighbor who had injured his leg, she "got stuck fast in the mud" and "had to cry aloud for help." Finally, "Charly Hockaday came to my relief, pulled me out and put down a plank to walk on."[74] Abbie Bright reported a similar incident on a trip to help a neighbor in Kansas. "There had been a log acrost the branch where I used to cross, it was gone and I had to take off shoes and stockings and wade. It was a miry place, and I went in over my feet, such ugly mud, had trouble to wash it off."[75]

If caregivers sometimes faced the perils of travel, at other times they had to cope with the tedium of confinement. "Staid at home all day," wrote Samuella Curd during her husband's long illness in 1862. "This is the fifth Sunday since I went to church, dont leave Mr. C at all."[76] Two months later she noted, "For a great rarity I sent for Mrs. Mc. to stay with Mr. C and I dressed up and started off . . . I felt so out of place fixed up."[77]

Caregiving also imposed economic costs. Although Sarah Gillespie had to forfeit her own income to nurse her mother, she and her brother paid the fees of at least one doctor. Mary Ann Webber's expenses included wages paid to both a neighborhood man who helped to dress and bathe her dying husband and a neighborhood woman who dipped the extra candles nighttime nursing required.[78]

Finally, caregiving involved "dirty work."[79] Many nineteenth-century medical interventions were "purgatives" that generated blood, vomit, and excreta. Surgeries and deliveries sometimes splattered assistants with various bodily fluids.[80] According to Emily Gillespie, a doctor brought a "rubber attachment for urinal purposes" to the house in November 1887; because Emily was extremely frail at this time, Sarah must have helped her mother use it.[81] Sarah's diary hints that she also had to clean up vomit, excreta, pus, and blood. Emily had believed that Sarah was too "fine" to participate in such "unpleasant" farm chores as milking cows and feeding hogs. Feminine delicacy, however, had no place in the sickroom.

The Content of Care

If caregiving disrupted women's lives and imposed serious costs, it also offered satisfactions. By analyzing the content of caregiving, we can better understand the elements women found gratifying.

Nineteenth-century caregiving encompassed a universe of activities, some very different from what we might designate as caregiving today. We have seen that instrumental services were an important component. Women cooked and cleaned, dressed sick people, helped them in and out of bed, and delivered what we now would consider skilled nursing and medical care. Although these activities often elicited complaints of overwork and exhaustion, they also could be a source of pride.

In a family letter written in 1868, Mary Ann Webber described the changes caregiving wrought in her daughter Alma. Because Alma's husband was failing in both "mind and body," she had to do all the farm work. Nevertheless, Mary Ann insisted that Alma's "present lot . . . is so much better than it was. I can see that her present position is doing her good, her self esteem and independence is increased. She is not narrowed down and humbled as she has been. She relies upon herself and feels that she possesses good powers of mind, as far as I can judge, should think she is well respected."[82] In overcoming challenges, some women discovered new resources. In 1857 Amelia Akehurst Lines wrote, "Went with sister to Dr. Campbell's office. Sister took ether and had eight or ten teeth taken out. She did not take enough to make her insensible to pain however, and suffered intensely. I stood by and held her hands through the whole. I did not know that I possess so much courage."[83] Grueling labor not only exhausted women but also demonstrated physical stamina. We saw that when Sarah Gillespie nursed her brother, Henry, she realized that she was "stronger than I thot I was."

Because caregiving began early in women's lives, it often provided one of the first opportunities to display competence in adult roles. According to an interviewer, Regan Wold later remembered "the great sense of responsibility" she had felt as a seventeen-year-old girl caring for her dying grandmother in North Dakota in the early twentieth century.[84] Regan also earned the respect of her aunt, who wrote to a friend, "She sure is a good girl if I do say it for John's niece. So quick to get around. Can harness horses, milk cows or most anything."[85]

The delivery of skilled care may have been especially likely to confer pride. A North Dakota woman wrote to a friend in 1899, "Cora has kept quite well for her this summer til a week ago yesterday she had a sick spell. She was taken in the night with a terrible pain in her head. We doctored her ourselves and got her all right in two or three days."[86] Sarah Gillespie gave her dying mother catnip tea, bathed her hip in smartweed water, and cleaned her bedsores. Emily Gillespie performed the equivalent of a surgical procedure when Henry cut his thumb "nearly off" with an axe. Maria D. Brown's son recalled, "I cut off three of [my fingers] one time when I was cutting sheaf oats for my pony in a cutting box. I rushed into the house with the ends of my fingers hanging by shreds. Mother washed them, fitted them together carefully, and bound them up so that they grew into perfectly good fingers again. Another time she saved my foot."[87]

Some women gained special recognition as healers. As Laurel Thatcher Ulrich writes of the early part of the century, "Caring for the sick was a universal female role, yet several women in every community stood out from the others for the breadth and depth of their commitment."[88] Although women rarely portrayed themselves as possessing exceptional knowledge, many children remembered their mothers as the first to be called in any emergency. Recalling her childhood in Nevada County, California, in the 1860s, Edith White wrote,

My parents were always ready to help their neighbors in trouble. Mother often spent night after night nursing the sick, especially during those terrible epidemics of diphtheria in the winter. It cost $10 to get a doctor to come from North San Juan, six miles away, and often the people couldn't well afford this. But they all had confidence in Mother and if she said "Get the doctor" they got him; if she thought that she could handle the case, they trusted in her skill. In those days everybody who died must be wrapped in a shroud to be properly prepared for burial. Mother made many a shroud for her neighbors, and sat up all night doing it. She washed and dressed them and helped to put them into the home-made coffins covered with black cloth. Those were sad times for the whole town.[89]

Domestic healing skills also had economic value. After Emily Gillespie's death, Sarah proudly noted that a local doctor offered to recommend her as a "skilled nurse."[90] Other women parlayed healing abilities into employment as midwives.[91]

Because sickness was likely to lead to death, caregiving also had an important spiritual component. Women sought to ensure that dying people were adequately penitent, "sensible" of their sins, and prepared to face death with equanimity.[92] In 1863 Eliza Webber, her sister Emma, and her brother Alpha left their home in Glover, Vermont, to sell children's books door-to-door in upstate New York. The project ended abruptly when Alpha contracted typhoid fever. In a letter notifying their parents of the disaster, Eliza wrote that she and Emma not only sat with Alpha at night and rubbed his body with alcohol throughout the day but also "read in the Bible everyday to him." The sisters summoned both a doctor and two ministers, who came "a number of times and . . . prayed with him." Perhaps as a result, Eliza was able to reassure her parents that her brother was "perfectly prepared to die."[93]

Samuella Curd considered herself successful in exerting a pious influence over a husband dying of tuberculosis. Sam had been married for two years to a Missouri merchant and had just given birth to her first child when her husband became seriously ill. She had other anxieties as well. Marriage had separated her from her family in Virginia. When the outbreak of the Civil War prevented communication, she worried about their well-being. Their absence also deprived her of the support that might have eased her grief. As her husband's condition deteriorated, Sam became increasingly disconsolate. After nursing him most of one night, she wrote, "Am feeling very much depressed. Mr. C had night sweats last night and is very feeble to day. Oh! I feel as if my heart would sink within me, when I see him look so badly."[94]

Sam's pleasure in her husband's growing faith helped to mitigate her despair. Even before his illness descended, she had expressed concern about his religious lapses. The death of a neighbor in childbirth in November 1860, for example, had prompted this remark: "Oh! that we all may profit by Bled's death. God grant my dear husband may be warned. Oh! the conversion of his soul, I desire above all earthly things."[95] As the gravity of her husband's illness became clear, Sam's fears intensified. After noting that she had heard "a most excellent sermon to the converted" on October 20, 1861, she wrote, "Oh! that Mr. Curd might be made to consider and not harden his heart."[96]

A few months later, her hopes began to be fulfilled. On January 18, 1862, she described "a talk with him upon the subject of religion" as "gratifying."[97] The following month she was even more encouraged: "Have had some satisfactory talks with him on the subject of religion and while his evidence is not as bright as I would hope yet I believe him to be a changed man. I pray God he will give him brighter manifestations."[98] She was able to proclaim her enterprise a success on March 17. After rubbing her husband's legs in the middle of the night, "We got to talking on religion to my great delight said he would join the church very soon. I believe him a genuine Christian."[99] Five days later he was "received into the church,"[100] and on March 30 Sam wrote, "A day long to be remembered by us all. Mr. Curd made a public profession of religion, there was a large congregation and many with whom he joined in sin, saw him make it God grant it may be blessed. Oh! it did delight my heart to see him in his weakness give himself up to God."[101]

The spiritual work caregivers performed had meaning for them as well. When Sam Curd discussed salvation with her husband, read the Bible to him, or accompanied him to church, she sought not only to prepare him for death but also to confront her own impending loss. On February 13 she wrote, "These are days when I need the Grace of God in great power oh! I feel as if my heart would burst; there is nothing but a gloomy future to me oh! God the idea of my dear husband being taken and I left almost crushes me; I cant be blind to his condition . . . Oh! God I am overcome. Give me grace or I die."[102] In order to accept, rather than "blind" herself to, her husband's growing frailty, Sam had to struggle against the despair that threatened to engulf her. She looked to the religion she offered her husband for the strength to engage in that struggle.

Deathbed scenes sometimes reinforced religious beliefs. As Katherine Ott notes, popular writers "portrayed deaths as ethereal moments that uplifted and enriched all witnesses."[103] Caregivers' diaries and letters often expressed a similar theme. Fanny Appleton Longfellow, for example, gave this description of the death of her brother Charles in 1835:

> He talked occasionally and his face beamed with the peace which earth knows not of . . . I shall never forget the strange look of wonder, almost pity, which he gave me as I was chafing his hands, as he saw the tears which I could not restrain streaming from my eyes. It was a silent rebuke that I could mourn for what opened to him happiness ineffable. He requested to be carried about, and he was conveyed in a sort of cradle of straw all over the house as he desired, suffering apparently very little except from difficulty to breathing, but even this did not disturb the serenity of his countenance for a moment. He at last put his hand to his eyes and exclaimed, "I can hardly see." These were his last words, and like a happy child he "went to sleep," to wake to those joys which are imperishable and eternal.[104]

Difficult deaths also had the capacity to instruct. Mary Ann Owen Sims recalled that in 1843 "uncle J. O[wen] one of Father's brother's (who had come to that State for his health—he had the consumption) died I shall never forget that death seane for he was a wicked man and oh the agonies of a lost Soul usher[e]d in to the presence of its Maker was truly heart rend[e]ring even to my youthful minde."[105]

Finally, caregiving had an emotional component. Some women found satisfaction in bestowing special attention on sick relatives and friends. "I had the great pleasure of supplying all her needs and fancies," wrote Louisa May Alcott when her beloved mother was ill in 1874.[106] After her mother's death three years later, Alcott wrote in her journal, "My only comfort is that I *could* make her last years comfortable, and lift off the burden she had carried so bravely all those years."[107] Alcott commented in a letter to a friend, "I could not let any one else care for the dear invalid while I could lift a hand for I had always been her nurse and knew her little ways."[108]

Sarah Hale was gratified to discover that her presence alone reassured her daughter-in-law Emily, who was anxiously awaiting her confinement. "I felt quite complimented," Sarah wrote to her son. "Nothing special for me to do, but Emily compliments me by saying she feels perfectly tranquil and safe now I am here."[109] Nineteenth-century attitudes about the importance of personal ties elevated this aspect of caring.[110] Because people believed that tensions and conflicts could produce disease, they thought that loving solicitude could restore health. Just as Emily Gillespie attributed her illness to her husband's violence and indifference, she insisted that Sarah's attentive care alleviated her emotional stress and thus facilitated healing. As Emily frequently stated, Sarah's kindness and sensitivity were the "best medicine."

Caring for family members, friends, and neighbors, women shared the distress of illness suffered by those close to them. Although women's writings often omitted the physical details of sickness, they dwelt on suffering and anguish. Larry Hirschhorn writes that the professions today "provide their members with professional 'armor,' with techniques and rules of action that allow them to minimize their emotional and psychological involvement with their clients. From the professions' point of view, such armor is essential to good practice . . . Professional codes sanction such distance on the grounds that excessive identification can limit the professional's capacity to give help."[111] But few nineteenth-century caregivers could remain emotionally distant. Intimate bonds tied many women to the recipients of their care. We saw that Sarah Gillespie experienced her dying mother's pain as if it were her own. Other women nursed children, siblings, spouses, and close friends. Moreover, the afflictions women witnessed often had enormous resonance for them. Some female attendants who watched women bleed to death in chidbirth were pregnant themselves. Women caring for seriously ill infants in the community often had children the same age at home. The tragedies of others provided occasions for women to assess their own preparation for life's contingencies—a major virtue in the nineteenth century. In September 1823 Sarah Hill Fletcher wrote in her diary that she had just "come from Mrs. Wick's who was very sick with the fever and felt very much distressed for her situation (asking myself whether I could [bear] things with as much fortitude or not). She certainly displais a g[r]eat [d]eal of philosophy."[112]

Caregiving also reopened wounds. Women who had endured intense physical pain during childbirth had to tend other women laboring in agony. During epidemics, mothers nursed neighbors' children through the same illnesses that had struck their own offspring. Those who had experienced anguish over the deaths of loved ones frequently were summoned to comfort others. As one bereaved mother wrote, "No one knows the feelings of a Mother when she sees her child in its last moments but those who have gone through with it."[113]

But if caregiving forced women to reexperience losses, it also provided a way to make sense of suffering. Albert Schweitzer knew suffering intimately, both from his missionary work in Africa and from his own serious illness after being imprisoned during World War I. In a famous passage, he wrote: "Whoever among us has learned through personal experience what pain and anxiety really are must help to ensure that those out there who are in physical need obtain the same help that once came to him. He no longer belongs to himself alone; he has become the brother of all who suffer. It is this 'brotherhood of those who bear the mark of pain' that demands humane medical services."[114]

Popular culture encouraged nineteenth-century women to view themselves as a *sisterhood* "of those who bear the mark of pain." The extensive "consolation literature" that arose in the middle of the century suggested that women could transcend suffering by reaching out to others. (Because caregivers continually dealt with loss, that literature had relevance for them as well as for mourners.) Wendy Simonds and Barbara Katz Rothman observe that "many of the poems and essays make the claim that a child's death can widen a mother's worldview and make her feel more connected with others in an all-encompassing net of Christian love."[115] For example, in "The Ideal and the Real," the author Mary Davenant wrote, "The sorrows she had experienced in the loss of her children, seemed to have awakened in her soul a more tender sympathy for the woes of others, and to know of suffering was with her the signal for its relief. Love was the element in which she lived, and upon her husband and her son it rested in its holiest earthly form."[116]

While Davenant's heroine responded to her loss by bestowing greater love and attention on her husband and son, other writers portrayed female characters who drew closer to other women. According to the biographer Joan D. Hedrick, Harriet Beecher Stowe's novels depict "an informal 'priesthood' of women who have suffered."[117] Stowe based that priesthood on her own experience. When her fifteen-month-old son Charley died of cholera in 1849, she turned for support to her friend Mrs. Allen, who had sustained a similar loss. After Stowe gave birth to another baby, she wrote to Mrs. Allen, "I often think of what you said to me, that another child would not fill the place of the old one that it would be another interest and love . . . so I find it—for tho he is so like I do not feel him the same nor do I feel for him that same love which I felt for Charley—It is a different kind—I shall never love another as I did him—he was my '*summer child*.'" She asked, "How is it with you in your heart of hearts when you think of the past—I often wonder how your feelings correspond with mine."[118]

Stowe used the authority derived from her experience to offer consolation to other bereaved mothers. Three years after suffering a second crushing blow—the drowning death of her son Henry—Stowe sent a letter to a friend who had just lost a daughter. "Ah! Susie," she wrote,

> I who have walked in this dark valley for now three years, what can I say to you who are entering it? One thing I can say—be not afraid and confounded if you find no apparent religious support at first. When the heartstrings are all suddenly cut, it is, I believe, a physical impossibility to feel faith or resignation, there is a revolt of the instinctive and animal system, and though we may submit to God it is rather by a constant painful effort than by a sweet attraction.[119]

We have seen that the strength Samuella Curd drew from religion enabled her to face her husband's approaching death from tuberculosis. Stowe, however, was well aware that religion could also deepen despair. Rather than sympathizing with their anguish, ministers counseled women to reconcile themselves to their losses by submitting to God's will. Stowe reassured her friend that submission could be achieved only through struggle. "I know all the strange ways in which this anguish will reveal itself—the prick, the thrust, the stab, the wearing pain, the poison that is mingled with every bright remembrance of the past—I have felt them all—and all I can say is that, though 'faint,' I am 'pursuing,' although the crown of thorns secretly pressed to one's heart never ceases to pain."[120]

Hedrick notes that Stowe's novels invested "real spiritual power" in women characters: "This reflected the realities of the women's culture in which Stowe herself had been an informal minister. Though not ordained or formally called, women carried out the functions of the ministerial office, preaching the gospel, comforting the afflicted, and burying the dead. Their spiritual power to comfort and counsel came not from a course of study at Andover or Yale, but from the power of sympathy born of experience."[121] As Stowe wrote in *The Minister's Wooing*, only people who had known "great affliction" were qualified to "guide those who are struggling in it."[122]

It is important not to romanticize the solace women gave each other. Elizabeth V. Spelman writes that "the history of woman's inhumanity to woman is a shameful aspect of the history of women."[123] Although Harriet Beecher Stowe claimed that the stunning grief that followed her baby's death enabled her to understand the horrors of slavery,[124] most white southern women failed to perceive the humanity of enslaved African American women who suffered. Wilma King notes that when the baby of Tryphena Fox's slave died shortly after the death of Fox's own child, Fox charged the mother with neglect but offered no commiseration. King comments, "The deaths of their children did not change the mistress-maid relationship since the women inhabited different spheres, separated by race and class."[125] Although Samuella Curd expressed enormous sensitivity to the agony of white, middle-class women in childbirth, she referred to a slave living in her house as "grunting" in labor.[126] Domestic servants who fell ill also received little sympathy.[127] When Ellen Birdseye Wheaton's servant Eliza became critically ill on August 8, 1853, Ellen twice summoned the doctor. On August 10, however, she wrote, "Eliza moved to her sisters . . . They are poor, and it will come hard on them, but there was no other way. I could not think it my duty to keep her."[128] A major function of nineteenth-century hospitals was to shelter servants bereft of family support. A speech delivered at the dedication of the Cambridge Hospital in Massachusetts in 1886 explained why that institution was needed:

> A young girl, the only servant in a large family, falls sick. She is in a remote room without fire. The mistress of the family, absorbed by her manifold duties, can give her but irregular and insufficient care, or perhaps she is cared for only by friends at service, who can ill be spared by those whom they serve. Whatever her medical attendant may advise there is no certainty that his remedies will be obtained or properly given, and what might have been with good care a mild sickness may become fatal. To such the hospital will give relief which will gladden all hearts.[129]

Compassion was frequently deficient even when it did not have to cross race and class lines. "I have often been struck with the feebleness and insufficiency of the consolations offered to us," wrote Mary Wilder Foote after her daughter's death in 1837. "Some will tell us that we must be comforted by the thought that the sickness was short, and did not produce much suffering. Another will remind us that God, in depriving us of these darling treasures, has still spared to us a more important life, and not taken our earthly all. And these reflections, my dearest Ann, have caused our hearts to swell with gratitude to our Father in heaven. But they would not console us for the losses we *have* sustained."[130]

When Amelia Akehurst Lines became ill in 1871, the coldness of her caregiver added to her distress. "I am feeling worse than usual to-day," she wrote in her diary,

> but I must bear all my sufferings in silence, for any complaints would be treated with indifference and contempt rather than sympathy and kindness. I wish Jane could feel for one half hour the pain which racks my poor back and the trembling weakness which almost prostrates me. I only want her to feel it long enough to satisfy her that *I suffer* and am not able to do or endure what those in full health and strength can. It is hard enough to suffer all the time and then to have no sympathy is rather more than I can bear with womanly grace and dignity . . . How little those in perfect health know the wants of the weak and suffering.[131]

Although we cannot estimate the proportion of nineteenth-century women who responded to the sick with empathy, we can discern the preconditions for doing so. It has become axiomatic to state that our society today denies illness and death, encouraging us to expect perpetual good health. We banish sick and dying people to institutions, where they receive care from professionals who armor themselves against suffering. Nineteenth-century caregivers, by contrast, could not easily shield themselves from the pain of the afflicted. Many nursed close relatives and friends whose troubles closely resembled their own. Moreover, empathic understanding received cultural sanction. Popular fiction suggested that women could transcend grief by responding to others in pain. At its best, caregiving both reflected and reinforced intimate personal bonds, rooted in a shared recognition of contingency and need.

"Supplying All Her Needs and Fancies"

Dominating the lives of nineteenth-century white women, caregiving exacted a heavy toll. It imposed overwhelming household responsibilities, disrupted public activities, encroached on sleep and leisure, and caused an array of physical ills. Nevertheless, the three major components of care—instrumental, spiritual, and emotional—sometimes conferred significant rewards. Because doctors could not demonstrate superior knowledge, women often garnered the satisfaction of making medical decisions on their own and honing and displaying skills; a few received special recognition as healers. Caregivers who assumed responsibility for the spiritual well-being of care recipients often deepened their own religious faith. At a time when medical beliefs assigned value to emotional connection, women were able to view themselves as restoring health when they provided empathy and solace. Some caregivers also achieved new levels of intimacy with the care recipients by acknowledging their common fate. And some believed that their encounters with disease, disability, and death gave them a kind of wisdom they could use to ease the sufferings of others. The second part of this book demonstrates how developments at the turn of the century undermined those features of care that nineteenth-century women found most fulfilling.

We turn next to enslaved African American women, whose experiences help to introduce the issue of resistance and struggle, another theme that is central to later chapters.

"Pretty Good At Doctoring": Enslaved Women in the Antebellum South

The caregiving experiences of enslaved women differed in important ways from those of the white women we have examined.[132] White women had many competing demands on their time and energy, but most were able to make caregiving a priority in times of crisis. By contrast, care for slaveholders' families invariably took precedence over care for enslaved women's kin. Most enslaved women could find time to nurse sick family and community members only when they returned at night, exhausted from working in the fields or the big house. Fannie Moore, a former slave, told interviewers that when her younger brother was dying, "Granny, she doctored him as best she could, every time she got way from the white folks' kitchen. My mammy never got chance to see him, except when she got home in the evening." When the mother learned one night that her son had died, she knelt "by the bed and cried her heart out." Shortly afterward, the boy's uncle buried him. The mother "just plow and watch them put George in the ground."[133]

White women were also much better able to take preventive measures to protect their families. Although some poor white women could not provide adequate food, clothing, and shelter, most were better able than enslaved women to keep their families safe and well. Very few white mothers had to surrender offspring as young as six to arduous labor. And virtually none routinely nursed the victims of brutal punishments.

Slave quarters were so overcrowded and lacking in basic sanitation and ventilation that one observer dubbed them "laboratories of disease."[134] Hard physical labor, combined with inadequate rest, diet, and clothing, heightened susceptibility to disease. Food allowances, consisting almost exclusively of rice, fatback, corn, and salt pork, provided ample calories but not basic nutrients.[135] The clothes distributed to slaves were often too flimsy to ward off rain and cold.[136] Going barefoot in all but the coldest months left people vulnerable to snake bites and nail punctures.[137] And work accidents and punishments caused serious disabilities. Whipping not only inflicted agonizing pain and skin lacerations but also produced shock, blood loss, and damage to muscles and internal organs.[138] Although slaveholders assumed some responsibility for ministering to sick slaves, they typically returned beating victims to slave quarters without providing any medical attention.[139] Joe Clinton recalled that slaves had to nurse a beaten man "for days and days" and "wash his wounds and pick the maggots out his sores."[140]

The inability of enslaved women to protect their children was one of the cruelest features of slavery. Almost 50 percent of slave infants died in their first year—almost twice the infant mortality rate among whites.[141] One cause of death among newborns was low birth weight, a factor Richard H. Steckel attributes largely to the arduous work required of enslaved women during pregnancy.[142] In addition, the quick return of women to the fields after childbirth frequently ended breastfeeding prematurely, and poor maternal diets meant that breast milk often lacked some essential nutrients.[143] The diets of children too young to work also were insufficient to safeguard their health. Such children, Steckel writes, "attained levels of net nutrition that approached those of the slowest growing population ever studied by auxologists."[144] In addition, children sustained serious injuries while their mothers worked, and some were subject to whippings and other punishments.[145]

It is likely that emotional trauma further undermined physical health. Nell Irvin Painter notes that the various forms of child abuse inflicted by slavery may have led to depression, low self-esteem, and anger, all of which can have somatic consequences.[146] One former slave remembered a woman comforting him as a young child when his mother was sold away. Nevertheless, he remained inconsolate: "Every exertion was made on my part to find her, or hear some tidings of her, but all my efforts were unsuccessful; and from that day I have never seen or heard from her. This cruel separation brought on a fit of sickness, from which they did not expect I would recover."[147]

Finally, white women had far more ability than slave women to choose treatments and providers. Viewing slaves as too ignorant, superstitious, and fatalistic to deliver decent care, owners demanded that all illnesses be reported to them.[148] Some responsibility for care fell on slave-owning women, who dosed with purchased drugs (especially quinine and calomel), along with traditional folk remedies.[149] Uncle Richard Carruthers recalled in a 1930s interview that his mistress "would use the kind of medicine she wanted to use on us."[150] In cases of very serious or persistent disease, slaveholders summoned local doctors, who employed the various "heroic" treatments fashionable at the time. Owners also occasionally removed victims of epidemic diseases to distant pesthouses. Many large plantation owners placed sick slaves in infirmaries.[151]

The great bulk of hands-on care in both infirmaries and slave quarters was assigned to elderly enslaved women known as "nurses."[152] Anna Lee later told an interviewer,

When we became sick . . . our master was awful good to us. He
first turned us over to our old negro mama . . . [who] got her hoe
and sack and to the woods she went gathering herbs to make our
medicine out of. Well she gathered cami weed roots, peach tree
leaves, red oak bark and privet roots; cooked or boiled them all
down to a thick syrup and gave to us for chills, fever, malaria and
so on. She used pine tree bark, onions and pure honey to make us a
cough syrup out of for our cold and coughs and it was real good,
son—better than anything these here doctors can give these
days.[153]

Although this nurse was able to exercise her own medical judgment,
most were expected to administer only the medications slaveholders
supplied.[154] "The nurses are never to be allowed to give any medicine without the orders of the Overseer or Doctor," advised a South
Carolina planter in 1857.[155] Infirmary nurses were also charged with
preventing patients from leaving and with compelling them to accept
unwanted treatments.[156]

Enslaved people complained that white medicine was less effective
than African American treatments,[157] had no power when diseases were
caused by supernatural forces,[158] and sometimes caused harm. One former slave reported that the calomel a white doctor administered
"would pretty nigh kill us."[159] It is hardly surprising that slaves feared
treatments chosen by the same owners and overseers who overworked,
whipped, and sexually exploited them. The use of medicine as punish-
ment may have deepened distrust.[160] Slaves also may have known that
white physicians experimented on them.[161] And even slaves who acknowledged benefiting from the treatment provided by owners understood the motive behind it. Eli Coleman, for example, told interviewers, "When we got sick, Master, he looked after us good and gave us the
best of care as we was too valuable to let stay sick or feeling bad."[162]
Several former slaves calculated how much their deaths would cost
their owners or compared their treatment with that of farm animals.[163]
And a few accused owners of engaging in triage based on patients' potential usefulness rather than the severity of their conditions. "My old
boss sure looked after you when you was sick," stated Jeff Calhoun. "If
you was a good hand you got good attention, but if you was just cus-

tomary you got attention as soon as they could get to you."[164] Slaves who distrusted their owners' care had a strong incentive to find ways to deliver their own.

In the past twenty years, historians have sought to recover the various forms of resistance and struggle that marked slavery in the United States. Women's defense of their children was often more subtle than the rebellions that typically engage historical attention.[165] Slave mothers' "weapons" included stealing food to supplement the rations owners supplied, encouraging offspring to run away, and telling folktales that offered alternative visions of the world.[166] Women's caregiving endeavors must be viewed within this context. Some women successfully concealed family illness and administered folk remedies and other treatments the owners forbade.[167] Moreover, women who found ways to render care sustained communal values, preserved the personal ties owners sought to destroy, and garnered respect.

Margaret Washington Creel writes that caregiving among the Gullah slave population of South Carolina fostered the community integrity that slavery assaulted. "The dying person was surrounded by the community, who offered comfort and support . . . Singing, praying, and pious conversation filled the cabin nightly."[168] Janey Landrum, a former slave in Texas, recalled, "The neighbors come in and help nurse when there was sickness in the family."[169] Crowded habitations facilitated the collective nature of caregiving. Moreover, a web of mutual obligations bound enslaved people to grandparents, grandchildren, aunts, uncles, nieces, nephews, and siblings, while "fictive kinship" linked unrelated individuals to each other, enhancing communal solidarity.[170] Collective care for sick and disabled people may, in turn, have reinforced the bonds of kinship and community that sustained whatever dignity and joy enslaved people achieved.

Caregiving was especially likely to solidify women's support networks. It was even more common for enslaved women than for white women to render care without male assistance. On the basis of her statistical analysis of slave households in twenty-six Louisiana parishes, Ann Patton Malone concludes, "In some stages and under some circumstances, more slave families were matrifocal than were contemporary white families because, under slavery, husbands, fathers, and adult males in general were sold, transferred, hired out, or otherwise removed from constituted family units more often than females. The female presence in the household was generally more durable and permanent in times of stress than was that of males."[171] Women managed by relying on each other. "Othermothers," including aunts, grandmothers, and unrelated community women, raised healthy children and nursed sick and dying ones.[172]

Women shared healing knowledge as well as responsibilities, and younger women learned from their elders.[173] Harriet Collins remembered, "Most of the old slaves was pretty good at doctoring and my Mammy, she taught me a lot herself. Some, she learned from the old folks from Africa."[174] Many other former slaves credited their African-born grandmothers with transmitting healing lore.[175]

Enslaved people's medical beliefs and rituals constituted an important part of what Lawrence Levine calls "the sacred world of black slaves."[176] Practitioners (many of them men) variously known as conjurers, root doctors, and hoodoos used spiritual forces to harm as well as heal. But religious beliefs also infused more routine forms of care.[177] As Sharla Fett writes, "Nursing, herbalism, and daily domestic care, most often practiced by women, were part of a continuum of African American healing resources which drew upon notions of spiritual power."[178] Such notions included the beliefs that illnesses stemmed from metaphysical as well as natural causes, that medicines had spiritual elements, that healers' powers represented divine gifts, and that healing rituals helped to link the living to their ancestors.[179]

Religious and healing beliefs, Levine notes, "actually offered the slaves sources of power and knowledge alternative to those existing within the world of the master class."[180] Elderly women who commanded such power enjoyed great honor and prestige. Harriet Ware, a northern woman teaching in the Sea Islands of South Carolina, wrote in 1862, "'Learning' with these people I find means a knowledge of medicine, and a person is valued accordingly."[181] A former slave in Georgia remarked that everybody respected his African-born grandmother "because she done accumulated so much knowledge and because her head were so white."[182]

We saw that white nineteenth-century women who gained renown as healers were able to translate their skills into economic independence. Claiming competence on the basis of experience, some obtained paid positions as nurses and midwives. Although female slaves who were hired out as midwives may have acquired important economic resources, elderly women who worked as nurses remained trapped in re-lations of domination.[183] They had no choice about assuming their roles, could not seek relief from overwhelming tasks, and were ex-pected to follow alien advice; slaveholders reaped the profit of their labor.[184]

Nevertheless, elderly enslaved women must have found the esteem of their own communities gratifying, especially in light of the con-tempt expressed by owners. Because slaveholders valued slaves exclu-sively in terms of work capacity, the loss of physical vigor negated their worth. A South Carolina overseer informing his employer of the death of an elderly woman wrote that she "has bin sick fur 2 years" and there-fore "was a Dead Expense to the Place."[185] Some owners flouted laws prohibiting them from freeing elderly slaves no longer able to work. Alex Lacy, a former slave interviewed in Texas, stated that his master "didn't have no old women on his place cause he got shed of them just like old mules."[186] Physical frailty did not, however, reduce the value of life to slaves, who revered wisdom, extensive family networks, and links to the African past.

⟨ To the extent that enslaved women caregivers strength-ened community bonds and garnered individual respect, they resem-bled the nineteenth-century white women discussed earlier in this chapter. In other ways, however, the caregiving experiences of slaves contrasted sharply with those of whites. Although many white women delivered care within severe practical and social constraints, most could at least give priority to their own family members during crises. Slave women invariably had to subordinate the needs of ailing kin to their owners' demands. Slaves also had far less control than whites over both the threats to family members' bodies and the choice of therapies. Vir-tually none could convert healing knowledge into financial indepen-dence.

Nevertheless, the caregiving work of enslaved women subverted the plantation regime in subtle ways. Women concealed children's ill-nesses, substituted herbal brews for calomel and quinine, bestowed lov-ing care and compassion on family members whom owners viewed only as labor power, and strove to preserve communities in the face of a sys-tem that constantly threatened their survival.

Although the theme of power and conflict emerges most starkly in the domestic healing work of enslaved women, we will see that political struggles surrounded the caregiving provided by many other women. Most scholars of caregiving today emphasize the various forces compelling women to render care, but poor women, especially women of color, historically have had to fight to be able to care for kin. Caregiving among many oppressed groups also traditionally has involved resisting alien health care services and asserting the unique worth and humanity of family members whom others valued only for their productive capacities. As we will see, even privileged women constantly negotiated the definition and control of medical knowledge. The following chapter returns to white nineteenth-century women, examining their contests with doctors for dominance at the bedside.

~3

"Tried at the Quilting Bees": Conflicts between "Old Ladies" and Aspiring Professionals

$\mathcal{M}$OST ACCOUNTS of the development of the medical profession during the nineteenth century focus on physicians' attempts to control access by establishing schools and campaigning to enact or maintain state licensing laws.[1] The quest for the rewards and privileges of professional status, however, depended less on those activities than on countless efforts to alter the balance of power at the bedside. Doctors sought to substitute peer review for women's evaluation of their performance and tried to exclude women from diagnosis and treatment. A particularly important goal was to extend jurisdiction to cover children's health care, a field previously ceded to mothers.

Institutional developments shaped the contests for control in individual sickrooms. Without the ability to regulate access into the medical profession, well-qualified practitioners could not easily distinguish themselves from their poorly trained counterparts. As the previous chapter noted, women sometimes concluded that all medical men were worthless after experiences with those who were inept or unethical. Moreover, unorthodox practices flourished. "Regulars" were challenged by groups such as the Thomsonians in the first part of the nineteenth century and by homeopaths and eclectics in the second. Women could thus choose from a broad range of providers when illness descended on their households. We saw that Sarah Gillespie consulted a magnetic doctor as well as an orthodox practitioner to treat her mother. Although the various irregular groups differed greatly among themselves, they shared a disdain for regular physician care and a belief in the efficacy of folk practice.

Nevertheless, to understand why professionalization remained an elusive goal throughout the nineteenth century, we have to examine not only organizational changes but also three factors that affected the physician-caregiver relationship even more profoundly—the locus of medical care, the timing of physician assistance, and the inability of physicians to claim unique competence.[2] The caregivers examined in this chapter are primarily white women and come from a wide variety of geographic areas. Although a few nineteenth-century doctors were women, the chapter focuses on male physicians.

Very few doctors worked out of offices or in hospitals in the nineteenth century; Paul Starr estimates that just 2 percent of American doctors had hospital privileges in 1873.[3] Instead of receiving clients in imposing and intimidating surroundings, physicians entered the family's turf. There they often worked without medical books, colleagues, or appropriate supplies. Sharing intimate space with family members also may have helped to erode differences of status. When physicians lived far from their patients and illnesses required attention over lengthy periods, doctors often boarded with client families. Even local doctors frequently slept at patients' homes and ate meals with the family when a difficult labor was prolonged. Dr. George S. King later recalled, "Many a night we slept on a couch or on the floor while the poor horse stood outside covered with a blanket."[4] In addition, physicians relied on relatives and friends for assistance, rather than on a staff of subordinates. In 1871 a physician operated on the thumb of a woman who was staying with a friend in Idaho. The friend later wrote, "By the time it came to the tying of the stitches she struggled so that the doctor asked me to tie them while he held her and I did."[5] Here the doctor and informal caregiver exchanged roles, the latter performing the more skilled task. Other women administered chloroform, checked the progress of deliveries, restrained patients during surgery without anesthesia, and helped to reduce dislocations.[6]

The site of care also exposed medical practice to lay scrutiny. Young doctors were especially likely to be intimidated. Dr. William Allen Pusey described an incident during his early years of practice:

One Sunday afternoon I was called by [a family] ten miles in the country to see a boy with a dislocation of the elbow, which the local doctors had been unable to reduce. I found the boy with a simple backward dislocation of the elbow. It was a typical country scene under such conditions. The boy was on a bed in a large room on the ground floor of the house, the neighboring women and—it being Sunday—the neighboring men to the number of a dozen or more were sitting around the room, with their eyes, as the sweating baffled doctor thought, upon him. Outside in the yard, were most of the other neighbors from miles around. I was a slip of a boy, none too impressive at any time and with an acute consciousness of my inability to live up to the appearance that the company expected of the doctor under those circumstances.[7]

Although doctors assumed that they alone were qualified to judge each other's work, career success depended on lay evaluation. Dr. Weir Mitchell, a neurologist, noted "the juries of matrons" that "do so much to make or mar our early fates."[8] Dr. Arthur E. Hertzler issued a similar complaint. Recalling his early years of practice in Kansas, Hertzler wrote, "The doctors . . . were tried at the quilting bees of the community."[9] In a book of advice to other physicians, Dr. D. W. Cathell warned, "No one can succeed fully without the favorable opinion of the maids and matrons he meets in the sick room."[10]

Like peer review, the ability to work without outside interference is basic to professional identity, but nineteenth-century physicians had to tread warily, deferring to the judgment of family and friends. Consider, for example, one physician's comment about the role of female assistants during childbirth: "The officiousness of nurses and friends very often thwarts the best-directed measure of the physician, by an overweening desire to make the patient 'comfortable' . . . Nothing is more common than for the patient's friends to object to [bloodletting], urging as a reason, that 'she has lost blood enough.' Of this they are in no respect suitable judges."[11]

The timing of physician assistance presented further challenges. I have noted that many women called on doctors only as a last resort, and transportation difficulties often delayed them from reaching the bedside. As a result, doctors were often the last to arrive on the scene. In addition, many entered sickrooms in the midst of emergencies. Some complained that they could not display their expertise to the best advantage in situations demanding speedy action rather than careful deliberation.[12]

The major factor undermining physicians' prerogatives was their inability to claim special competence. We take for granted an enormous chasm between professional and lay knowledge and skills, but throughout most of the nineteenth century little distinguished the ideas and practices of physicians from those of family caregivers. Harold Wilensky argues that "if the technical basis of an occupation consists of a vocabulary that sounds familiar to everyone . . . then the occupation will have difficulty claiming a monopoly of skill or even a roughly exclusive jurisdiction."[13] Nineteenth-century physicians lacked an esoteric body of knowledge. Lay people had similar concepts of disease and bodily structures and could easily comprehend doctors' language.[14]

Doctors and family caregivers also employed many of the same diagnostic and therapeutic practices. In the absence of thermometers, X rays, and, in the beginning of the century, stethoscopes, doctors relied primarily on observation of patients. As Charles E. Rosenberg writes, "A flushed face and rapid pulse, a coated tongue and griping diarrhea would be apparent to laymen just as to physicians; and grandmothers as well as senior consultants could and did make reasoned prognoses."[15]

Lacking special diagnostic tools, doctors were restricted to therapies that could elicit swift and dramatic symptomatic change. In the first half of the century, doctors employed such heroic remedies as bleeding, cupping, and purging. Family members readily observed the results. Six days before her husband died in 1844, Elizabeth Duncan wrote in her diary that "he suffered agony all Night and when I went in the morning quite early I sent over for Dr. Pierson and for Dr. Jones and they bled him 1 Quart and his colour which had forsook the cheek seemed to come back."[16] In an account of her husband's death in 1855, Mary Ann Owen Sims wrote, "He requested me to examine the blister (that the Drs. had put on his thigh during the night) . . . I toled him it was not drawing."[17] Although after 1850 doctors increasingly sought to stimulate, rather than deplete, the body, their treatments continued to be aimed at eliciting visible physiological responses.[18]

In many cases, doctors and family members assumed similar responsibilities. Before the advent of asepsis and antisepsis at the end of the nineteenth century, surgical care consisted largely of dressing wounds, setting broken limbs, and lancing boils.[19] As we saw in Chapter 2, some women felt competent to perform these procedures on their own. The overlap was even greater in the area of pharmaceutical care. Doctors carried powders in their saddlebags and concocted different remedies at their patients' homes. Because doctors charged only for drugs in nonsurgical care, they had a strong incentive to provide drugs to the great majority of patients. Many case notes of the era record the medicines dispensed rather than the nature of the problem.[20]

But physicians did not have a monopoly on the administration of medications. Many women kept a stock of herbs, which they picked in the woods or from their gardens during the summer and "put up" each fall, along with preserved foods. A Missouri woman interviewed in the early twentieth century remembered her mother's remedies:

> The nearest doctor was 20 miles away and there was no way to travel *only* horseback and no money to pay with if he did come . . . Mother watched over us carefully. There wasn't money to buy medicine. In the spring she would make sassafras and sage tea to condition our blood. In the summer and autumn we would eat . . . anything we found growing wild without washing it. Naturally, we would get "wormy." [Mother] knew the symptoms. Some mornings before breakfast she would stir up a mixture of wormfuge [vermifuge] in a skillet of molasses . . . Before night we were rid of our worms. If one of us needed a tonic Mother went to the woods peeled off some bark from a wild cherry tree, dug some sarsaparilla, some blackroot, and other herbs (I have forgotten), boiled a brew out of it and gave it in regulated doses . . . She made tea of pennyroyal, mullein, and tansy for our stomach cramps; slippery elm she made poultices of and applied to boils.[21]

One of the first tasks of many women who migrated west was planting the "starts" they brought with them.[22] Others asked relatives to send the herbs that were unavailable in their new homes.[23]

Like many other forms of production, drug manufacturing moved out of the home in the nineteenth century. Even such potent medications as mercury were available in many local stores and could be administered without physician oversight. "I expect this will smell of calomel, oil ct.," wrote Abbie Bright in her journal, soon after arriving at the home of her brother and his family in Indiana in 1871. "The children have been quite sick with lung fever, are a little better but very restless."[24] When Maria D. Brown of Iowa found her nephew "sick with bloody flux," she "went to the drug store and bought some slip-

pery elm and laudanum."[25] Various entrepreneurs began to market patent medicines, and advertisements for their compounds soon filled the
pages of women's magazines. These nostrums, too, helped women cir-
cumvent physicians' authority. "I am giving both children Scoville's
Blood and Liver Syrup now—regularly," wrote Mary Abell from Kansas to her mother in New York in 1868. "It may take a dozen bottles—
but that is a comparatively small doctor's bill—and it may be the means
of saving their lives, for Scrofula is a terrible malady."[26] The following
year, Mary extolled "Sage's Catarrh Remedy," which she used for her
own eyes. "It is the greatest thing I know of," she wrote.[27] In 1871
she again expressed confidence in a patent medicine administered to a
child: "We are all well at present, though Robbie was sick last Sunday
afternoon vomiting. I was afraid he was going to be real sick, but a
few doses of 'Jayne's Tonic' made him all right."[28] When Robbie was
"croupy" in 1874, she gave him "Arnold's Cough Killer," which she had
bought on a visit home.[29]

Although women's competence as healers impeded medicine's quest
for professional status, some doctors increased caregivers' capabilities
by writing popular health guides. One of the harshest critics of those
works testified to their power. "What can be more annoying," wrote
Walter Channing, a Harvard professor of obstetrics and medical juris-
prudence, "than to be met at the chamber door of a patient by a friend,
a female friend, with book in hand, welcoming us by reading the history of the disease, and then telling us of remedies and results, adding
that calomel and bleeding were now necessary, but she really was unwilling to meddle with mineral poisons, or with edged tools."[30]

Publications by practitioners who departed from the tenets of orthodox medicine enabled some women to dispense entirely with physician
assistance. Maria D. Brown noted that she summoned a doctor to vac-
cinate the family during a smallpox scare and to "usher" three babies
into the world. "But the rest of the time I ministered to the family
myself. That is, with the help of good Dr. Gunn. Dr. Gunn was the author of a big book . . . which told how to care for the sick and make
them remedies from the herbs that grew all around us. Whatever the
ailment, from hiccoughs to tapeworms, I consulted Dr. Gunn."[31] Although John Gunn was trained as a regular physician, his enormously
successful *Domestic Medicine*, first published in 1830, included botanic
and folk treatments along with learned ones.[32] Homeopathic doctors

distributed "domestic kits" containing pills as well as guides to their use. A native of West Virginia who followed her husband to a Montana cattle ranch in the 1880s, Nannie T. Alderson wrote,

> In all the years of our life on a ranch, we never had a doctor for the children but twice . . . On one of my visits east, a friend in Kansas had given me a kit of homeopathic remedies to take home to the ranch saying he had raised his family on it. I certainly raised mine on it. The kit contained a number of bottles of little white sugary pills, and a book of directions telling you which to use in case of colds, fever, stomach trouble and so forth. Whenever one of the children was ill I simply consulted the book and gave a pill from the proper bottle.[33]

Mary Edgerton left Tallmadge, Ohio, to move with her husband to a small mining camp in Bannack, Montana. She wrote to her sister in 1865,

> The baby was taken sick Sunday night with a cold and has almost had lung fever. She was quite sick until Friday when she commenced getting better . . . Tell Lucy [Edgerton's sister-in-law] that I "doctored" her with homeopathic medicine that she gave me. If I had been in Tallmadge I should hardly have dared to have "prescribed" for her, but did not like to send for a new doctor. (The one we have always employed was not at home), so thought I would go by the "book" and she has got along very well.[34]

Had family caregivers derived healing knowledge only from medical sources, physicians might have had greater success in exercising control. But women drew on information from many channels, combining those elements that seemed most relevant in particular cases. Most household manuals written by lay authors contained healing information along with instructions about preparing food and managing servants. For example, *The Southern Gardener and Receipt Book*, published in 1860, included cures for cholera and consumption, as well as for less serious afflictions such as bee stings and colds.[35] Advice about disease and treatment also could be found in such popular women's magazines as *Godey's* and *Peterson's*.[36]

In addition, women shared remedies among themselves. Mary Ann Owen Sims wrote that when her father "was quite sick" in 1843, "Mother had [recourse] to the remidees usually used in all families for caughs and it improved his health very much."[37] A letter from Mary S. Paul, a mill worker, to her father in 1855 illustrates women's confidence in the treatments they learned from each other:

> Oh there is a remedy for rheumatism that a lady here told me of, I was telling her about your case and she told me to tell you to take steam baths, in this way. When you feel the lameness coming on, have a sheet wrung out of hot water and wrap it about you. Then over that put flannel blankets and dont spare the clothes. The object is to produce heavy perspiration and thus throw off the disease. Half an hour is long enough to remain in the sheet. In coming out of it take a warm bath and rub till the flesh is dry.

Mary concluded, "I have never heard of this remedy before but I have a great deal of faith in it, and I do wish you would try it."[38]

Knowledge and skills were also acquired experientially. Girls learned to brew herbal remedies and prepare poultices the same way they learned other domestic skills—while helping their mothers at home and accompanying them on visits to ailing neighbors. Sarah Gillespie may have considered herself a competent caregiver because she had assisted her mother in nursing her brother, Henry. An early-twentieth-century example also illustrates this pattern. Hallie F. Nelson was in high school in Nebraska when the nursing of her brother, suffering from pneumonia, fell to her. Although a local doctor told Hallie how to make turpentine and lard poultices, she also drew on the knowledge she had absorbed while watching her mother. "I had seen Mama do this dozens of times," she later wrote, "so I felt quite confident."[39]

Instruction often was inseparable from practice. Recalling the various types of help available to birthing women in Nebraska in the 1880s, Dr. Francis A. Long wrote, "An instance occurred in this area when there was no one available but the twelve year old daughter. The labor was precipitate. The mother called the girl and told her what to do and together they managed to tie the cord, get the baby dressed and the mother's toilet arranged."[40] A history of nursing in Kansas by the Work Projects Administration (WPA) noted that during nineteenth-century home births, "Daughters of fourteen or more were considered old enough to stay at home and assist . . . If the mother needed special attention the girl might be told to 'clean up the baby,' the mother and nurse directing her anxiously at each step."[41] Many also must have received instruction while working alongside their mothers. Because caregiving frequently was a social endeavor, mature women as well as young girls had many opportunities to observe others administer treatment and learn from them.

It is important not to overstate the trust women placed in the healing lore embedded in female communities. Just as women recounted horrendous tales of physicians' ineptitude, so they cited egregious errors committed by female relatives and neighbors. A Vermont woman told her sister and brother why she had suffered a nearly fatal hemorrhage after a miscarriage: "I probably would have been well in a short time if I had had a physician to begin with. I thought I would do well enough, Mrs. Watson [a neighbor] was with me, and I supposed all was right, but the whole difficulty was the placenta, or afterbirth, which did not come away. Mrs. Watson thought it had and told the Doctor so when he came, so he did not understand the trouble and supposed it all weakness."[42] Effie Hanson of North Dakota wrote to a friend, "Anna E. has another boy, was born the 4 of August. Weighed 8 lbs. They nearly lost him as the 2 women was afraid of him and wouldn't go near him. It was Ed's mother and another woman. They laid him away till the next day and never as much as washed him. So Anna found him soaked in blood."[43] The WPA history of Kansas nursing reported a similar incident:

> Slow transportation and poor communication gave rise to emergencies, and inexperienced or stupid women had to be pressed into service. In a small town on one of the first railroads to push across the State was a woman who expected each day for a month that delivery might be at hand. No relatives or competent women were available to help and the nearest doctor lived nine miles down the track . . . One morning . . . the baby arrived suddenly with only a frightened woman from across the street at hand. She stood by helplessly, too paralyzed to bring even the supplies asked for by the patient. The mother saw her baby slowly turn blue. When the neighbor saw it was unable to breathe, she dropped it

on the bed and began crying hysterically, "Oh, Lordy, Lordy, what shall I do!"[44]

What distinguished the nineteenth century was not a belief that all women could deliver competent care but rather the respect accorded practical experience. The philosopher Lorraine Code writes that we currently make a "distinction between knowledge and experience, in whose terms knowledge is valued more highly than experience and confers authority where experience cannot."[45] Nineteenth-century women, however, were able to gain credibility as experts on the basis of experience alone. When a Vermont woman's infant son lay dying, she called not only a doctor but also a neighbor, Mrs. Ware, because "she is used to the croup." Mrs. Ware "brought up a bottle of Nicens Syrup" and helped the mother cover "the babe's lungs and throat and feet with an onion poultice."[46] A Kansas woman wrote to her parents two weeks after her confinement, "I had two most excellent women here when I was sick—one of large experience, and more to be trusted than half the doctors."[47] Another woman described her own birth on an Idaho homestead in the 1880s: "They thought my mother was dying. She was only seventeen years old. I was slowly dying myself, too, and so was my mother. There was an old lady in the neighborhood who had been around births and she knew something about it. Finally she heard about it and here she come. She walked several miles. She said, 'We're gonna get that baby.' She got busy, and I was born."[48] We will see that doctors routinely belittled female healers as "old ladies," a term encoding a growing disdain for the elderly. But age was a positive attribute to those who rooted authority in accumulated experience and tradition.

Doctors had little success touting the superiority of their educational credentials. Suspicion of book learning was widespread throughout much of the century. Moreover, theoretical education was often irrelevant to medical practice. In his study of twentieth-century doctors, Eliot Freidson writes, "The clinician is prone in time to trust his own accumulation of personal, *first hand experience* in preference to abstract principles or 'book knowledge.'"[49] Nineteenth-century medical beliefs reinforced that orientation. Because disease was believed to arise from the particular interaction of individuals with their environment, universalistic knowledge of physiological processes was considered less important than personal knowledge of patients and the contexts of

their lives. As an editorial in the *Boston Medical and Surgical Journal*
wrote in 1883, "No two patients have the same constitutional or mental proclivities. No two instances of typhoid fever or of any other disease, are precisely alike. No 'rule of thumb,' no recourse to a formula
book, will avail for the treatment even of the typical disease."[50] This belief encouraged doctors not only to respect family caregivers' intimate
understanding of patients but also to seek such an understanding themselves.[51]

Another reason doctors could not marshal a convincing argument
about the utility of a medical education was that they were well aware
of the deficiencies of their own. Many nineteenth-century medical
schools were poorly funded commercial enterprises, staffed by part-
time instructors; some even lacked laboratories and libraries.[52] A 1906
survey conducted by the American Medical Association found that the
quality of only half of all medical schools could be considered acceptable.[53] Dr. Francis A. Long recalled an experience from his early years
of practice in Nebraska in the 1880s:

> Among the early settlers the physician was also the dental surgeon,
> for resident dentists were scarce and the smaller communities did
> not afford enough work to support dentists. In medical school we
> received no instruction in dentistry of any kind whatever. When
> the first patient came to have a tooth extraction I did not know
> enough to take the armhold the dentist takes around the head and
> face of the patient. I made a sorry mess of it, but I got the tooth.[54]

He had greater luck at his first confinement:

> The patient was the wife of the section foreman. As soon as I en-
> tered the bedchamber the husband said, "Doc, have you had any
> experience in handling such cases?" I had schooled myself for just
> such a question and unhesitatingly, but shamefully, replied "Oh,
> yes!" (My total college experience was with a manikin, you re-
> member). Luckily for me, the child was born about ten minutes af-
> ter my arrival, else I might have fallen into grave disrepute.[55]

A female physician in rural California wrote, "A young doctor, fresh
from medical college, can pass many embarrassing moments in the

presence of the neighborhood midwife. Country people have been through the stress of illness, without trained medical assistance so often that they have an astonishing knowledge of human ills gained in the school of experience."[56]

Some doctors confessed that they listened to female attendants not only under duress but also out of respect for their judgment. One wrote that he "got through" his first delivery "with the help (and truth compels me to acknowledge), advice and instruction of some good women who knew much more of the practical side of obstetrics than I did."[57] Although I have emphasized the information flowing from physicians to women, it is important to remember that the knowledge exchange sometimes went in the other direction.

Dr. J. Marion Sims, a famous surgeon, described the profound sense of incapacity with which he approached his first case. A recent graduate of the Jefferson Medical College in Philadelphia in 1837, he "had had no clinical advantages, no hospital experience, and had seen nothing at all of sickness."[58] Summoned by a prominent community member to visit his sick baby, Sims "examined the child minutely from head to foot . . . But, when it came to making up a prescription, I had no more idea of what ailed the child, or what to do for it, than if I had never studied medicine. I was at a perfect loss what to do, but I did not betray my ignorance."[59] Telling the mother that he would have the prescription ready in an hour, he

> hurried back to my office, and took out one of my seven volumes of Eberle, which comprised my library, and found his treatise on the "Diseases of Children." I hastily took it down, turned quickly to the subject of "Cholera Infantum," and read it through, over and over again, to the end most carefully. I knew no more what to prescribe for the sick babe than if I hadn't read it all. But it was my only resource. I had nobody else to consult but Eberle.[60]

When Sims visited the home later in the day, he was "very much surprised to find the baby very much as in the morning; no better and no worse. I saw that as the medicine had done no good it was necessary to change it . . . I turned to Eberle again, and to a new leaf. I gave the baby a prescription from the next chapter. Suffice it to say, that I changed leaves and prescriptions as often as once or twice a day."[61]

An "old nurse" hired by the family to tend the child added to Sims's unease. "This old nurse seemed to scrutinize me, and very particularly watched everything I said and did. Nothing escaped her, and I felt very uncomfortable in her presence. I wished that she had never come here."[62] While Sims examined the baby one night, the nurse said,

> "Doctor, don't you think that this baby is going to die?" I said, "No, madam, I did not think so, not at all." Externally, I was very calm and self-possessed; but internally I was not, for I really did not know what that child would do. Presently the child stopped breathing, and I thought it a case of syncope. I never dreamed that it would die. So I jerked the baby from the bed, and held its head down, and shook it, and blew into its mouth, and tried to bring it to. I shook it again, when the old nurse laid her hand on my shoulder gently, and said: "No use shakin' that baby any more, doctor, for that baby's dead!"[63]

Two weeks later, Sims attended another sick child, who also died. "I was then so demoralized, and so disgusted with my beginning in the profession, that if I had had money enough, or any money at all . . . I would not have given another dose of medicine. But there was no other alternative for me. Being obliged to continue in the profession that I had started in, I was determined to make up my deficiency by hard work."[64] Realizing that expertise could derive from experience, Sims decided that such work would involve, not "reading books," but rather "observation and diligent attention to the sick."[65]

Insecure about the value of their training and confronting women who assumed the right to judge medical skills and direct treatment, physicians responded in various ways. Many routinely disparaged women's knowledge and skills. Although Sims eventually acknowledged the nurse's superior insight, other doctors frequently complained about "ignorant old ladies." Dr. Samuel J. Crumbine condemned "the old grannies who thought they knew more than the physician. To us doctors on the frontier these ancient know-it-all's were often a positive curse."[66]

After Dr. Hiram Rutherford moved from Millersberg, Pennsylvania, to eastern Illinois in 1840, he wrote to a friend, "I am enabled to persue a much better and bolder practice here than in M. The people here call in time and take medicine as it is prescribed. There is no clique of old Dutch women over the patient, laying the medicine aside."[67]

Doctors portrayed the bedside gathering of friends and family as a threat to the patient rather than a source of comfort and support. "The lying-in-room is no place for a crowd," proclaimed Dr. Thomas Bull, explaining, "The patient . . . is much disturbed by their conversation, and what is a much greater evil that this, by their imprudent remarks they frequently diminish her confidence in her own powers, or in the judgment and skill of her necessary attendants. The mind in a state of distress is easily excited and alarmed, and whispering in the lying-in-chamber, or any appearance of concealment, quickly produces an injurious impression."[68]

In an account of his father's medical practice in the 1870s and 1880s, William Allen Pusey wrote, "He knew from his own experience when ill how trying were the friendliest visitors to ill and nervous patients. But this control of visitors to the seriously sick was a difficult problem in those days. Country people think it is neighborly—which it is—to call upon the sick and the custom was to come and sit around the sick room."[69]

Nonorthodox physicians also discussed the harm caused by informal caregivers in the sickroom. Joel Shew, a leading proponent of hydropathy, complained, "At home the patient is often annoyed by the fears, importunities, and meddlesomness of friends."[70] Many doctors sought to limit the size of the bedside circle. Pusey noted that "in very important situations," his father "would keep [neighbors] cleared out."[71] Other doctors gradually shifted their practices to offices.[72]

Doctors who could not alter the context of care shaped their behavior to inspire confidence. Some sought to present a semblance of authority. Dr. Hertzler noted that the visibility of performance "made it necessary for the doctor to make a display of great activity, a show staged for the benefit of the relatives."[73] When summoned to treat a woman with convulsions, Dr. Long "assumed a very sober and severe attitude [and] ordered the members of the household about."[74] Doctors also were quick to claim credit for all signs of recovery, even those that bore no relationship to their interventions. They blamed poor outcomes on delays in seeking medical help, and they explained misdiagnoses by arguing that the illnesses had changed.[75]

Finally, doctors tried to restrict the medical information supplied by household guides. Beginning in the early nineteenth century, some manuals by physicians omitted instructions for tasks such as bleeding or administering toxic drugs, asserting that they were too difficult for women to perform. As the century advanced, some authors of domestic health guides went further, seeking to relegate women entirely to prevention and nursing care.[76]

These various strategies laid the groundwork for the medical profession's campaign to consolidate its power and privilege in the early twentieth century. We will see that physicians continued to belittle women's healing knowledge, criticize the emotional support they provided, attribute all good outcomes to medical interventions, blame caregivers for waiting too long to summon professional assistance, and limit the information dispensed to the public. Subsequent chapters examine the extent to which such efforts eventually enabled physicians to usurp women's authority at the bedside.

Before the transformations wrought by the bacteriological revolution and the rise of hospitals, however, these strategies achieved little success. Throughout the nineteenth century, women derived their knowledge largely from sources separate from physicians. If women lacked the reassurance derived from believing that doctors knew best, they retained the self-respect that came from speaking with their own authority and making autonomous decisions.

Part Two
1890–1940

4

A "Terrible and Exhausting" Struggle:
Martha Shaw Farnsworth, 1890–1924

$\mathcal{D}$ESPITE THE WEALTH of recent studies charting the metamorphosis of the formal health care system during the late nineteenth and early twentieth centuries, we know little about the changes wrought in informal care. Assuming that professional medicine absorbed family healing and nursing, most historical accounts follow care out of the home into physicians' offices and hospitals. James H. Cassedy justifies this approach by arguing that family care was shorn of medical significance: "The care and support provided by the family circle itself remained crucially important to the general well-being and morale of the seriously ill or dying person in America, but some of the family's traditional roles gradually diminished during this period. A major factor in bringing this about was the shifting of the locale of much medical care . . . from the home to the hospital."[1] Ruth Schwartz Cowan expounds the substitution thesis even more unambiguously. After tracing the growth of the nursing profession, she asserts that "every hour of care" that nurses "offered to patients was an hour that would earlier, and under other circumstances, have been offered by a housewife."[2]

But family caregiving is not a timeless and static endeavor, changing only through the gradual loss of its medical component. Nor does an hour of professional care translate directly into an hour of relief for family members. Rather than assuming that families withdrew their services during the late nineteenth and early twentieth centuries, we should ask how the revolution in medical knowledge and practice transformed the content and meaning of the care that continued to be delivered at home. To what extent did the development of revolutionary new surgical and diagnostic techniques convince family caregivers to relinquish control over medical decision-making? And to what extent did the growth of formal services create new responsibilities for caregivers?

In any case, the rise of the health care industry was not the only factor affecting family care. This period also witnessed profound changes in transportation and communication technologies. Although a few historians have investigated the effects of railroads, automobiles, and telephones on the practice of medicine,[3] the impact of these developments on the work of family caregivers has been ignored. Changes in domestic technology are also absent from the accounts of medical historians. During the late nineteenth and early twentieth centuries, large corporations began to mass-produce goods and services for the home.[4] Electricity, gas, indoor plumbing, and store-bought foods also helped to transform family care and likewise demand our attention.

This chapter examines the ways in which such changes shaped domestic healing by examining the diary of Martha Shaw Farnsworth, a Kansas woman who was both a giver and a recipient of care. Martha began keeping a diary in 1882, at the age of fourteen; by the time of her death in 1924, she had written over four thousand pages.[5] A reader of popular romantic novels, Martha drew heavily on them to construct this account of her life. She dramatized her troubles, emphasized morality rather than psychological insight, and wrote in what we now consider an excessively florid style. Keeping in mind the literary form Martha emulated can help us understand not just the nature of her caregiving relationships but also the sense she made of them.

Martha was born on April 26, 1867, the oldest of three daughters of an Iowa farmer. Her mother died in childbirth in 1870. Two years later, Martha's father remarried and moved the family to a Kansas village near Winfield. Her subsequent childhood recollections included herding cattle while watching out for wolves.

As a teenager Martha portrayed herself as high spirited, independent, and fearless. She played baseball, rode bareback, and engaged in a series of flirtations, despite her stepmother's disapproval. On January

23, 1883, Martha wrote, "My step-mother says if I don't quit letting the boys walk home with me, she will put us all to bed." Nevertheless, she continued to frequent dance halls, walked home alone with young men, and sat talking with them on the veranda after other members of the household had gone to bed.

Martha sought release from her parents' authority by living apart from them. In April 1883 she moved to a neighbor's house, taking the first of a series of positions as a hired girl. Martha occasionally held other jobs as well. In 1885 she briefly taught school; the following year she worked in a hotel in Medicine Lodge, a town about ninety miles from Winfield.

But illness frequently impeded Martha's quest for independence. On August 26, 1883, she wrote that she was home "to stay" because her stepmother was sick and needed help. Although Martha resented the summons, "for I was having such a good time and my stepmother is none too kind to me," she hoped to be "a little better treated, now I'm needed." We will see that one way Martha retained her dignity throughout her life was by demanding respect and consideration in return for responding to the needs of others.

The next serious illness occurred in Martha's absence. She was working at the Medicine Lodge hotel when she learned that her sister had been stricken with typhoid fever. The disease was common in Kansas at that time because of the poor water quality.[6] On August 24, 1886, Martha wrote,

> At 9 A.M. received a *Telegram*, telling me my *poor darling sister* was dead. Oh! how *cruel* the folks have been, not to send me word, so I could have gone home, in time. God *have mercy. How can I ever bear it.* I *loved* and *worshipped* my darling sister, above *everything* else in the whole world. She died at 5:30 this morning. I took the 11 o'clock A.M. train for home.

Before the advent of telephones, it was easy to remain uninformed about the existence of illness in the family. But some technological developments already had begun to affect Martha's life. She received news of the death by telegram and, thanks to the network of railroads recently constructed, was able to arrive in time for the funeral.

Martha's own sickness also drew her home. Although she returned to

Medicine Lodge on August 30, she was back in Winfield two months later. "At Pa's, feeling so sick: Have 'Typhoid-fever,'" she wrote on October 30. "Dr. Stine, who boards with Pa is doctoring me." Martha's experience as a patient reminds us again that nineteenth-century caregiving often fell short of its romantic ideal. On November 3 she wrote, "Wish I was back in Medicine Lodge, for my stepmother is so cross to me." Martha began to improve in early January 1887 but soon suffered a relapse. On February 2 she wrote, "My stepmother says I '*have to go*' as soon as I am strong enough." Although Martha was "not *strong yet*" on February 14, she moved to a neighbor's house because her "step mother doesn't want me at home." When the family departed for Colorado in March, Martha remained behind.

In September 1887 Martha moved to Topeka and two years later married Johnny Shaw, a twenty-eight-year-old postman. It was above all in relation to this marriage that Martha portrayed herself as the heroine of a romantic novel, facing adversity with unvarying courage and cheerfulness. Their troubles began almost immediately. On November 1, 1889, Martha wrote, "In bed most of day. Mis-carriage: missed just one mo: feel awful bad." The next day she reported that Johnny verbally abused her, and on November 7 he arrived home drunk.[7] Her husband's illness had the most profound impact on the course of the marriage. On November 23 Martha noted that Johnny "came home at noon" with a fever; on November 27 she "went to the Doctor's in the evening for Medicine." Two days later, she summoned another doctor, returning with Henry Roby, a prominent homeopath.[8] Although fetching medicine and doctors typically was men's work, women took over when men were incapacitated. The task could be long and arduous, even in urban areas. In the late 1880s, Topeka's streets were unpaved and frequently muddy;[9] Martha's long skirts must have added to her difficulties. The absence of streetlights meant that walking alone at night could be dangerous.[10]

When Roby returned on November 30, he pronounced Johnny improved. Roby enjoyed a substantial reputation in the community,[11] but Martha had little confidence in him. "I don't exactly like him," she wrote. "He seems to know all about him, without asking anything about his previous condition." It is unclear what "previous condition" Martha thought the doctor should have inquired about; her diaries do not mention a prior condition that may have troubled Johnny. Moreover, in the late-nineteenth-century, patients' medical histories were considered less important than their habits and general lifestyles.[12] As we shall see, Martha herself later attributed Johnny's illness to his personal behavior.

On December 1 Roby's assistant, Dr. Charles F. Menninger, arrived. According to Martha, he "gave Johnny a thorough examination." "We are *very* much pleased with him," she wrote. Because Menninger remained Martha's physician off and on for almost thirty years, he merits some discussion. Although she preferred him to Roby, it is unlikely that he would have impressed her initially as very different from any of the doctors she had known as a child in rural Kansas. A recent graduate of Hahnemann Medical College, a small homeopathic medical school in Chicago, Menninger had been practicing less than a year when Martha first consulted him. He was well aware of the deficiencies of his education. Hahnemann had recently established a small laboratory and library, but it still did not teach new developments in medicine and provided little clinical experience.[13] Nor was Menninger entering a secure or highly paid occupation. Earning just $40 a month, he relied on his wife's income from teaching to make ends meet. They lived in just two rooms in Roby's office building.[14]

This period of sickness introduced Martha not just to Dr. Menninger but also to the problems Johnny's poor health would create throughout their marriage. Illness appears to have aggravated his irritability and impatience. On December 8, she complained, "He got so very angry at me this eve and cursed me so hard, and was so mad he wouldn't take his medicine, because he thought I took more time than I needed, to eat a lunch." The following day she wrote, "He hardly lets me take time to breathe." Johnny's condition also interfered with his ability to fulfill the role of breadwinner. On January 6, 1890, Martha remarked that Johnny had returned to work after a four-week absence. But he continued to "lay off" some days. It may not be coincidental that Martha's diary also included the information that she had taken in two roomers. Although keeping boarders was a common way for women to contribute to the household economy in the nineteenth century,[15] the precariousness of Johnny's health may well have increased Martha's determination to find her own source of income.

With Johnny still sick on February 11, Martha wrote that they were "studying his case and trying to learn what would be best to restore his health." Although Martha does not define the nature of their study, it is likely that they read popular medical literature. Martha and Johnny also critically evaluated the medical assistance they obtained. When physicians offered advice, Martha felt competent to challenge it. "Doctors here . . . want to operate on Johnny for a Fistula," she wrote on February 12, "but I don't want them to: I am afraid it is Tuberculosis." This was a sensible diagnosis. Tuberculosis was a leading cause of death in the late nineteenth century, and Martha must have known several people who suffered from it.[16] She also may have been aware that even the most experienced doctors frequently missed its signs, especially in the early stages.[17]

On February 17 Martha announced a new decision: Johnny would "go to Chicago to be doctored." No overriding medical imperative compelled Johnny to travel to a distant city to seek care from strangers. Unlike Cook County or Walter Reese, the hospital he entered in Chicago was a fledgling institution with only a local reputation. Founded in 1883 by the German American community, the German Hospital opened its doors in 1884; in 1890 it had just sixty beds and served an annual patient population of 550.[18] Christ's Hospital, a comparable institution in Topeka, also admitted its first patients in 1884 and grew slowly during the remainder of the decade.[19] The explanation for Johnny's trip probably lay more with Menninger's background than with any special treatment available in Chicago. As a newcomer to Topeka and a member of an irregular medical sect, Menninger lacked ties to the local medical community. He did not gain admitting privileges at Christ's Hospital for another eight years.[20] If he remained outside the medical establishment, however, he was firmly rooted in the German American community. The son of German immigrants, Menninger had grown up in Tell City, Indiana, among a large German population; he did not begin to learn English until he entered school at the age of five.[21] His wife, Flo, was also the offspring of German immigrants.[22] It is likely that nationality had influenced Menninger's choice of medical school. Samuel Hahnemann, the founder of homeopathy and namesake of the school, was a German doctor, and the sect enjoyed a large following among German immigrants throughout the nineteenth century.[23] Menninger apparently found it easier to admit a Kansas patient to a German hospital in Chicago than to a hospital in his own town of Topeka.

Johnny left for Chicago on February 18, 1890. Although Martha acknowledged feeling "hurt" by his demand that she stay behind, she assuaged her pride by insisting to herself that she alone could tend him properly. "He needs me so much," she noted. When he wrote that he had undergone surgery and "came very near dying," she commented, "Now I *knew* I ought to have been with him" (February 26). On March 11 she invoked the ideal of the loyal wife to defy Johnny's authority: "I have made up my mind. I am going to Chicago and see my husband." Borrowing money from her roomers, she departed two days later.

Although Martha portrayed this journey as an expression of wifely devotion, it was also an adventure. She "saw some pretty places, passing thro' Illinois." After reaching Chicago, she interspersed sight-seeing with bedside visits. Having never been "in a real City before," she found "so much to see." One afternoon was spent "going thro' some big stores," and another walking to the shore of Lake Michigan, getting her "first look at a large body of water." The hospital also fascinated her. "They have almost every *Nationality here*, and surely every kind of disease and surgical case," she wrote. "A Hospital is most interesting." When rain prevented her from venturing outside, she busied herself "'picking up' many German words and getting so I understand lots of it" (March 17–25).

Joan E. Lynaugh points out that historians have tended "to telescope the story of the changing American hospital so that it seems as if hospitals were transformed directly from shelters for the chronically ill and homeless poor into highly technologic, medically dominated curative institutions." Lynaugh describes "a critical intermediate stage," which she dubs "the 'domestic era' of hospital development."[24] Martha's account suggests that the German Hospital was such a "domestic-era" institution in 1890. Although Johnny received an operation, surgery apparently had not replaced custodial care as the hospital's central function. Many patients Martha met on the ward were well enough to leave the premises during the day. Johnny, too, remained at the hospital for seven weeks, a lengthy stay by present-day standards.

The transitional nature of the institution shaped Martha's experience there. Because the German Hospital had acquired little of the bureaucratic rigidity which characterizes medical institutions today, it easily incorporated Martha's presence. The matron invited her to board at the hospital, sharing a room with a few convalescent women. When she developed a sore throat, she received medical care. If Martha was treated more like a patient than a visitor, however, she was reminded of her caregiving obligations as Johnny's discharge approached. On March 28 she wrote, "They tell me I can take Johnny home now whenever I learn to dress the wound, made by operating, so I went into the Operating room with the Doctor and Nurse this morning but it looked so badly, I could not bear to touch him." Just as the hospital staff casually accepted her as a patient, so they allowed her access to space now the exclusive province of medical personnel.

Martha must have overcome her squeamishness, because she and Johnny left the hospital on April 3. Their relationship soon reverted to its earlier pattern. Back in Topeka in mid-April, she wrote that Johnny's health was better but he was "cross as a bear." On September 4 she wrote, "Our *first Wedding Anniversary*, and the year has been *so full* of tears . . . I *know* he loves me, is *proud* of me, but he lets his temper rule him and make him unkind." When she had another miscarriage the following month, she complained that her suffering elicited little sympathy.

The improvement in Johnny's health proved ephemeral. On October 14 Martha wrote, "Thro' the Summer, Johnny seemed to have regained his health, but now that Fall has come he is not real well and I feel he *never will* be well." The return of his cough confirmed her suspicion that he was "*going into Consumption.*" Excessive drinking, she asserted, had undermined his health.

On November 24, 1890, Martha wrote, "We have *made up our minds* to *visit* my people in *Colorado.*" In the late nineteenth century, it was widely believed that the western climate had a beneficial effect on tuberculosis sufferers. As Billy M. Jones notes, "Faith in climatic treatment became so universal, that most patients accepted with unreserved approval a physician's charge to seek a more favorable climate."[25] Known as "the World's Sanatorium," Colorado was an especially popular destination for invalids. In 1881 a railroad advertisement proclaimed that "nearly one-half, of all the people now residing in Colorado were influenced in coming here, either directly or indirectly, by considerations of health."[26] Family ties also may have influenced Martha and Johnny's choice; they could save money on room and board by staying with Martha's parents, who had moved to Colorado in 1887. Nevertheless, the train fare was a financial strain. The trip also exacted a psychological cost. *"Breaking up housekeeping* and *we had only just begun,"* she complained on December 2, the eve of their departure.

Most late-nineteenth-century health seekers in the West initially penned optimistic accounts of the value of the air they found.[27] Martha wrote in a similar vein on December 31, shortly after reaching Colorado: "Johnny is much better than when we came. We brought ten dollars worth of medicine with us and I don't believe he will need any more."

Martha's diary is silent about why the couple decided to go back to Topeka in late March. She noted, however, that Menninger considered their return premature. "Met Dr. Menninger on street this morning," she wrote on March 30, 1891, soon after their arrival. "He says, Johnny *is not yet strong enough,* to live here and must go back at once and stay at least three years." Although Martha took this advice seriously enough to record it in her diary, she and Johnny disregarded it for six months. On April 1, 1891, they moved into a new house in Topeka.

Johnny's instructions were more difficult to disregard. On June 18 Martha wrote, "I went to town this afternoon and bought me a new dress of French mull-Lavender. I always have to ask Johnny's consent before I buy anything for myself and take him along or show him a sample." Her inability to exercise control over her reproductive life was even more troubling. The previous month she had begun to suspect that she was pregnant again. When the time for a miscarriage passed, Johnny demanded that she have an abortion. After granting permission for the pregnancy to continue, he complained about her morning sickness.

Johnny soon imposed new hardships on her. In the fall he began to "cough considerably" and decided to heed Menninger's counsel. Menninger now added that Johnny should travel in a covered wagon. Martha beseeched Johnny to let her stay behind. She was in the middle of a difficult pregnancy and feared she would be unable to withstand the journey. The trip also would separate her again from her circle of friends and place her beyond the reach of medical help during her confinement. As she wrote on October 1, "We *will be fifty miles* from a Railroad and *there will be many deprivations. I can have no nurse. no doctor. no help,* when *my little* [one] *comes.* I *beg* Johnny to *let me stay,* as . . . I could *have the care that is a woman's right at such a time."*[28]

When Johnny refused to allow Martha to remain in Topeka, she wrote, "I am *willing* to make the sacrifice, if it will but restore my husband's health. Our friends think him very selfish to *compel* me to take such a trip in my condition . . . Woman will sacrifice everything for the man she loves, why will *he* not do *half* as much for her" (November 12). Richard Sennett and Jonathan Cobb write that sacrifice is "the last resource for individualism, the last demonstration of competence . . . It is the most fundamental action you can perform that proves your ability to be in control; it is the final demonstration of virtue when all else fails."[29] A woman who continuously strove to remain in control, Martha now sought the moral high ground. Her cheerfulness in adversity contributed to her sense of superiority. The trip lasted four weeks and was extremely grueling. Although she railed against the injustice of it in the privacy of her journal, she took pride in keeping her complaints to herself. "I never quarrel with him and he *never sees ought but a smiling face*" (November 7).

Martha grew no more reconciled to the lack of medical attention as her confinement approached. When the labor began, shortly after she moved into her new home, she sent Johnny to summon her sister May, her stepmother, and Mrs. Gordon, a neighborhood woman who was the mother of fifteen children. While waiting for their arrival, Martha commented, "Mrs. Gordon is *all* I can have to help me thro" (January 23, 1892). Even the joy of a healthy baby did not convince Martha that she had received adequate care. "Today, at 12 minutes past 1 o'clock P.M. my *Precious*, 'wee girlie' came to her mother. The *dearest, sweetest,* little, *treasure, ever* a mother had," Martha wrote on January 24. "But *what a time we had, to get her:* there are no doctors near here and *motherhood* was *all* but impossible . . . Mrs. Gordon, *tore me*, with her fingers and *pulled* baby *away, scratching* the little *forehead* and *almost crushing* the *head until* was a *great ridge across* the *top, big* as my *finger* and the darling was *black* with *strangulation*." Martha concluded her account with yet another allusion to the absence of medical personnel. "Mrs. Gordon, Johnny, Ma and sister, were only ones with me."

As a postpartum patient, Martha chafed at all the restrictions imposed on her, just as she had as a teenager. "I would love to get up, but they won't let me," she wrote four days after giving birth. "There has been no time, I have felt the least bit weak. My unusual health and strength is a surprise to everyone." Trusting her own knowledge rather than that of her stepmother and Johnny, she "*shocked*" them the following day by walking across the room.

Motherhood meant that Martha now had another duty she considered equivalent to her duty to Johnny. She wrote on March 3, "I *bless God every day, for the little life* He has *given into my care* and *I pray always that I may live worthy [of] such love.*" On the twenty-fourth, she proclaimed Baby Inez "the *sweetest, dearest, cutest, blessedest* baby ever a mother had." Each new development was a source of wonder: "She can sit alone and crows and coo's so sweet."

Martha's marriage, however, continued to deteriorate. As Johnny's growing infirmity limited his ability to farm, she blamed him for imposing an onerous workload on her. "I wonder," she wrote on March 10, "if a woman is supposed to kill herself for a man, who has a temper like a Bear." Martha also worried that Johnny exerted a negative influence over the baby. "I sometimes wish I could take her and go away off, where we would never see her father—he curses me so and is so ill tempered. I am afraid she will learn to do the same, when old enough" (March 22).

In May a new worry arose. Baby Inez began to cough and became fretful. At a time of high infant mortality, any sickness could presage disaster. Because infectious diseases were rampant and antibiotics nonexistent, infants and children frequently became ill and died.[30] In 1890, 58 percent of all burials in Leavenworth, Kansas, were for children under the age of five.[31] In nursing Inez, Martha was participating in one of the most common and emotionally wrenching forms of nineteenth-century caregiving. Martha tried to reassure herself that the baby suffered from nothing more serious than a cold but acknowledged on May 9 that "sometimes it makes me heart-sick." On May 17 she wrote, "I am convinced she is 'teething,' tho' many say 'too young.'" This was a reasonable, if terrifying, diagnosis. According to medical beliefs of the time, dentition was a dangerous passage that could precipitate several fatal illnesses.[32]

Martha was as dismissive of traditional healing practices for her ailing baby as she had been for herself during childbirth. "How I wish there was a good Doctor in this part of the country," she wrote on May 20, "that I might consult him for my little 'joy-girl,' instead of using *all* the remedies, *all* the old 'grand-mothers' can think up, for *all* the 'diseases,' one ever heard or dreamed about." Although some feminists wax nostalgic about networks of women exchanging information on children's health care, Martha had no use for such sources of knowledge. A wide variety of nonorthodox healers practiced in the Midwest in the early 1890s,[33] but Martha was nearly as wary of them. On May 28 she decided to consult "Mrs. M. E. Martin, a sort of 'Home-made' Baby doctor." After a second visit on June 7, however, Martha grew skeptical: "Mrs. Martin thinks Baby's trouble is her lungs and I'm just as sure it's her teeth."

The following day Martha resolved to return to Topeka "to get a good doctor." Although Martha presented herself as acting primarily for the baby, she also acknowledged that the trip advanced her own interests. "If [Inez] gets well," she declared, "I'll be in no hurry to come back to a cross man. I shall at least take a good, long rest and am packing my trunk, with that in view."

Arriving by train on June 11, she immediately summoned Dr. Menninger, who corroborated her diagnosis. "It *is* her teeth, as I suspected." In addition, Menninger stated, the baby suffered from "Brain-fever." Menninger continued to visit the baby regularly during the next few weeks. When Inez went into "spasms" on June 25, he "stayed some time" and returned the next day with medicine.

Despite Martha's confidence in Menninger, it is unlikely that he had much to offer. Discussing Menninger's first years as a physician, Winslow writes, "The most disheartening part of medical practice at that time was the diseases of children: meningitis, diphtheria, scarlet fever, typhoid, and the like. Too often the doctor was entirely helpless; the best he could do was to soften the blow that was about to fall on the parents. At such times Charles would silently pray, asking God to lead him further into the light of knowledge and proficiency."[34] Menninger also had not acquired the rewards of professional status. Having left Roby's practice in August 1890, he struggled to attract an adequate paying clientele and remained dependent on his wife's income.[35]

Although Martha stayed with Johnny's mother and his sister Retta, she initially refused to accept their help with the baby. "I do not undress, day or night and trust my child to no one," she wrote on June 14. "I only sleep with her in my arms." By the twenty-second, the stress of care had taken its toll. "Had to call Dr. Menninger to see *me* for I am all worn out with loss of sleep and rest, and care and anxiety and I have a very sore breast: in fact I am *sick*, all over, and had to give up awhile this afternoon and go lie down and sleep and leave my darling to the care of her Aunt Retta Shaw." As the baby worsened, Martha marshaled a broader network of support. On June 26 she reported, "Eva Herman and Mrs. Wm Baker helped me all day." The following day she commented, "Mrs. Pettit and Mrs. Ed Johnston were with me when baby died."

Throughout the summer, Martha poured out her anguish in the pages of her journal. "Oh! the emptiness of my arms, the loneliness of my heart. Oh! God, ease this terrible heart-ache," she wrote on June 29. An entry on July 17 read, "I am so weary of heart I could die. I do not see how I can ever live without my Babe."

Martha had telegraphed Johnny when the baby was dying, and he arrived soon afterward. Although they continued to live together, first in Topeka and then back in Colorado, she insisted that the terms of their relationship had changed. "I stay with him, simply because I believe as a Christian, it is my duty to do so," she wrote on November 4.

In the fall of 1892, Johnny's illness again preoccupied her. Because he had become too sick to farm, he decided to seek a cure in Los Angeles. Despite worries about the harmful effects of ocean fog, the coastal cities of Southern California drew large numbers of tubercular patients during the late nineteenth century.[36] With a new move looming, Martha complained about her nomadic life. "This settling in a new home, and so soon 'tearing up' and going again takes the heart out of me" (November 28).

Nevertheless, when Johnny offered her a divorce, she declined. On November 14 Martha wrote, "Johnny says he will divide with me what little we have and I can go my way and he will go his." She "could shout with very joy at the thought of freedom from such a life," but "duty" commanded her "to stay with him." Furthermore, she told him that "if he was to get sick, he would need me, and not every one would stand by him." She repeated this over and over. "No one wants me to go away with him," she wrote on November 28, "but if *he* insists on going, I feel it my duty to go with him; no one else would look after his welfare as I would." In such passages Martha portrayed caregiving as a choice, rather than the natural and inevitable reflection of her gender. Her willingness to accompany Johnny to California and nurse him as his condition worsened was an achievement, in her view, demonstrating her special worth.

The move proved as disruptive as she had feared. Arriving in Los Angeles, she felt adrift in a new land. "Christmas Day, and what a mockery it seems to me," she wrote. "Strangers, in a strange land, among strangers, more than a thousand miles from home, is not conducive to a very happy Christmas." On New Year's Day, 1893, she commented, "Johnny and I went for a walk after dinner, but how could it be pleasant, when you know not a soul to say 'Howdy-do' to."

Other members of the invalid community eventually helped to assuage her loneliness. On March 3, 1893, she wrote, "I have met some very wealthy people here and made some very pleasant friends. Mrs. Morey, whose hands are covered with diamonds—she wears *ten fine* diamond rings on one hand—has just about such a husband as I have: he is about the same size and looks much like Johnny: *he* also has consumption and is cross and cranky as can be. Well, *she* and I are *friends* and sympathise fully, with one another."

Johnny's deteriorating condition also compelled her to reenter the labor force. On January 22 she reported that she had been hired to serve meals at a boardinghouse. She was "thankful" for the job, although "pride made it embarrassing." Had they remained in Colorado, she noted, she would have been able to earn higher wages and avoid the indignity of waitressing. The demands of care also narrowed her options. Because she had to return home to tend Johnny in the middle of the day, she could not work as either a nurse or a clerk. But the flexibility of her hours meant that she bore a double burden. On February 20 she described her daily routine: "To work at 6 A.M. Home again at 2 P.M. back to work at 4 P.M. and home at 7 o'clock for the night. 17 blocks to the [boarding house] walked four times a day, is 68 blocks, or more than five miles a day."

Nevertheless, work had its compensations. Martha found some companionship among her coworkers, including a Chinese dishwasher to whom she gave Bible lessons. Although she previously had complained about having to consult Johnny before buying anything for herself, she wrote on May 30, "After the Breakfast hour, I went to town and bought a *nice Guitar*, in a *Pawn-shop, for $5.00* [using] some of my *tip-money.*" Employment also offered relief from the stress of care. On February 19 she wrote that if her job was "hard," it was also "a blessing, in that I do not have to be so much with Johnny and run the risk of taking consumption, for he coughs dreadfully and the smell from his body is sickening: smells like his body was dead." The entry ended with the "wish" that she "did not have to sleep in same room with him."

Four years earlier, Martha had nursed Johnny without worrying about her own risk of infection. Now, fear of contagion mingled with revulsion at his body, increasing the burden of care. Sheila M. Rothman notes that after Robert Koch's discovery of the tubercle bacillus in 1882, educated Americans "slowly began to reckon with the fact that proximity to a person with tuberculosis could be dangerous."[37] Kansas did not launch an extensive health education campaign about tuberculosis until after the turn of the century.[38] But in Los Angeles, Martha associated with patients and their families and may well have learned about the communicable nature of the disease from them. Another woman who had accompanied a tubercular family member later recalled her morning ritual in southern California in 1893: "I began to empty the cuspidors. Every room except mine had at least one cuspidor partly filled with water . . . I knew cleaning the cuspidors was dangerous work."[39]

Martha's anxiety about Johnny's impending death grew throughout the spring and summer. "Johnny sick—in bed most of time," she wrote on March 31, 1893. "I am so afraid I will come home some evening and find him dead." On July 22 she wrote, "Death is so near my home, I shudder." Two days later she announced that she had "quit work" and was "home to stay, for Johnny has grown so much worse, it is not safe to leave him alone any more." On August 1 they received money from Johnny's mother and the following day boarded the train to Topeka. "I *return* home, with a heavy heart," she wrote, "for again, I am leaving many dear friends and most of all because I know, just ahead a little way, death is waiting to claim the one to whom I'm bound."

For the second time in fourteen months, Martha arrived back in Topeka with a dying family member. Once again, she complained that the burdens fell most heavily on her. Although they stayed with Johnny's brother and had other relatives and friends around, Johnny insisted that she alone care for him. "Johnny slowly grows weaker and I am with him day and night," she wrote on August 16. "Have not undressed to go to bed, since I left Los Angeles. He won't let anyone else care for him, so day and night I sit by his bed-side, getting what sleep I can in a rocking-chair, and I never seem rested." The stifling summer heat must have added to her difficulties.[40] Moreover, some of her care involved hard physical labor. Because Johnny could no longer "raise himself up in bed" by the end of August, she had to "lift him so much and turn him." On October 5 she described her martyrdom thus: "Two months this afternoon, since we came home and not *once* in all that time, have I had my clothes off, only to change to others, nor have I been in bed. I sleep in a chair beside the bed, that I may minister to his every want. Several times I have lain down on the floor on a pallet, but he does not like to have me do so."

Observing the customary reticence of the period, Martha wrote nothing about the intimate aspects of care. She must have fed Johnny, washed blood, excrement, and sputum from his body, and changed his clothes and bedding. She previously had recoiled from the sight of his surgical wound and the smell of his ailing body; the new information about contagion had added an element of fear. We therefore can assume that she found the tasks she performed in the summer and fall of 1893 extremely distasteful. We can only speculate about what the confrontation with physical frailty meant to her. Was she able to distance herself emotionally from Johnny's deterioration because she assumed that it stemmed from moral failure? To what extent did she dwell on the possibility that her own health, too, could fail at any time?

Like many nineteenth-century women, Martha assumed responsibility for her husband's spiritual well-being. "I wish he was a Christian," she wrote on August 24. "It is hard to see him dying an unbeliever, an *Infidel.* I pray God to change his heart."

Johnny's death on October 26, 1893, generated turbulent emotions. "*Tonight I am entirely alone and miserable,*" she wrote. "*Tonight I am a widow. I am free. My heart* would *cry out in very joy, because it is freed from a wretchedly miserable life,* and *my heart is breaking with pain, heart-ache and utter desolation.*" Although she claimed to "miss him more than anyone can know," she burned many of his possessions on October 30 "that I may have no reminder of my unhappy life."

The period following Johnny's death also provided an occasion to reflect on the meaning of the care she had rendered. Again, she insisted that she had acted primarily out of a sense of duty, not from warmth or affection. "I have striven to do what God would have me do," she asserted the day after Johnny died. On March 8, 1894, she recorded a comment by one of Johnny's former coworkers that had been reported to her: "Sam Robinson, an old Mail-Carrier . . . said I *was a good, true woman, or I would not have staid by John Shaw as I did;* said *not one woman in a thousand would have staid with him.*" Martha's self-denial previously had enabled her to consider herself more virtuous than Johnny; now she was able to view herself as morally superior to other women.

Johnny's death also thrust Martha back into the working world. "I must be looking about me for something to do," she wrote on November 2, "because Johnny left me no means of support." On November 19 she reported, "Fred Farnsworth came for me this morning and took me up to his Mother's, to make arrangements to stay with her as a nurse, as her daughter must go to her home in Calif." As Susan M. Reverby writes, "Marriage to a very poor man, divorce or abandonment, or widowhood were often preconditions for nursing. Widowhood, in particular, appears to have been an important, if cruel, pathway into nursing. With no need for formal credentials, a woman could offer her experience of caring for a dying husband as her qualification to nurse."[41]

In entering the Farnsworth home, Martha was resuming the type of position she had held prior to marriage. Like a hired girl, she received room and board and little pay. Moreover, the social status of her employers was not greatly superior to her own. Although three Farnsworth sons had embarked on high-paying careers, Fred, who lived with his parents, was a postal carrier and had been a close friend of Johnny Shaw. And just as Martha probably participated in the life of the household when she worked as a hired girl, so now she ate her meals with Mr. Farnsworth and his son Fred and spent her free time with them.

The job was a welcome change from the work of nursing Johnny. "Oh! how good it seems, to have everyone kind to you, how restful," she wrote on December 1. "I never hear a complaining, nor unkind word and I feel as if I had been let out of prison." As Mrs. Farnsworth's condition deteriorated, Martha's workload increased. On December 20 she wrote, "Mrs. F. is failing so, that she takes almost my constant time, and each night I must stay in her room over night." An entry three days later read, "Both Mr. and Mrs. Farnsworth very sick and I go constantly from one room to another . . . I barely got a doze last night."

Less than three months after presiding over Johnny's death, Martha held another bedside vigil. On January 1, 1894, she noted, "I did not go to bed at all last night, but sat alone all through the night, in a rocker, beside the bed of Mrs. Farnsworth, holding her hand. I slept when she slept. She just will not let me out of her sight." Mrs. Farnsworth died five days later.

This death brought little change in Martha's life. Because Mr. Farnsworth still needed care, she agreed on January 11 to "stay . . . some time yet, as nurse and housekeeper." Moreover, Fred had begun to press her to marry him, and in April she finally agreed. After their marriage on May 2, 1894, Martha and Fred continued to live with Mr. Farnsworth. In November 1895 they moved to their own house, leaving the elder Mr. Farnsworth in the care of a daughter.

Martha's second marriage was generally harmonious. Unlike Johnny, Fred did not demand wifely subservience, and Martha could retain her dignity and autonomy without a struggle. The major constraint on her life was responsibility for onerous domestic and farm chores. Fred's wage, like that of many working men, was insufficient to support the household. Instead of seeking paid work, Martha raised poultry and sold eggs and milk. As late as 1922, when she was fifty-five years old, she still had sixty-six chickens. Her housework, too, was far more grueling than that of most middle-class city women. Long after others had begun to send out laundry, Martha devoted much of one day every week to washing and another to ironing. She also baked the bread and canned the vegetables and fruit that better-off women bought in stores. Later, when the demands of care were again added to her responsibilities, Martha's burdens were staggering.

Like many other midwestern women in the early twentieth century, Martha delighted in the new goods and services that gradually lightened her tasks.[42] On March 30, 1911, she noted that the Edison Company "sent men out . . . to 'wire' our house for Electric-lights." The installation of electricity made various appliances possible. On February 3, 1912, she waxed lyrical about her new "suction sweeper," which she called "the finest thing *under* the sun." When indoor plumbing arrived on August 12, 1916, she pronounced herself "glad" to have it.

Martha's encounters with medical developments must be viewed within the context of her positive response to science and technology generally. It is reasonable to assume that her enthusiasm for the new consumer goods and services facilitated her acceptance of the innovations in diagnosis and treatment that she experienced as both a patient and a caregiver.

There was, however, one technological advance Martha greeted with ambivalence. On November 13, 1905, she wrote, "Men here stringing wires for a Telephone which I don't want but my neighbors want me to get, so as to visit over the Phone." As we will see, even after the telephone enabled her to obtain medical assistance in emergencies, she remained unconvinced of its advantages.

Three episodes during Martha's second marriage reveal the impact of medical and technological changes on care. Although the first incident involved her as a patient rather than as a caregiver, it illuminates her attitude toward medical achievements. Her entry for February 16, 1906, reads,

> Went to *Roller Skating Rink* this morning for an hour's skate with cousin Belle Van Orsdol, and just as I was taking my last round, I *fell* and *broke my left arm* at *wrist. Also dislocated it. I didn't faint but my! how it hurt, tho' tooth-ache* is *worse*. They called a hack and sent me to Dr. S. A. Johnson's Office, where I was *examined under X-Ray*, by *Dr. Johnson. Dr. J. C. McClintock* and *Dr. W. F. Bowen* and *two X-Ray or Coil Photos* taken of *my arm*, which shows a *very bad, oblique fracture* of the large bone.

McClintock and Bowen were prominent Topeka surgeons with whom Menninger worked closely.[43] As the number of specialists grew rapidly, patients increasingly consulted them directly rather than asking general practitioners for referrals.[44] Radiology was another innovation. Wilhelm Röntgen announced his discovery of X rays in January 1896, and by 1897 several Kansas doctors had acquired the new technology. At a meeting of the state medical society in 1904, some physicians mentioned using X rays to diagnose bone fractures.[45] Offices equipped with X-ray machines had clear advantages over patients' homes as the site of medical care. For the first time, there was a reason for Martha to visit a doctor's office rather than summoning him to her house.

Although diagnosis was now made in an office, treatment remained at home. There the doctors administered chloroform and then set Martha's bones in a two-and-a-half-hour operation. Two days later, the doctors returned to her house to remove a splint and put her arm in a cast. But because "the bones had slipped apart," she was told that she would have to go to the hospital for surgery. Martha agreed but decided to consult an alternative practitioner as well. "Mrs. Goddard *is going to give me 'Christian Science' treatment and says they will not cut nor wire* my arm as they intend to do," she wrote on February 20. The following day she proclaimed that therapy a success. Although the doctor had warned he would have to "*saw out an inch of bone,*" she awoke from the anesthesia to discover that her arm had not been operated on. "*Christian Science triumphed,*" she wrote.

Back home on February 22, Martha mentioned the expense of medical care for the first time. The cost of hospital services remained relatively low throughout the early twentieth century;[46] Martha's hospital bill was just $17.14. The surgeons, however, charged her $100, a sum she considered "pretty steep." The total medical bill was slightly more than Fred's monthly salary of $116.

Martha's troubles continued throughout March. "*I'm praying I may not have to* go back to Hospital," she wrote on the first of the month, "but Doctors have *given me no hopeful word yet.*" An X ray taken a few days later showed "something wrong." Although the doctors summoned her for another examination on March 10, "they do not tell me what they mean to do." Fearful of surgery, she again consulted Mrs. Goddard. On March 12 the doctors gave her another X-ray examination. As she reported, "They called me down *to break my arm over again* but after *today's examination, decided it would not be best to do so,* tho' found bones had slipped ⅛ of inch and my arm is *to be allowed to* heal *in this manner:* it *being broken in three pieces.*" The cast was finally removed on April 6.

This episode illustrates the power of medical technology to alter authority relations between physicians and patients. The doctors made at least one critical treatment decision when Martha was under anesthesia. The impact of the new visualizing technology was even more profound. As a postpartum woman, Martha had been able to rely on embodied knowledge to challenge her stepmother's instructions. But X rays produced data that rendered her physical sensations irrelevant. She did not doubt that the doctors knew more about her broken arm than she did.

Moreover, as Stanley Joel Reiser points out, physicians "who possessed an X-Ray picture could ponder and debate the medical problems of the patient, and subject his anatomical flaws to searching review— without requiring his physical presence."[47] In this case as well, the medical gaze occurred in the patient's absence. Instead of discussing treatment options with Martha, the doctors selected a course of action on their own and did not inform her of their decision. As she wrote on March 10, "They do not tell me what they mean to do."

It is not clear that this episode bolstered Martha's overall respect for medical expertise. Paul Starr argues that the "growth of medical authority" rested, above all, on "the growing recognition of the inadequacy of the unaided and uneducated senses in understanding the world."[48] Martha, however, refused to view medicine as the only legitimate source of knowledge. Even while complying with her doctors' instructions, she invested faith in other types of knowledge. Christian Science was one of the sects thriving in Kansas during the early twentieth century that aroused the greatest rage in the orthodox medical community.[49] Martha's reliance on Mrs. Goddard thus constituted a direct challenge to her doctors' authority.[50]

Martha's openness to inconsistent beliefs and practices may have been far more common than Starr assumes. He cites a survey conducted between 1928 and 1931, which found that "all the non-M.D. practitioners combined—osteopaths, chiropractors, Christian Scientists and other faith healers, midwives and chiropodists—took care of only 5.1 percent of all attended cases of illness." As a result, Starr concludes, physicians "had medical practice pretty much to themselves."[51] But that study appears to exaggerate the triumph of physicians. Recent research reminds us of the syncretistic nature of popular medical beliefs even today and of the broad array of medical practices that continue to attract large and loyal followings.[52] A 1997 study found that more than a third of adults in the United States use some form of alternative therapy.[53] We can assume that people in the early twentieth century were at least as likely to subscribe simultaneously to a variety of beliefs about illness and treatment.

Martha's ability to distance herself from medical authority can be explained in various ways. She brought to her encounter with X rays not only her independent nature but also extensive experience caring for the sick and dying, and she had reason to trust her skills. When Johnny first became ill, she suspected tuberculosis and was proved right. Her diagnosis of her baby's "teething" also eventually received corroboration. The use of X rays did not weaken her confidence in her ability to exercise judgment.

Anxieties surrounding medical technology may have reinforced Martha's desire to seek other forms of assistance. She later wrote that she almost died as a result of an overdose of the chloroform administered during her arm surgery in 1906. Although she did not mention any fear of X rays, she may have heard reports of their dangers as well. In Kansas, as elsewhere in the nation, the early X-ray machines were improperly used, and both doctors and patients occasionally suffered serious injury.[54] If medical technology increased doctors' authority, it may also have provoked fears that propelled patients to seek alternative remedies, thus, ultimately, undermining physicians' control.

Martha's next major experience with medicine similarly incorporated both new and traditional elements. On February 2, 1913, she wrote, "About 8 o'clock this evening Aunt Kate Van Orsdol Phoned from Silver Lake, that Freda had just been taken with appendicitis, and I told them to call a doctor." The town of Silver Lake was approximately eight miles from Topeka. The youngest child of Martha's sister, May, Freda enjoyed a particularly close relationship with Martha. She had been born on the anniversary of the death of Martha's baby, and she had spent much of her early life with Fred and Martha. Two years after May's husband died in 1896, May had left Colorado and moved with her children into the Farnsworth home. Although May moved to her own house in Topeka in 1903 and returned to Colorado in 1908, Martha continued to feel responsible for her niece's well-being, occasionally sending her money and advice. Although Freda was visiting other relatives in Silver Lake when appendicitis struck in 1913, she was again living with the Farnsworths.

Martha's relatives seem to have felt competent to diagnose appendicitis without consulting a physician. Moreover, the doctor they eventually called appears not to have recommended immediate surgery. When Martha phoned early on February 4, she learned that Freda "was doing alright, but wanted me." Martha therefore made arrangements to travel by train to Silver Lake and bring Freda back to Topeka. A phone call later that day abruptly altered her plans. Martha's relatives now informed her that "Dr. Dudley of Silver Lake said I must bring an Automobile and come get her at once and bring her to Hospital for operation." Martha phoned the owner of a local garage, who drove her to Silver Lake. "What a hard race with death," she commented. "I hope I never have to take another." Arriving at her aunt's house, Martha

found the poor, dear child suffering agony: we soon had her in the Automobile and Dr. Dudley too and began our terrible race— death kept close beside and it seemed at times, as if he *must* win. My heart bursting with grief, I held her close in my arms, across my body all the way, to make it easy, but she suffered terribly and when within four miles of Topeka, I saw the whiteness of death driving back the purple fever, I thought my heart would break. But at last we reached Stormont [Hospital], where everything was in readiness.

Twenty-seven years earlier, Martha had not learned of her sister's illness until it was too late; now she could receive immediate news of family illness by phone. The telephone also saved essential minutes in the crisis. Martha phoned both the garage owner and the hospital, allowing the staff to have "everything . . . in readiness." The transportation revolution enabled Freda to have emergency surgery in a hospital several miles away. But automobiles were still not commonplace; although physicians were among the earliest car owners,[55] the Silver Lake doctor apparently did not have one. Ambulances also were unavailable. Martha was thus compelled to hire a car in Topeka and travel to Silver Lake before the race to the hospital could begin.

When they reached the hospital, Martha watched the surgery and later gave a graphic description of the diseased organ: "I saw the appendix, a greatly enlarged, ulcerated and perforated rotten thing. Gangrene and also just a starting of peritonitis."

Appendectomy was a powerful symbol of medical prowess. Before the development of antiseptic techniques, surgery had been restricted to bodily extremities.[56] According to David Rosner, "The successful removal of the appendix was perhaps the most dramatic testament to the ability of surgeons to operate and prevent infections."[57] But once again the marvels of scientific medicine did not blind Martha to other forms of knowledge. Because Freda remained in danger, Martha again called in Mrs. Goddard, the Christian Science practitioner.

After waiting to see Freda "come out of Anaesthetic," Martha returned home to eat and do her work. "I needed a moment of rest," she explained, "for I was exhausted from the long ride in the cold and with heart breaking grief." She was back at the hospital by eight o'clock in the evening and stayed until almost ten o'clock. Returning to the hospital at half past eight the following morning, she "waited on Freda all day." Her report for February 7 was similar: "With Freda all day at Stormont Hospital. The Hospital is full, with only 16 nurses, so they neglect Freda's bathing and I had to make a kick." That evening Martha "went home by car as I was too tired to walk. I did not get to sit down five minutes during the day, but work over her constantly." On February 8 she wrote, "Another hard day at Stormont Hospital with

Freda. I've eaten nothing but cold lunch, and little of that, since Freda's operation." Because the snow had melted, the walk home in the evening was not "so hard," but Martha was "so very tired and worn."

Martha's account lends some support to the familiar argument that the transfer of medical care to institutions relieved family members of critical obligations. When nursing Johnny, Martha had sat up through the night to watch for troublesome symptoms. Now she could leave Freda in the hands of institutional staff and return home to sleep. Nurses also relieved her of responsibility for at least some aspects of personal care. Nevertheless, Martha's diary suggests that change may not have been as rapid or absolute as previous accounts claim. In her history of childbirth, Leavitt argues that when parturient women arrived at the hospital, they "found themselves abandoned to the impersonal routines of impersonal institutions."[58] But Martha not only tended Freda on the ward, she also accompanied Freda into the operating room and remained with her throughout the procedure.[59] It is true that Martha was an observer, not an assistant. Unlike previous generations of women, she had no responsibility for holding basins, supplying instruments, helping with sutures, or cleaning up afterward. And whereas women did not have to request permission to watch the surgery performed in their own kitchens, Martha's admission to the hospital operating room occurred at the discretion of doctors.[60] Nevertheless, her experience raises questions about the extent to which family members relinquished jurisdiction over hospital patients in the early decades of the twentieth century.

If hospitalization of a family member freed Martha from some tasks, it created others. For the first time, she was responsible for monitoring the work of paid caregivers. When the nurses' care fell short of her standards, she made a "kick." She also had to travel back and forth between home and hospital. Although she once returned home by car, she typically walked, often through snow. Because she could not intersperse caregiving with farm or household work, her chores accumulated. And hospital care was expensive. Although we can assume that Johnny received free care in 1890,[61] Freda was a private-pay patient. When Martha subsequently had reason to tally the various sacrifices she had made on Freda's behalf, paying the hospital bill occupied a prominent place on the list.

Martha's caregiving obligations were not confined to Freda. Martha's sister May and May's daughter Zaidee moved into Martha's house soon after Freda entered the hospital, and on February 22 Zaidee required assistance. "I went as usual to Stormont Hospital to take care of Freda," Martha reported,

> but at 1:30 P.M. was called home to help Zaidee thro' confinement . . . Well, I ran as much of way home, as I could thro' deep snow, and had to "get busy" at once, and the baby (a ten pound boy) came at 2:33 P.M. I got hold of the little fellow and pulled him away, let him lay 30 minutes, then cut the cord, rolled him in a blanket and laid him aside: not a soul but her mother and I with her. Dr. Jeffries was called, but did not arrive for one hour and two minutes after baby was born.

As long as birth remained at home, family members rather than hospital staff substituted when doctors were late.

Martha brought Freda home on February 25, three weeks after the surgery. During the early decades of the twentieth century, the length of the average hospital stay dropped sharply.[62] Although Freda's stay was long by present-day standards, it was much shorter than Johnny's seven-week hospitalization in 1890. Freda's discharge was a relief to Martha. "Another stormy day and it seems like Paradise, to be able to stay at home," she wrote on February 27. "I *am* resting; at least it seems like rest, to be at home." But she also noted that her hands were "more than full"; her house was "a Hospital," with "Freda in one room and Zaidee in another and neither one able to go in to see the other." Freda continued to require skilled nursing care; the day she left the hospital her wound still contained "pus," and Martha was responsible for applying dressings.

Martha could not have delegated any of this work to paid nurses. The first Kansas nursing schools were established in 1888.[63] The great majority of graduates worked as private-duty nurses, providing care to patients in individual households,[64] but hiring a nurse was not an option for Martha. In at least some parts of the country, credentialed nurses earned an annual wage of approximately $950,[65] and even the weekly or monthly equivalent would have been a sum far beyond the reach of the Farnsworths.

Martha's last major caregiving experience occurred in 1915. On November 14 she wrote, "My good Teddy [Fred] went to see Dr. Menninger this afternoon, about his heel and finds he has Erysipelas and badly—caused by bruise from hard walking with heavy load of mail." This time a doctor's office was the site for the delivery of routine health care, not just services requiring sophisticated equipment. Although Menninger still did not expect patients to make appointments, he increasingly saw them in his office rather than their homes.[66]

In other ways as well, Menninger's practice had changed fundamentally in the twenty-two years since he last had ministered to a member of Martha's family. As medicine had consolidated into a privileged and powerful profession between 1890 and 1915, Menninger gradually had incorporated the precepts of scientific medicine into his practice. His reputation grew.[67] In 1898 he gained both admitting privileges at Christ's Hospital and acceptance into the Shawnee County Medical Society. Two years later he was elected president of the society.[68] His private practice also flourished, and by the second decade of the twentieth century, he had become one of the most popular physicians in Topeka.[69] It must have been reassuring to Martha to be able to rely on a physician who commanded such respect among both his professional colleagues and the lay public. We will see, however, that although she regularly sought his assistance during Fred's long illness, she assumed that she alone made medical decisions.

Erysipelas—a bacterial infection called Saint Anthony's fire—was known to be a highly contagious disease in the early twentieth century,[70] but just as Martha had blamed her first husband's tuberculosis on his drinking, so now she viewed Fred's problem as an occupational injury. She may have been especially ready to do so because she had often complained about his working conditions, particularly the length of his working day and the weight of his load. Unfortunately, Martha's diary does not tell us whether she took special precautions to safeguard her own health.

With Fred still out of work on November 27 and no indication of when he could return, money became a source of concern. In one respect, however, the Farnsworths were better protected against sickness than most working-class families, for they had purchased an "Insurance and sick allowance Policy of $10.00 per week." Fred's illness also underscored the critical role Martha played in the household economy. "We are not starving," she wrote, "for we have the cow and chickens and a cellar full of fruit and vegetables."

On November 29 Fred's condition suddenly deteriorated. "Beautiful sunshine outdoors, but all darkness in our home," Martha wrote. "All last night and today *Death* has tried to come in and take my good Teddy: the struggle has been terrible and exhausting." (Menninger later explained that the cause of the problem was an embolism in the lungs.) Although Fred insisted he did not need a doctor, she "ran down stairs and phoned Dr. Menninger, who being out to Christ's Hospital, had not far to come and was here in about ten minutes." Technological progress had eliminated the onerous task of fetching the doctor, and the time it took a physician to reach the patient's home had drastically declined. In the early years of his career, Menninger had traveled around Topeka by a combination of streetcar, bicycle, and buggy.[71] After he purchased a car in 1910, however, at least some trips to the sick could be made in a matter of minutes.[72]

Concluding a "hurried examination," Menninger asked Martha to phone another doctor "to come at once." Although she "had trouble 'getting' Dr. Owen," she "finally succeeded." Martha also mobilized nonmedical forms of assistance. Just as birthing women in the nineteenth and early twentieth centuries frequently gathered female relatives and neighbors along with physicians, so Martha phoned her "good friend Mrs. A. E. Jones." She arrived shortly after the doctors and spent the night at the Farnsworth house. The following day Martha wrote, "Mrs. Jones will go home tonight and Mrs. Wilcox come up. Any way *some* one will stay in house with me, so I won't be alone."

It was still customary in the second decade of the twentieth century for serious illnesses to be treated at home.[73] Despite the proximity of Christ's Hospital, no one appears to have considered moving Fred there. One consequence was that the doctors relied on Martha, rather than on institutional staff, for assistance. She helped Menninger "give Teddy five 'Hyperdermics' in the veins" and wrapped him in clothes she had heated with irons to ward off chill.

On the evening of December 5, "a most agonizing attack came on." This time it was more difficult to summon help. Menninger had hired a receptionist to answer his telephone soon after establishing his own practice,[74] but as long as he continued to make house calls, there was no guarantee he could be located in an emergency. Failing to reach Menninger by phone, Martha "raised a window called at the top of my voice for help and blew a whistle." Although her neighbors appeared to be at home, they did not respond. Martha therefore "gave up and worked over Fred for a time, then tried again and got Mrs. Wilcox who stayed at Phone until she got the Doctor." When Menninger finally came, "he could do nothing, as he had given the limit of medicine." As he was about to depart, Fred suffered another attack. "For five hours, he walked thro' the 'Valley of the Shadow' and we did not know whether he would come back: it would have been easier to have seen him die then to sit by and see him in such agony and powerless to give him relief. At midnight he got easy, but at 3:30 A.M. he had another spell, which only lasted about an hour."

Martha's nursing responsibilities expanded as a result of this second crisis. On December 7 she noted that she "rubbed" Fred's leg and wrapped it in "hot Witch hazel woolens" every three hours and give him medicine "every hour day and night." Although Fred improved during the next two weeks, he suffered yet another setback on December 20. Menninger diagnosed phlebitis, instructing Martha to "go back to the hot witch-hazel pack every three hours." "Well I could almost give up in abject despair," she confessed to her diary. "Will complications *never* cease to set in? We thought Fred would soon be up and now this—one of the most tedious and slowest of *diseases:* it is dreadful."

During the long convalescence that followed, Menninger continued to call regularly at the Farnsworth house. But Martha welcomed advice from other sources as well. On January 10, 1916, she reported,

> Mrs. Calvin came over and spent the evening with us and gave me a new recipe for Fleabitus (milk leg) which Dr. Weston of Chicago gave her (and which cured her after having it for four years) and she helped me put it on Fred. "Put cabbage thro' a meat grinder, making it very fine and put on a cloth and bind on Varicose vein, with five yards of bandaging, at bed-time: next morning take off and sponge limb with good rich buttermilk and bind on fresh cabbage—use about ¼ cup of buttermilk—the milk may be used quite cold."

Leavitt argues that "the price of the new science was a growing separation between expert and layperson . . . The knowledge gap produced when medicine became increasingly technical put the uninformed in awe of medical science."[75] But not all therapies were technically sophisticated. Mrs. Calvin's treatment resembled the remedies contained in the domestic manuals circulating in the mid-nineteenth century; it relied on common household implements and food and was simple enough to be administered by family members. Although the treatment originated with a physician, it could be disseminated through lay networks.

Martha did not inform Menninger of the new therapy until five days after introducing it. "Dr. C. F. Menninger came out this morning and was fairly amazed, and greatly pleased, with Fred's improvement due to Cabbage poultice," she wrote on January 15. If Martha appreciated Menninger's stamp of approval, she felt enough confidence in her own judgment to disregard the modification he suggested. "He was thankful to know about the Cabbage treatment and said to continue its use: but he sees no merit in using the buttermilk—but as it is part of the treatment, we will continue *its* use also."

Although Fred's inability to work did not force Martha into the job market, she again faced competing demands. She could integrate her regular round of chores with her nursing responsibilities because care took place at home. On December 15, for example, she noted that she "took the usual care" of Fred, doing her weekly washing "between times." Her workload, however, may have been as grueling as when she nursed Johnny in 1893. Electricity and assorted household appliances had lightened her tasks, but she still lacked indoor plumbing. Bathing Fred and washing his bedding and clothes must have involved considerable drudgery. The bitter Kansas winter added to her difficulties. "A howling Blizzard—15° below zero, 43 mile wind from North West, blowing sleet and snow," Martha wrote on January 12, 1916. "But I was out early, and cleaned the barn, fed the cow and chickens, carried water and coal and kept everything 'snug and warm,' took care of my good Teddy and did my usual house work." Although snow fell the following day and the temperature dropped still lower, she still "did *all* the usual rush of work."

Martha's complaints also fastened on her lack of support. Friends who had initially rallied around them seemed to lose interest as Fred's illness lingered. "I stay alone with Fred, all the time now," she wrote on December 13. "My neighbors all got tired quick." As the holidays approached, the absence of visits was especially painful. "We seldom see anyone any more, but the Doctor—everybody calls by phone and it's the Holiday season and everybody *rushed*." She expressed even greater

bitterness on December 30: "We are all alone all the time now and being Holiday week, everyone so busy with his plans for the New Year, no
one comes in." During the blizzard in the middle of January, she wrote,
"Not a neighbor came in to see how we are 'making it,' these bad days."

We can interpret Martha's complaints in various ways. As we have
seen, Martha tended to dramatize slights and slurs. By accusing her
neighbors of neglect, she could again cast herself as a self-sacrificing
martyr, a role she had assumed frequently during her first marriage. It
also is possible that Martha gave mixed messages. Because she prized
her strength and self-sufficiency, she may have rebuffed offers of help
that she desperately wanted.

Martha believed that the telephone was at least partly responsible for
her plight. "All our Calls are by Phone and I almost wish I had no
phone," she wrote on December 30, 1915. Susan Strasser notes that
"telephone conversation . . . constitutes a wholly different kind of communication from face-to-face conversation, in which participants read
each other's faces, watch each other's hand gestures, and have an opportunity to really touch."[76] The telephone can weaken instrumental,
as well as emotional, aspects of support. When communication is restricted to phone calls, undone chores remain invisible, and friends
may be less likely to lend a hand.

The nature of Fred's disease may have been an additional factor. It
was one thing to respond to Martha's pleas for help during emergencies; it would have been a very different matter to provide sustained
support over a four-month period. As caregiving has focused increasingly on chronic ailments, it has become a much lonelier endeavor.

Finally, Martha may have based her expectations of support on the
patterns of mutuality she had observed as a child in rural Kansas.[77] By
1915 various factors, including geographic mobility and urbanization,
had weakened bonds of interdependence among many women. Like
other Kansas towns,[78] Topeka grew rapidly during the late nineteenth
and early twentieth centuries, making many of Martha's neighbors relative newcomers. She herself had led a peripatetic existence during her
first marriage, moving a total of six times. Her sister's departure in
1908 left her bereft of close relatives, and even her most loyal friend,
Mrs. Jones, moved away from Topeka shortly after Fred's recovery.
The laborsaving devices that eased Martha's daily burdens may have
further attenuated her support networks. Instead of coming together to

share household tasks, women increasingly performed their chores in isolation.[79] Although these changes affected women of all social classes, Martha's experience reminds us that the repercussions were especially serious for those with limited financial resources. Unable to hire servants or private-duty nurses, Martha remained dependent on community ties for support. When these proved tenuous, her responsibilities became overwhelming.

As Fred began to recover, Martha focused on her own health problems, which she attributed to the stresses of care. On February 7, 1916, she reported that her nerves were "trying to go to pieces," her sleep was erratic, and she found herself "dropping things." On the nineteenth she wrote, "My nerves are all *unstrung* today . . . I wish I could just let go of myself, and *scream*, and *scream*, and *scream*, and *scream*."

Fred's illness also imposed serious financial burdens. Although he did not require technical equipment, the services of specialists, or hospital care, his medical bill was sizable. In April Martha recorded that she paid Menninger $75 and the drug store $17. A recent study by Joel D. Howell and Catherine G. McLaughlin of the medical care purchased by selected urban working-class families in 1917 helps us evaluate that expense. When Fred worked regularly, his annual income was $1,392, which placed the Farnsworths exactly at the median of the families Howell and McLaughlin studied. The $17 drug store bill was only slightly higher than the average medicine expense for households that purchased medicine during the year. The doctor's bill, however, was double the mean physician expense of $37.77 for families in the study that had paid doctors.[80] Starr notes that income lost because of illness during the early twentieth century tended to be "two to four times greater than health care costs."[81] During Fred's four-month absence from work he forfeited a total of $580 in earnings. The combination of wage losses and medical costs was $672, but Fred received just $205 from the insurance company. After settling their outstanding grocery bill on April 4, Martha reported that they had "nothing left."

Martha defined her role as maintaining, as well as restoring, health, and Fred's working conditions remained a source of anxiety. On June 1, 1916, she wrote, "A very hot day and Fred had so large a mail, he could not come home to dinner. One of the 'Subs' helped him with three blocks of his heaviest mail this morning, telling him to 'keep it secret' or it would anger the other 'Subs' who had all agreed to stand together, against Fred—not to help in any way and so if he was not strong enough, he could not work, would lose his job, and they would get it." She was even angrier with Fred's employers, writing on December 31, 1918,

> Deep snow and heavy mails and my poor Teddy had to work all day with no time to stop to get anything to eat. His foot is very sore and the P.O. authorities won't let him off to take care of it. I wish it were possible to make the Postmaster and the various Superintendents work as the Carriers do—that there could be a law passed, compelling *them* to go out and wade the deep snow, the same long hours without food, with the heavy loads on their backs, sick and hurt or injured—what a lesson in mercy it would teach these Government *task masters.*

A woman who sought control over many aspects of her life, Martha remained powerless to reduce the hazards that threatened Fred at work.

Martha had experienced trouble with her eyes for many years, and in January 1920 doctors recommended surgery. The prospect terrified her. Recalling her previous experience with chloroform, she began to prepare for death; when the doctors subsequently advised against operating, her relief must have been enormous. On March 25 Martha again expressed her faith in alternative medical practices. "We went to Grace Cathedral this evening to hear James Moore Hickson who heals disease by 'laying on of hands,'" she wrote. "I *do not doubt* for a moment, that God uses him as a channel, to heal all who came in faith."

In December 1923 Martha began to complain of illness, and on February 2, 1924, she entered the hospital, where she died eleven days later of malignant hepatitis.[82]

⌒ IT HAS BECOME commonplace to note that the growth of social institutions such as schools, prisons, and hospitals removed important functions from the home. Martha's diary tells a different story. Her obligations, rather than disappearing, changed form. As Laura Balbo points out, the growth of a vast health and social service system increasingly has required numerous women to engage in "servicing work."[83] When Martha's niece entered the hospital, much of the time

Martha previously might have devoted to personal care now was spent mediating between Freda and formal health providers.

Many factors other than the expansion of the health care delivery system affected the amount and type of family responsibilities. The containment of infectious diseases meant that women spent less time ministering to seriously ill and dying infants. By the time of Martha's death in 1924, both malaria and typhoid fever had been virtually eliminated in Kansas, and the incidence of tuberculosis had declined. The early decades of the twentieth century also saw the decline of the climate theory, which had kept Martha on the move during her marriage to Johnny Shaw. But not all changes alleviated family care. Had tuberculosis struck Martha's household in the 1920s, public health measures directed against the disease might well have augmented her tasks. Moreover, as chronic diseases replaced infectious diseases as the major cause of death, responsibilities for care shifted to the latter part of the life course.

In addition, Martha never relinquished control over medical decision-making. Although she repudiated many traditional practices, she felt fully capable of assessing her doctors' competence and challenging their recommendations. Her encounter with some of the most dazzling advances of modern medicine failed to persuade her to surrender authority to physicians. We saw that new diagnostic techniques enabled doctors to position her as a passive object rather than a self-determining agent. But even after experiencing doctors' new power to see inside her body, she continued to trust her own knowledge and judgment. Nor did Menninger's growing eminence transform their relationship. While Martha relied on Menninger throughout Fred's illness in 1915, she also used other channels to acquire medical knowledge, and she made at least one important treatment decision without his approval.

Issues that tend to escape the purview of medical historians shaped the content and meaning of Martha's caregiving responsibilities. Her workload was partly determined by gender norms. Subscribing to prevailing notions of womanhood, Martha assumed that her duty to provide care transcended the particularities of her relationships. For four years she nursed Johnny Shaw, a man she described as abusive. Her self-abnegation contributed to her sense of moral ascendancy. During Martha's second marriage, a variety of new, mass-produced goods and services eased some of her household responsibilities. Telephones eliminated one task entirely. Here, too, the impact may have been complex and contradictory. Martha was convinced that the telephone weakened the support networks that had lightened the caregiving burdens of previous generations of women.

Martha's diary also highlights the slow and erratic pace of change. Many late-nineteenth-century features of caregiving remained intact well into the twentieth century. Because birthing women and seriously ill patients frequently remained at home, Martha continued to deliver skilled medical care. When surgery took place in a hospital, she accompanied the patient into the operating room and remained throughout the procedure. Although cars and telephones greatly facilitated access to formal health care providers, doctors continued to spend many hours on the road and, thus, were frequently unavailable in emergencies.

In addition, change occurred unevenly, affecting different groups of women in different ways. The weakening of the bonds of kinship and community inflicted the greatest hardship on women who could not rely on personal servants or private-duty nurses to replace the support networks of their mothers' day. The rising cost of health care similarly had the most serious impact on low-income women. Martha's bill of $117 in 1906 and Fred's bill of $92 in 1915 represented enormous outlays to a household getting by on $116 a month. Although Martha does not specify the amount she paid for Freda's hospital stay in 1913, she indicates that it imposed an excessive burden. And consumer goods and services reached Martha relatively late. She was still lugging pails of water inside to bathe Fred and wash his bedding and clothes long after more affluent women had gotten indoor plumbing.

The various changes that transformed the nature of Martha's caregiving work profoundly affected the experiences of many of her contemporaries as well. Subsequent chapters explore how caregivers in diverse social positions responded to the altered understandings of disease, the growing demands for servicing work, the gradual spread of domestic technologies, the development of new diagnostic and surgical techniques, and the vastly increased prominence of the medical profession.

~5

"Just as You Direct": Caregiver
Translations of Medical Authority

$\mathcal{T}$HE RISE of the formal health care system during the late
nineteenth and early twentieth centuries reduced the status of the care
family members delivered at home. This era enshrined the virtues
of rationality, objectivity, neutrality, and universality. Knowledge accorded the honorific title "science" received special veneration. Developments in medicine both contributed to the growing faith in science
and shared in its prestige. An accumulation of breakthroughs, including the isolation of the pathogens causing major infectious diseases and
the development of dramatic new diagnostic technologies, dazzled the
public.

Various health care providers gained social legitimacy by allying
themselves with these developments. Hospitals conformed surgical
procedures with discoveries about asepsis and installed X-ray machines
and clinical laboratories, which publicity photographs prominently displayed.[1] As the reputation of hospitals rose, growing numbers of physicians sought to affiliate with them, participate in their governance, and
fill their beds with patients. A nationwide survey conducted in 1909
found 4,359 hospitals with a total of 421,065 beds.[2]

Allopathic, or "regular," physicians capitalized on advances in laboratory science to assert their dominance over competing schools.[3] They
reorganized the American Medical Association by linking it more
closely with local and state medical societies; by 1910, over half of all

119

allopathic physicians had become members.[4] This newly reconstituted body then sought to limit access to the profession. In 1910, together with the Carnegie Foundation, it produced the Flexner Report, which called for a drastic reduction in the number of medical schools. Within the following decade, the number fell from 155 to 85.[5] As a result, entry into medicine was restricted to those who had completed a standardized university curriculum based on the principles of scientific medicine.[6]

Although nurses never achieved equal power or prestige, they, too, sought professional status by donning the mantle of science. The first nursing schools opened in 1873, and their numbers grew rapidly, reaching 1,600 by the outbreak of World War I.[7] As the number of graduates multiplied, nursing leaders increasingly defined their occupation in terms of technical skills and abstract knowledge.[8]

The various claims to scientific expertise were not always justified. Joel D. Howell's study suggests that the laboratories and X-ray machines pictured in hospital marketing literature sometimes remained unused.[9] Although the germ theory of disease dramatically increased public confidence in medical care, it initially had negligible effect on physicians' armamentarium.[10] Nursing schools dispensed little formal instruction, and the activities of many graduates were often hard to distinguish from those of noncredentialed nurses.[11] Nevertheless, doctors found that the rhetoric of science could bolster the reputation of the formal health care system, even when its real achievements lagged behind.

The idealization of scientific rationality made it easier to disparage women's traditional healing practices. I have noted that physicians had long engaged in power struggles not just with "irregular" practitioners but also with family caregivers, whom many doctors regarded as ignorant. We will see that doctors who identified with medical science had a stronger basis for belittling lay knowledge. Elite nurses, too, emphasized their superior training to distance themselves from family caregivers. Edna L. Foley, superintendent of the Visiting Nurse Association of Chicago, wrote,

> Perhaps patients alone appreciate the well-taught nurse and understand the many fine distinctions that fill the gap between her and the untaught. There are a good many women and some men

also, who, for love's sake, can give quite wonderful care to their own sick, especially when this care is given under the supervision of the best physicians and surgeons obtainable; but there are a great many more who, notwithstanding the fact that they put every bit of affection possible into their work, invariably do the wrong thing and harm the patient far more than they help him.[12]

In describing family caregivers as "untaught," Foley dismissed the informal transmission of knowledge and skills by which women for generations had learned to heal. According to another nursing leader, even the most competent family caregiver fell short of the ideal of science: "When I was a girl, nursing care was either considered a gift, like a good voice, or an occupation, like cooking. Every family had some member or friend who was always known as a 'born nurse' and whose help was called on in an emergency. In many cases, she certainly deserved her name, and the care she gave was much better than none at all, but it was anything but scientific."[13]

Formal health care providers increasingly denigrated the emotional aspects of care. Chapter 3 argued that nineteenth-century physicians viewed the emotional component of care from two competing perspectives. On the one hand, prevailing medical beliefs encouraged physicians to value personal relationships both to alleviate stress and as a source of knowledge. Assuming that disease arose from the interaction of people with their environments, doctors sought information about individual patients and the contexts of their lives. On the other hand, self-interest prompted many doctors to belittle the solicitude and comfort informal caregivers offered. Arguing that family and friends disturbed and alarmed patients, doctors sought to disperse bedside attendants and sickroom visitors. In addition, doctors differentiated themselves from informal caregivers by touting the superiority of universalistic, as opposed to particularistic, knowledge.

Attitudes toward emotion in popular culture encouraged physicians to discard the first view in the early twentieth century. As Jan Lewis and Peter N. Stearns write, that period witnessed "an emphasis on the management of emotions and an outpouring of prescriptive literature instructing Americans on how to control their emotions."[14] Discovery of the bacteriologic causes of specific diseases made it more acceptable for physicians to maintain distance from patients and treat them as indistinguishable. Biological reductionism rendered irrelevant the patient's emotional and moral state, interaction with providers, and physical surroundings.[15] The shift to offices and hospitals further increased the impersonality of care by preventing doctors from observing patients' homes and relationships.[16]

New therapeutic approaches stressed the importance of controlling patients' bodies and emotions. Chris Feudtner notes that Elliot Proctor Joslin, the foremost diabetes specialist from 1916 to the 1950s, believed that a "rigorous style of managing the diabetic life" represented the best care. "Even before insulin was first used in 1922, Joslin had believed in patient education and self-control." After the introduction of insulin, "he thought that disciplined diabetics could attain mastery over their disease."[17] An 1887 book titled *Anaemia* declared that "a complete control" of chlorosis patients "is essential."[18] We will see that tuberculosis specialists similarly counseled patients to regulate their lives and adhere closely to their doctors' orders.

This emphasis on control helped to devalue the attentiveness and responsiveness traditionally associated with family care. In the writings of turn-of-the-century physicians, nurses, and other health professionals, those traits existed only in exaggerated form. Sensitivity became indulgence and pampering. Family members demonstrated "excessive consideration" or "over kindness"; patients relying on family care were "spoiled" or "coddled too much."[19] "It can be put down as one of the advantages of a hospital," intoned an administrator in 1900, "that the relatives and friends do not take care of the patient . . . It is much better for [patients] not to be under the care of any one who is over-concerned for them."[20] The 1887 book on anemia quoted above argued that the "seclusion" of chlorotic girls was "of great importance, for by it an important obstacle to recovery is at once removed, to wit, the demoralizing sympathy of injudicious friends."[21] Leading authorities on tuberculosis advocated that patients be placed in sanatoriums, in part to enforce the discipline sufferers needed. Edward Otis, for example, wrote, "In some homes, the patient could never be controlled sufficiently to make the cure."[22]

Patients remaining at home were enjoined to place themselves under the control of credentialed nurses, if at all possible. As a sanatorium staff physician wrote in 1907, a trained nurse "is beyond price" for "a patient who insisted upon being treated in his own home—surrounded by a devoted family, always ready to help him break through prescribed lines."[23] We will see that private-duty nurses repeatedly complained about overly affectionate family members who undermined the therapeutic regime.

Nurses congratulated themselves on their emotional detachment from sickness and death as well as from individual patients. Chapter 2 demonstrated that popular nineteenth-century fiction encouraged women to use the sufferings of others to make sense of their own tragedies and prepare for future ones. But where nineteenth-century writers found opportunities for spiritual and emotional growth, twentieth-century nursing leaders saw only mental instability. Barbara Melosh notes that although the supervisors of student nurses "tacitly acknowledged students' emotions in the face of death," they "insisted on self-control. One nurse's memoir described her lonely watch with a young dying patient and her overwhelming emotion as the end approached. She resolved, 'I must steady myself. It will never do to go to pieces like this at the last moment.'"[24] A nursing student who later confessed that she "became totally unstrung" after a patient died also noted that she eventually learned to restrain her feelings of vulnerability.[25]

Physicians also praised nurses as a unique group of women who had learned to prevent passion from overwhelming their reason. John Brooks Wheeler, a University of Vermont professor of surgery, told the graduating class of the Mary Fletcher Hospital Training School for Nurses that the value of their education lay as much in the self-control they developed as in the technical knowledge they acquired. He gave the cautionary example of an uncredentialed nurse who "lost her head" when a patient began to hemorrhage. "The nurse snatched off the bedclothes, caught a glimpse of blood on the sheet, threw up both hands with a wild whoop and rushed yelling into the street." Wheeler concluded that "if she had been thoroughly trained, she would have become accustomed to such emergencies and, what is of much more importance than familiarity with any situation in particular, she would have been taught to practice self-control and not to go into hysterics when things suddenly look alarming."[26] The highest tribute Wheeler could confer was that nursing graduates had traveled far from untrained family caregivers.

The proliferation of nursing schools also weakened the link between women's informal craft and paid healing work. A family in Ann Arbor,

Michigan, provides a case in point. Like Sarah Gillespie and Martha Farnsworth, Emily Jane Green Hollister claimed competence as a nurse on the basis of her experience as a family caregiver. When an economic crisis compelled her to seek employment in 1887, a local doctor deemed her eminently qualified to work as a nurse because she had cared for her eleven children during various illnesses. "You are just the woman we want here," he stated and immediately sent her to nurse six children with typhoid fever.[27] She continued to receive cases regularly throughout her thirty-one-year career. But it was much harder to market domestic healing skills by the time Hollister's youngest daughter decided to become a nurse. She thus followed the new route into the field, graduating from the University of Michigan Training School for Nurses in 1903.[28]

Formal instruction also increasingly supplemented and replaced experience and apprenticeship in midwifery. In a study of four Wisconsin counties, Charlotte G. Borst found that by the early twentieth century, even women in the most isolated rural areas turned to birth attendants without formal training only when school-educated midwives were unavailable.[29] Midwifery changed in the South as a result of the Sheppard-Towner Act of 1921, which authorized funds for midwife training programs and empowered public health nurses to license qualified graduates.[30] The number of midwives fell during the 1920s from 6,000 to 4,339 in Virginia, and from 4,209 to 3,040 in Mississippi.[31] Although some lay midwives may have pursued their practices underground, others appear to have abandoned the occupation.[32]

The transition to physician-assisted birth further reduced the economic value of informal care. Throughout the nineteenth century, growing numbers of women had called on physicians for assistance during delivery. The pace of change accelerated at the turn of the century, as public health reformers, general practitioners, and obstetricians called for the elimination of midwives because of their "ignorance." That term, we have seen, had been applied to family caregivers throughout the nineteenth century. Numerous historians have pointed out that immigrants and women of color constituted the overwhelming majority of midwives by the early twentieth century and that the campaign against them encoded racial and ethnic biases.[33] It is less frequently noted that this campaign also transmitted powerful messages about the worth of healing skills acquired through practice and experience.

The changes I have outlined occurred slowly and unevenly across regions and populations. We will see that hospital care reached different groups at different times. Rosemary Stevens writes that doctors in 1918 "were a very mixed bag of individuals, ranging from eminent professors and highly paid city specialists (sometimes topflight experts, sometimes organized into affluent private groups which offered the latest fads to well-heeled patients) to poorly trained and marginally paid hacks, looking for all the practice they could get."[34] Many family caregivers thus interacted with physicians whose claims to scientific practice might be no greater than their own.

Nurses, too, remained a heterogeneous group for many years. Excluded from the new training schools, women of color continued to work as "professed" nurses.[35] White women without formal credentials found employment in the many white households that could not afford the high fees of nursing graduates.[36] And some trained nurses remained proud of their occupational roots in traditional family and neighborhood exchange, arguing that technical expertise should not eclipse personalized care.[37]

Data from various geographical areas demonstrate that female immigrants and women of color attended births well into the twentieth century. Although physicians supervised 90 percent of the deliveries of native-born white women in Waterbury, Connecticut, between 1913 and 1915, midwives assisted 70 percent of the confinements of Italian women. In rural Mississippi, midwives delivered 88 percent of African American babies, while doctors delivered 79 percent of white babies.[38] As late as 1936, midwives also presided at 95 percent of all births in San Miguel, a predominantly Hispanic county in New Mexico.[39] Despite the hostility of doctors and nurses, midwives who were immigrants or women of color earned recognition and respect from those they attended. Susan L. Smith notes that African American midwives in the South were, "along with teachers, the female counterparts to preachers as the most influential people in rural areas. They were at the center of traditional healing networks . . . and served as advisers and spiritual leaders."[40]

Just as the health care system changed slowly and erratically, so family caregivers responded in complex and contradictory ways to its growing power and prestige. Martha Farnsworth's diary suggests that women could simultaneously revere and reject medical authority. Martha considered herself deprived when she had to give birth without physician assistance, and she repeatedly spurned the advice of "grand-mothers." Nevertheless, she continued to draw on a range of therapeutic traditions when nursing her niece and second husband in the early twentieth century. Even after her physician became one of the most prominent members of the Topeka medical community, she made at least one major treatment decision without consulting him.

What factors encouraged other caregivers to relinquish control of medical decision-making or to continue to trust their own knowledge and skills? To begin to answer this question, I first examine professional advice on child rearing, which was an important early site for medical intervention. Such advice reached a broad population, advocated expert guidance on matters previously within women's domain, and gained legitimacy from its association with science. I then explore the interactions between family members of tuberculosis sufferers and a prominent physician who demanded strict obedience to his methods.

Advice for Mothers

Thousands of women wrote to the Children's Bureau in the early twentieth century. Many were responding to an outpouring of advice that reflected and reinforced physicians' claims of expertise on children's health care. Although correspondents often sought information about child rearing rather than care for the sick, their letters reveal both the reasons women submitted to medical authority and the complexity of women's relationships with individual doctors. Moreover, women who became accustomed to relying on physicians for routine child care may have been especially likely to defer to them when illness descended on their households.

Established in 1912 by Lillian Wald, founder of the Henry Street Settlement, and Florence Kelly, who had led the campaign against child labor, the Children's Bureau was expected to "investigate and report upon all matters pertaining to the welfare of children."[41] In its first two decades, it could point with pride to a number of notable achievements. It published several major studies of the causes of infant mortality, launched a drive for birth registration, helped to implement a federal child labor law, organized a series of national conferences on maternal and child health, participated in the movement to expand widows' and mothers' pensions, and spearheaded a successful campaign to pass the Sheppard-Towner Maternity and Infant Protection Act.[42]

The Bureau's unusual administrative style partly explains why mothers solicited its advice. Julia Lathrop, the first chief, was a former Hull House resident, and she brought the ideals of the settlement movement with her when she entered public life. She believed that the development of close personal relationships between members of different classes could promote social harmony.[43] Although the Bureau received a total of 125,000 letters in one year alone,[44] Lathrop and her staff replied to every correspondent with warmth and concern. Many women penned only a few short sentences requesting information, but others seem to have assumed that the Bureau was interested in the details of their lives and wrote extensively about themselves and their children.

Women also consulted the Bureau because it published *Prenatal Care* in 1913 and *Infant Care* in 1914.[45] Subsequent editions of both bulletins appeared every few years. The first 30,000 copies of *Prenatal Care* quickly sold out.[46] Almost 1.5 million copies of *Infant Care* were circulated between 1914 and 1921.[47] In 1929 the Bureau staff estimated that half of all infants in the United States had benefited from their child care advice.[48]

The Children's Bureau publications were part of a broad campaign to transform maternal practice. Advice manuals proliferated. Such mass-circulation magazines as *Good Housekeeping* and the *Ladies Home Journal* were filled with recommendations about feeding and disciplining infants and children. National women's organizations, such as the National Congress of Mothers (later the Parent-Teacher Association), the Child Study Association of America, and the American Association of University Women, helped to make maternal education an issue of national concern.[49] Social workers and public health nurses spread the new information to poor mothers in tenements, settlement houses, milk stations, and clinics. Home demonstration agents carried it to rural communities. And secondary school and college teachers instructed young women in home economics classes. Although advice literature for mothers had long been available, it had never before reached such a broad segment of the population or been presented in such a standardized format.[50]

The explosion of maternal advice stemmed from various factors, including the growing faith in professional expertise of all kinds, the emphasis on Americanization, the rise of the home economics movement, and perhaps most important, pediatricians' professional project. Pedi-

atrics emerged as a distinct medical specialty in the late nineteenth century. Lacking a particular body part over which to claim jurisdiction,
pediatricians asserted authority over child welfare and development.[51]
Pediatricians wrote many of the popular new advice books on child
rearing, and even lay writers emphasized that they were popularizing
the theories of leading pediatricians.[52] Andrew Abbott notes that advice
columns are "familiar vectors" of professional claims: "By revealing to
the public some of its professional terminology and insights, a profession attracts public sympathy to its own definition of tasks and its own
approach to solving them."[53] The advice industry also helped to create
demand for pediatric services by telling women to disregard the advice
of other mothers and rely entirely on medical experts, not just for
treatment of physical ailments but also for guidance on routine aspects
of child care.[54]

I have noted that turn-of-the-century medical practitioners frequently couched their activities in the language of science, even when
they had little justification for doing so. Advice givers similarly described themselves as promoting "scientific motherhood," despite the
absence of studies to support many of their recommendations.[55] The
precision of the advice also lent it authority. Writers specified the exact
amounts of milk required by babies of different ages and the intervals
that should elapse between feedings.[56] According to *Infant Care*, bottle-
fed babies should receive milk from Holstein cows; Jersey or Guernsey
cows would not do. The temperature of an infant's room should be
sixty-five degrees. Colicky babies should be bathed in hundred-degree
water. A soda bath should have two tablespoons of soda for each gallon
of water.[57] Early-twentieth-century advice givers left no room for individual judgment because they assumed that uniform standards were ap-
plicable to all infants; mothers' empathic knowledge about individual
children was thus irrelevant.[58]

Experts also denigrated the intimacy that might form the basis for
such knowledge. John Broadus Watson, whose theories underlay the
editions of *Infant Care* published in the 1920s and 1930s, titled a chapter of his book "The Dangers of Too Much Mother Love."[59] Just as
physicians, nurses, and social workers criticized caregivers as "over-
concerned," so experts reproved mothers and grandmothers for being
"doting," "over-solicitous," and "blindly fond."[60]

Because maternal affection resulted in irrational actions, these experts claimed, it caused mothers to inflict various types of harm. Those who refrained from curbing infants' "strong and dangerous impulses" produced little tyrants.[61] Rocking, cuddling, playing with, or singing to infants overstimulated them.[62] Dr. Isaac Apt, later the first president of the American Academy of Pediatrics, wrote in 1923, "Infants and young children suffer from the attention showered on them by the parents, numerous friends and relatives. They are picked up, hugged, kissed, caressed, shouted at, sung to and exhibited to friends and neighbors by unthinking parents until the babies show symptoms of nervous exhaustion."[63] The nineteenth-century advice literature for mothers had similarly exhorted them to follow reason rather than emotion.[64] What was new was the mass dissemination of this message and the eager reception it received from women.

Alison M. Jaggar writes, "If childrearing is a science, it is one that changes with extraordinary rapidity."[65] As early as the 1930s, Freudian psychology had begun to influence American experts, and a few stressed the need to foster children's growth and development rather than to control their physical and emotional impulses. Flexibility replaced rigidity as the sign of the good mother. As the new ideas spread, references to "inferiority complexes" began to appear in letters to the Children's Bureau. But psychoanalytic concepts influenced only a minority of mothers in the period we are examining.[66] I therefore emphasize the attitudes of those mothers who sought to apply the tenets of scientific mothering, not those who subscribed to the newer, more child-centered doctrines.

This section examines the letters that women wrote to the Bureau between 1914 and 1936.[67] The letter writers came from groups that tend to be especially receptive to expert advice. Although the correspondents included mothers from a wide variety of backgrounds, native-born white women predominated. According to Robyn Muncy, African American, American Indian, and European immigrant women frequently expressed contempt for authority derived from formal education rather than personal experience.[68] The new advice was also foreign to the white southern tenant farmers Margaret Jarman Hagood studied in the 1930s. "In terms of conventional standards of habit formation an evaluation of the infant's raising is low," Hagood reported.[69] Such women also relied on traditional home remedies and patent medicines when children fell ill.[70]

Almost by definition, the correspondents accepted the legitimacy of professional expertise. Many had read not just *Infant Care* but also the advice columns of the popular women's magazines; some noted that they had enrolled in special courses on scientific mothering to perfect their skills. Women's networks also helped to spread the advice. Some letter writers requested new copies of *Infant Care* to replace the ones they had passed on to friends; others provided lists of names of new mothers to whom the agency should send its publications; and still others noted that they were writing on the recommendation of neighbors or kin.

The letter writers revealed their faith in the advice literature in various ways. Mother after mother claimed to comply with the new rules about feeding, sleep, fresh air, discipline, and training. "I follow the government schedule on page 75 of 'Infant Care,' feeding him milk, oatmeal water and boiled water and sugar," wrote the mother of a five-month-old in 1926.[71] Other women boasted that they followed the new advice "conscientiously," "religiously," and "minutely." Even the most mundane aspects of child care elicited questions. How long should cereal be cooked? Which shoes were best for toddlers? A Maine woman asked in 1915, "On page 42 you speak of Barley Flour to be given in water and cooked 20 minutes and added to the milk. Now do you mean 'Robinsons Barley' bought at drug store?"[72]

Women ascribed considerable power to the new methods. "I thank you very much for sending me the pamphlet on 'Infant Care,'" wrote a Nebraska woman in 1915. "It seems to me if a baby were taken care of according to your instructions in 'Infant Care' it would surely be a normal child."[73] Others offered their own experience as proof that the methods worked. A woman who had relied on the government publication for help with a premature infant asserted, "Now I have a splendid baby with a great sense of humor."[74] An Illinois woman declared that because her baby "has been raised absolutely on schedule," he was "very little trouble."[75] Comparison with the offspring of less well informed mothers often reinforced the writers' faith in the superiority of the advice they followed.

Women who were dissatisfied with their children's progress sought to modify their scientific child rearing techniques rather than abandon them entirely. Ignoring the multiplicity of forces affecting children's development, one Ohio mother asserted in 1916, "Our first baby (now

6 years) was brought up exactly by Dr. Holt's book, and while fairly well she is far from strong, and I am determined to try another method with our second baby."[76]

The language the women used also revealed the influence of expert advice.[77] Many women writing to the Children's Bureau before 1920 described health problems in extremely vague terms. They spoke of their children as "sickly," "puny," "poor," "run down," or "falling away," or noted that the children needed "beefing up" or "starching up." Such terms rarely appeared in letters written in the 1920s and 1930s. By that time, of course, many more diseases, such as diabetes, asthma, and allergies, had been identified.[78] But the changing language of the letters also may indicate growing acceptance of a basic assumption of modern medicine, that ill health results from specific disease pathogens and processes rather than expressing a general disequilibrium.[79]

Women adopted other types of rhetoric from the advice literature as well. Advice givers exhorted mothers to produce offspring who conformed to certain specifications. "My baby is a No. 1 Baby by physician's records," boasted a mother in 1930.[80] Others described their offspring as "splendid" or as "perfect specimens." Women also described their own behavior in the language of the literature. They aspired to act "intelligently" and to fulfill all the prescribed "scientific and hygienic duties."

We can explain in several ways why mothers embraced the new advice. Some letter writers confessed that they felt ill equipped for motherhood. "I am so ignorant about babies," wrote a woman in 1931.[81] Many approached maternal tasks with trepidation because they were young and inexperienced. Isolation often intensified insecurity. Although some women obtained the new literature from other mothers, several letter writers explained their need for professional advice by noting that they were living among "strangers." The popular advice literature may also have shaped attitudes. By dismissing folk remedies and experiential knowledge, the manuals may have undermined women's faith in their own judgment.[82] And by urging mothers to spurn the advice of neighbors and friends, experts may have increased women's sense of isolation.

In addition, the advice literature addressed some of women's deepest fears. Although the infant mortality rate began to decline at the turn of the century, it remained alarmingly high for several years. Between 1915 and 1919, nearly one-tenth of all babies died before their first birthdays.[83] Letter writers before the mid-1920s often stated that death had struck their nurseries; several had buried more than one child. The loss of a child made the surviving ones seem especially precious. A woman who wanted to help her sister "give more nurse" for her baby explained her concern this way: "I lost my baby the day it was 6 weeks old and hers must be spared to us all if possible."[84]

To women who had experienced the death of a child, the illnesses of subsequent offspring were especially terrifying. A woman whose first child died at the age of ten months wrote about a second ailing infant, "The fear that this baby will continually get worse haunts me day and night. So in sheer desperation I've written this."[85] Many women who had not themselves lost children surely knew others who had; many also must have witnessed the death of siblings in childhood.

The drop in death rates may have encouraged mothers to embrace scientific mothering during the second half of the period we are examining. As Julia Grant writes, "Falling infant mortality rates both promised that science could lead to recognizable improvements in children's behavior and provided middle-class women with additional time and energy to concern themselves with their children's psychic well-being."[86]

The new advice not only reduced women's feelings of helplessness in the face of dread diseases but also enhanced their personal sense of mastery. Just as many nineteenth-century women derived satisfaction in honing healing skills, so also many correspondents to the Children's Bureau expressed pride in their ability to adhere to the new rules about child rearing. Contrary to the belief that women's reliance on expert advice increased their subordination,[87] the letter writers presented themselves as eager pupils developing new competencies, not as workers who had been robbed of a skilled heritage.

If the advice literature gave women new confidence in their abilities, however, it also instilled new anxieties. "Life was simpler for mother," stated a Middletown woman interviewed by the Lynds in the 1920s. "In those days one did not realize there was so much to be known about the care of children. I realize that I ought to be half a dozen experts, but I am afraid of making mistakes and usually do not know where to go for advice."[88] Women who consulted the Children's Bureau expressed similar concerns. One, for example, wrote, "I am very ignorant concerning the rearing of babies and although I am nursing him quite successfully so far I feel that there are so many things I do not know that I might unknowingly do many things which might have bad effects on our baby."[89]

Because advice manuals decreed that there were critical periods for children's emotional and physical development, even minor errors were believed to have lasting consequences. A woman who had been "absolutely unsuccessful" in her attempts to make a thirteen-month-old infant drink from a cup asked, "What are the dangerous results that might attend his using a bottle after fourteen months?"[90] Several women worried that they already had caused "irreparable harm." The distribution of standardized charts for height and weight bred fears that children were deviating from the norm. Some letter writers sought reassurance that their offspring were developing appropriately; after providing information about children's measurements, they asked the Bureau staff to tell them whether the children were "normal" or "right." The new worries the child care manuals produced could be alleviated only by strict obedience to the precepts of professional advice givers. Nineteenth-century caregivers had relied extensively on the advice of their elders, but now mothers, as well as doctors, wrote contemptuously about "old ladies" who knew nothing about the fears besetting young mothers and therefore had little to offer.

Nevertheless, the letter writers did not accept without question all the advice bestowed on them. Some acknowledged being torn between old and new. One woman described her conflict this way: "As people advise me this and that, [I] don't know who to listen to."[91] Another wrote, "I have a little boy one year and nine months old, and some people insist on giving him cake, pie, cookies, doughnuts, etc. in spite of my objections. They have even said he could have pickles . . . I was shocked beyond measure when after my baby swallowed a prune seed, a lady said, 'It wont hurt him, it's good for him, the rough surface will hold particles etc.'" The letter concluded, "I am trying to raise my baby to a strong healthy boy, but it is hard to always know the right thing when older people say such things as I have mentioned."[92] Others asked the Children's Bureau staff to evaluate recommendations from friends and relatives. Was it safe to give a baby calomel? castoria? wormseed tea? Could "black gum powder" cure children's eye problems? Would ripe bananas help cure a child's eczema? Should mothers refrain from cutting babies' fingernails before the first year? Just as Martha Farnsworth used a neighbor's cabbage remedy even while relying on her physician, so these mothers retained at least some faith in the treatments recommended by other women. Although the letter writers subjected such suggestions to expert scrutiny, they seemed reluctant to reject them completely.

Several women appeared to be unaware of the contradictions in their beliefs. Although they expressed a determination to abide by expert advice, they also mentioned the patent medicines they administered or the folk remedies they employed.[93] And a few women looked to the Children's Bureau as a source of traditional lore rather than scientific medical advice. A woman in 1935, for example, requested directions for making a tonic from beets.[94]

Women's attitudes toward individual doctors further demonstrate the limits of medicalization. Although it is commonly assumed that confidence in medical expertise translates directly into faith in doctors, many correspondents who fully embraced the tenets of scientific medicine distrusted the doctors they saw. The Bureau continually exhorted women to have confidence in their physicians; suspicion of the medical profession, however, was a key reason for writing to the government. Women asked the agency staff to pass judgment on the advice physicians dispensed, provide information that doctors had withheld, and listen to a long list of complaints. Many had taken their children to several doctors before turning to the Children's Bureau in despair. A typical comment read, "I have carried him to several doctors and they dont seem to help him much."[95]

Two caveats are necessary. First, as already noted, the medical profession was of mixed quality in the period we are examining. The proportion of specialists grew rapidly during the 1920s and 1930s,[96] but both geographical distance and inadequate income prevented some women from obtaining their services. Second, dissatisfied women may well have been overrepresented among the letter writers; mothers who were pleased with the care their children received had little reason to solicit additional advice. If we must be cautious about generalizing from this group of women, however, their correspondence does reveal the expectations women had of doctors at the time.

One common criticism was that doctors dismissed children's problems as trivial. A woman concerned about her four offspring wrote in

1933, "I think you will tell me to see a Doctor I have, and he never gave me any satasfactory remedy. He didn't seem to think it was any thing serious."[97] Other letters accused physicians of ignoring such varied problems as sties, nightmares, decaying teeth, bowed legs, asthma, bad breath, diarrhea, and masturbation.

Another recurrent complaint was that doctors provided insufficient information. Advice manuals had convinced mothers of the need to consult doctors about even the most mundane aspects of children's upbringing, but women found their providers ill equipped to handle many requests. "I can't seem to get any satisfaction by asking physicians so will write to you," wrote a California woman in 1918. She wanted "to know if Fletcher's Castoria, which is so widely advertised is advisable, and if the so-called pacifiers injure babies mouth or throat."[98] A Texas mother beseeched the Bureau in 1920, "Please read this letter through as it means so much to me." Her physician was "supposed to be an excellent baby specialist," but he "did not give me any advice at all" about infant feeding.[99]

When doctors rendered advice, it could conflict with the recommendations of other authorities. "I notice in your book on 'Infant Care' that the baby's eyes should not be exposed to the sun," wrote a New York mother in 1927. "My doctor has told me to place the carriage in the sun with the hood *down* and let the sun get at his face."[100] Eight months later she wrote again: "I notice in your book on 'Infant Care' on page 40 you describe bananas as being an unsuitable food for a young baby. I have one fifteen months old and his baby doctor has prescribed *that* fruit as part of his diet."[101]

And doctors disagreed among themselves. Mothers reported receiving conflicting advice about applying boric acid to a baby's infected eyes, placing a truss on a three-month-old with a rupture, giving a baby Eagle Brand milk, rubbing the legs of a girl with infantile paralysis, removing adenoids and tonsils, performing circumcisions, taking a two-year-old with sinus trouble to a new climate, and inoculating children against diphtheria and whooping cough. Although some women looked to the Children's Bureau to resolve controversies, others insisted that the final decision rested with themselves. As a Montana woman noted in 1923, contention among experts undermined their authority. "When authorities and experts disagree to such an extent, how can a mother have confidence in them?" she asked rhetorically.[102]

Women challenged their doctors' competence for other reasons as well. Rather than simply deferring to expertise, many letter writers assumed responsibility for evaluating the advice they received. But some medical pronouncements appeared to violate common sense. One mother explained why she could not accept her doctor's assertion that a neighborhood dog was responsible for her daughter's pinworms: "As I have been keeping her away entirely from my friend's dog that had worms the infection must be coming from some other direction."[103] Others used their own knowledge of the new methods to challenge doctors. Thus, a mother in 1921 criticized the various practitioners she had consulted this way: "They don't believe in [feeding at] regular intervals, and, believe me, thats what I insist on most firmly."[104] Mothers also complained about "old fashioned" doctors who knew nothing about the significance of eyedrops for newborn babies or cod-liver oil for growing children.

Women who refrained from criticizing their children's medical care occasionally revealed distrust of the medical profession by asking the Children's Bureau to evaluate recommended treatments. "Could you tell me whether or not it is advisable to correct bow-legs in a baby by putting them in a cast," inquired the mother of a sixteen-month-old girl in 1929. "I took the baby to a physician and he suggested putting them in a cast."[105]

Recommendations for surgery provoked the greatest unease. Over one-fourth (27.5 percent) of all hospital admissions between 1929 and 1931 were for tonsillectomies or adenoidectomies, many of them performed on children.[106] Rosemary Stevens writes that surgery was one of the two fields that "paid doctors best and produced the most dramatic results and the most grateful patients: a child whose throat was no longer swollen from inflamed tonsils; an appendicitis victim brought back from expected death; a patient with a mended bone; a healthy mother with a new baby. Patients were happy to pay for the privilege."[107] But the women who wrote to the Children's Bureau were well aware that all operations posed risks, and few willingly entrusted their children to surgeons. Several consulted the Bureau in the hope that the staff would be able to suggest nonsurgical alternatives for their children's maladies.[108]

Obtaining adequate information was particularly important when surgery loomed. One woman was weighing a recommendation for an adenoidectomy for a nine-year-old girl. "I am trying to get all the information I can Maybe that will help to decide," she wrote.[109] It has become common to state that the growing complexity of medical care during this period meant that women lost access to healing knowledge and surrendered authority to physicians. But the letters suggest that some women sought the information they needed to participate in medical decisions. When doctors failed to provide such information, mothers looked for it elsewhere.

Completed operations did not necessarily restore trust. One mother gave this account of her seven-year-old daughter's progress: "Over a year ago we had her tonsils and adenoids taken out, but I can't see that she has been any better since the operation. We are always so distressed to find she rattles and seems to smother so when she has the slightest cold."[110] Others charged that surgery aggravated their children's problems. Although successful surgeries could bolster confidence in physicians' authority, the comments of some women remind us that the new therapeutics were not invariably effective and that poor outcomes could shatter illusions about the capabilities of the medical profession.

Not surprisingly, bereaved mothers had the most serious complaints. Several blamed physicians for their losses. One wrote, "My baby was sacrificed thru mere ignorance. This happened in the capital of Illinois . . . I soon found that not only mothers of large families knew nothing about the scientific care of babies, but the best Doctors in the city knew less."[111]

Although many women faulted doctors for making serious mistakes, some blamed doctors for failing to resolve irremediable problems— leukemia, the sequelae of polio and encephalitis, "bad temper" in a two-year-old girl, and even pimples on a teenager. Believing that science had promised them perfect children, some mothers were angry when told that doctors could not remove such blemishes as birthmarks or freckles. In other ways as well, many women measured physicians against an impossible ideal. They expected the doctors they consulted to be as detached and objective as the science the professionals claimed to represent; these women were shocked and dismayed when their doctors proved to be ordinary humans with their own needs, interests, and desires.

Although medicine succeeded in transforming itself into a high-status profession by identifying with science, the process of establishing dominance over individual clients may have been far more complex and contradictory than previously assumed. The prestige of science could undermine a doctor's standing with patients as well as bolster it. Many women who wrote to the Children's Bureau had an image of medicine that was too exalted for any individual to fulfill. Some turned to the Bureau for advice because they considered it an invisible, anonymous voice of the authority they sought. Thus, one mother stated that she was reluctant to place her two-year-old son "at the mercy of some specialist" until she had received "sound, impersonal information" from the government.[112] Another asked the Bureau for "unbiased advice."[113]

Other comments suggest that women brought the habits of consumers to medical encounters. One, for example, wrote in 1935, "It seems when you take a child to a doctor they give you no satisfaction. I know now he had worms . . . but doctor said he was all well."[114] A father whose four-year-old child suffered from chronic intestinal trouble wrote in 1921, "I would appreciate very much if you could advise me what to do towards helping this poor childs condition as I am terribly disgusted with the way these physicians have treated this case, after spending every dollar I possessed for their services and obtained no results."[115]

The culture of consumerism flourished in the 1920s as large manufacturers hired advertising agencies to stimulate demand for their products.[116] Stevens writes, "As hospitals assimilated their image to the consumer-oriented society of the 1920s, they engaged in increasingly sophisticated marketing techniques, including offering lines of credit that enabled Americans to purchase surgical operations or supervised deliveries as easily as they purchased dishwashers, refrigerators, or automobiles."[117] Such inducements implied that medicine was a consumer good like any other. The ethic of professionalism assumes that professionals alone have the power to judge quality.[118] As consumers, however, correspondents to the Children's Bureau insisted that they retained the right to determine whether they had received their money's worth.

If women's extravagant faith in scientific medicine caused them to look more critically at individual practitioners, however, their skepticism of particular doctors did not disabuse them of the notion that modern medicine had miraculous powers. Women who were dissatisfied with their children's medical care frequently asked the Bureau to recommend "the best doctor" in the field. Assuming that medicine had a cure for every affliction, they attributed poor outcomes to the personal inadequacies of their physicians rather than to the limitations inherent in a field they were determined to trust. Like other forms of belief, such as religion, magic, and law, medicine remained impervious to falsification.

Advice for Families of Tuberculosis Sufferers

Advice about the care of tuberculosis patients also changed dramatically in the early twentieth century. In the 1890s, Martha and Johnny Shaw had twice moved west in search of the climate that was believed to facilitate a cure. They also exercised considerable discretion over Johnny's treatment. Although they consulted a physician as soon as they suspected tuberculosis, they felt free to disregard his principal recommendation for several months. Martha never mentioned a doctor's visit during the long periods she and Johnny lived in the West. Even when he lay dying in Topeka in 1893, Martha nursed him without professional supervision. During the first decades of the new century, however, many physicians lost faith in the climate theory. At the same time, increasing numbers of physicians began to follow Peter Dettweiler, a German physician, whose ideas were introduced to Americans by Paul Kretzchmar. "The smallest details of the patient's life," Kretzchmar wrote, should be "controlled by the supervising physician and nothing of any importance . . . left to his or her judgment."[119]

In this section I explore the ways in which such attitudes altered the relationship between caregivers and physicians. I examine 114 letters from family members of tuberculosis patients to Dr. Lawrence F. Flick between 1906 and 1925.[120] A Philadelphia physician who had himself suffered from the disease in the early 1880s, Flick not only treated large numbers of private patients but also played a leading role in the early-twentieth-century tuberculosis control movement. His accomplishments included the establishment of the Pennsylvania Society for the Prevention of Tuberculosis, the Henry Phipps Institute for research on the disease, two nursing schools for tubercular women, and the White Haven Sanatorium, the first tuberculosis sanatorium in the state.[121] Whereas many women writing to the Children's Bureau complained about "old fashioned" doctors who were ignorant about scientific methods, family members consulting Flick could draw comfort from his stature as a major authority in the field. But just as Martha Farnsworth kept some distance from Dr. Menninger despite his growing prominence, so some of Flick's correspondents felt free to challenge his judgment.

Fresh air, rest, moderate exercise, and proper diet constituted the core of Flick's therapy. He recommended that patients have one large meal a day, at least six quarts of milk, and six raw eggs. In addition, Flick instructed patients to rub an oily form of iodine "into the armpits and into the inside of the thighs once or twice a day" and take creosote in hot water before each meal.[122] Flick also prescribed various tonics containing strychnine, arsenic, phosphorus, and iron. When the disease affected the lungs, Flick recommended fly blisters (irritants derived from beetles), plasters, and dry cupping.[123]

Flick's advice owed little to the recent bacteriological revolution. Although Koch's discovery of the tubercle bacillus in 1882 galvanized the world, it had few practical applications. Lacking a vaccine or cure, Flick, like other physicians, continued to rely on remedies that had been current long before Koch's announcement. Since the 1830s, popular health reformers had advocated diet, fresh air, and exercise to build resistance. Blisters and cupping also had been fashionable in the early nineteenth century. Despite Flick's disdain for the expertise his patients and their caregivers claimed on the basis of personal experience, his dietary instructions derived from measures he believed had proved successful in his own case.[124] Physicians now conclude that most of the activities and foods Flick recommended were totally ineffective and that a few, such as the consumption of large quantities of eggs and milk and the ingestion of various tonics, probably harmed some patients.[125]

But any doubts Flick may have harbored about his therapeutic regime did not appear in his writing. He continually asserted that obedience to his methods would result in a cure. Reports of reversals did not shake his confidence. He dismissed some patients' setbacks as unimportant and blamed noncompliance for others, which he said would abate as soon as behavior changed. Only when death seemed imminent did Flick acknowledge the possibility of therapeutic failure.

Flick's message had important implications for caregivers. By continually fostering expectations of recovery, he undercut the spiritual dimension of their work. Pat Jalland notes that in nineteenth-century Britain, tuberculosis was "idealized . . . as a blessing in disguise which allowed time and mental clarity for spiritual reflection and improvement."[126] In the United States, as we have seen, caregivers throughout the second half of the nineteenth century took advantage of the long period of decline from the disease to help sufferers purify their souls. Flick's program, however, provided little opportunity for spiritual preparation.

Other features of Flick's message transformed the emotional component of care. Instead of catering to patients' wishes, family members were supposed to monitor their behavior. The task of enforcing the diet must have been especially onerous. In the 1880s, Sarah Gillespie had been able to view herself as providing the best possible care by supplying the oysters her dying mother craved. But under Flick's regime, fulfilling an invalid's gustatory desires was a fault rather than a virtue.

The focus on regulation and control also strengthened arguments for the superiority of formal care over informal. Like other leading authorities on tuberculosis, Flick advocated institutionalization to enforce the discipline sufferers needed.[127] Nurses supervising Flick's patients often complained about interfering family members. One wrote to Flick that the patient's wife "has annoyed me greatly for the last month because there is no sick room rule here . . . You have supported me in saying Mr. M. must have rest and quiet. But frequently Mrs. M. insists on my leaving the room 'as she knows very well how to care for him.' When I return I find that she is either in his bed, or demonstrating her affections, and expressing pity for him, so that he would unconsciously derive some bad effects from it in his present condition."[128] That nurse stressed her "duty" to "not yield to the authority of a patient's relatives or their kindness."

In another case, a mother was faulted for undermining professional authority. The nurse had instructed an eighteen-year-old boy to sleep in a shack behind his house. "His mamma," the nurse reported, "is very nervous and afraid it might be too damp out in the shack, and she is afraid of the wind blowing on him, and if he is left out in the shack when we go to bed she is most likely to have him back in his bed-room by morning."[129] In a letter to the father, Flick asserted not only that the boy must "not be permitted to judge what is best for him either in the way of exercise, diet, or medical treatment," but also that "these things must not be under the control or subject to the wishes of those who are tied to him closely by bonds of relationship." The boy "should be subject entirely to the directions of his physician in every detail under a competent nurse and no one else should have any voice in the interpretation and execution of the physician's directions."[130] Far from being a source of comfort to the sick, family solicitude and devotion were represented as dangerous laxity hindering the fight for recovery.

A primary reason family members wrote to Flick was to seek his reassurance that patients would recover. In addition, many letter writers were either responding to his request for regular reports or consulting him about the treatment administered at home. Correspondents whose relatives resided in a sanatorium typically sought patient information. Some wanted to alert Flick to the need for special considerations. A few sought to hasten discharge.

Most letter writers presented themselves and the patients as adhering closely to instructions. A woman nursing her niece assured Flick that "no one has adhered to your treatment more strictly than she has to the letter."[131] A husband wrote, "You can feel assured that your prescribed treatment will be carried out to the smallest detail."[132] Many other correspondents insisted that they were complying with advice "faithfully" or "just as you direct." Such expressions of fealty may have been part of the price paid for relying on Flick's expertise. We will see that he threatened to dismiss any patients or family members who betrayed the slightest doubts about his regime. An important caregiving responsibility, therefore, was to frame acceptable portraits of the patients and their families.

But even if correspondents occasionally exaggerated their loyalty to ensure Flick's goodwill, there is no reason to doubt their acceptance of his methods. Several letter writers had made enormous sacrifices to comply with Flick's directives, reorganizing their households, spending a great deal of money, and enduring lengthy separations from loved ones. Correspondents caring for family members at home often wanted to observe Flick's treatment plan punctiliously and plied him with questions about the minutiae of his instructions. Could patients occasionally have poultry or oysters with their one large meal? Could they take a spoonful of whiskey with a pint of milk? Could cream substitute for milk, and if so, how much? Was it permissible to sprinkle cinnamon on raw eggs to mask their taste? Could patients ever eat candy? When patients left their beds, could they engage in exercise, or must they sit quietly? How much oil should be rubbed under the armpits? Correspondents also relinquished major life decisions over such matters as schooling, work, and travel to Flick. A few expressed a sense of betrayal when rigorous adherence to Flick's instructions failed to result in a cure.

The widespread faith in medical science in the early twentieth century can partially explain correspondents' subservience to Flick's dictates. Although Koch's discovery had few practical applications, it had greatly enhanced medicine's prestige, especially in controlling tuberculosis. The precision and certitude of Flick's advice further endowed it with a nimbus of scientific authority. Just as maternal advisers specified the exact times of infant feedings, so Flick told one man that his wife should take one pint of milk at 6:00 A.M., another at 7:00 A.M., and the third at 8:00 A.M.[133]

Caregivers' responsibility for record keeping may have further socialized them to certain assumptions and beliefs. Flick expected family members to take patients' weight, temperature, and pulse several times a day and carefully chart the results. Theodore M. Porter argues that "quantification is not merely a strategy for describing the social and natural worlds, but a means of reconfiguring them. It entails the imposition of new meanings and the disappearance of old ones."[134] To the extent that family members accepted such "objective" measures of reality, they may have been especially likely to defer to Flick's judgment.

In addition, both patients and family members must have derived considerable psychological benefit from acquiescing to Flick's authority. Although the trust they placed in his regime was not clearly deserved, it did provide a sense of control and efficacy in the face of a terrifyingly unpredictable and, ultimately, unmanageable disease.

Nevertheless, not all letter writers accepted Flick's program uncritically. A few lodged very serious complaints. One woman wrote, "I shall take my daughter from the sanitarium to-morrow, and will also make known my reasons for so doing. I will not hesitate to say to you now that I consider you were entirely mistaken as to her symptoms when you examined her, there has been absolutely no trace of a cough from the day she reached [the sanatorium], and I am not alone in thinking you very far out of the way or a complete quack on the subject."[135]

Others must have terminated Flick's services without explanation. Many who continued to demonstrate enormous respect for his expertise refused to yield completely to his authority. Some made important life decisions on their own, informing him only after the fact. Some modified the treatment plan without consulting him, discontinuing prescribed foods, tonics, or rubbings. Some rejected his recommendations for sanatorium placement. And some had the temerity to make their own therapeutic suggestions. "Why not try this," one husband wrote. "Insist on as many eggs and as much milk as she can stand; get her up and out of bed, even if for only 15 minutes per day." Although the letter writer acknowledged that "this may be in direct opposition to the ordinary rules in such cases," he feared that continuing the forced diet would have serious adverse consequences.[136] Five letter writers suggested that sick family members seek a climate cure in the West rather than remain under Flick's care in Pennsylvania.

Correspondents who retained some distance from Flick's authority often drew on other medical advice. As Barbara Bates notes, "The care of consumptives did not shift abruptly from home to resort to institutions . . . During the first two decades of the twentieth century, well-to-do patients sampled one method of taking the cure, and then another."[137] Some families were especially likely to hear conflicting advice. Patients who lived too far from Philadelphia to visit Flick regularly often consulted local doctors, many of whom did not subscribe to all aspects of his program.

Correspondents also continued to trust their own judgment because they had information Flick lacked. Many observed the troublesome side effects of his treatment. The special diet frequently induced nausea. Cold milk produced chills on early winter mornings. Some letter writers pointed to idiosyncrasies that influenced patients' responses to the therapeutic regime. The daughter of one sanatorium resident complained that her mother was "uncomfortably cold in the tent" during the early morning. "She has always suffered from cold feet."[138] Other correspondents noted that patients had sensitive stomachs even before being forced to ingest large quantities of milk and eggs.

The letter writers were especially likely to value their own psychological insights. Because tuberculosis is a chronic disease, such issues loomed very large. As weeks and then months passed, homebound patients increasingly chafed at the constraints Flick imposed. They wanted to eat more varied diets, stay up later, visit friends, attend to business, and go to school. Institutionalized patients hated the food, the cold, and the regimentation; deaths on the wards depressed them.

Above all, sanatorium inmates suffered terrible homesickness. Although Flick discounted the significance of family warmth and concern, several letter writers asserted that loneliness exacerbated the disease. One man insisted that his daughter "would Die from Home Sickness" if she were institutionalized.[139]

The letters also discussed the anxiety, frustration, and demoralization of patients both at home and in institutions. Many had abandoned their hopes and plans. When new symptoms arose or old ones were exacerbated, patients became "despondent" and "melancholy." In addition, correspondents sought to convey their own distress as the disease progressed.

Letter writers reported practical, as well as emotional, problems. The task of rubbing patients for at least an hour a day exhausted some caregivers. Sanatorium fees caused financial hardships. Some homes were too damp or dark for patients to comply with Flick's directives. One letter writer could not locate any scales with which to weigh his wife within two blocks of his home.[140]

Some correspondents wanted to influence Flick's interactions with patients. Several letters asked him to talk to patients who despaired of recovery and encourage them to remain in the sanatorium. The father of one sanatorium resident commented, "My reason for writing at this time is to give you a little advance information. In H.'s last letter to me, just received, he says that he has just about reached the limit of his endurance away from home and he intends to ask you on Saturday about the probability of coming home next month, and knowing him as I do I feel that it would be wise for you to encourage him as you no doubt know best how to do."[141] The convoluted language in this letter suggests trepidation about offending Flick by claiming superior knowledge of the patient.

Three men wrote asking Flick to conceal the diagnosis from their sick wives, whom they described as extremely sensitive. "Whatever you do," wrote a Connecticut physician seeking an appointment for his wife, "don't let on to her that she has or ever has had tuberculosis, as it would place her in a very nervous state."[142] In a subsequent letter the physician described his wife as suffering from "hysteria."[143] Five women urged Flick to warn men who were too cavalier about their health. A mother, for example, wrote, "N. tells me you will see us next Thursday. If N. has not gained this past month, and I *fear* he has not, won't you please frighten him a *little*, so he will take *better care* of himself."[144]

Other correspondents similarly sought to use Flick's authority with their relatives. The mother-in-law of a recently institutionalized man noted that her daughter was "completely worn out after the long vigil" of nursing her husband through the winter. "Now if you will emphatically tell G. he must have a nurse, whether he wants one or not," the letter continued, "and that his wife positively cannot do any more nursing, you will confer a great favor upon us all. Arguing with my daughter accomplishes nothing, and it is a delicate subject to broach with her husband. But your word is law with him."[145] This woman seemed to be motivated less by respect for Flick's medical authority than by a desire to use it to implement her own decision.

In his brief responses to forty-eight of these letters, Flick attached the greatest importance to physical conditions, focusing whenever possible on quantitative measures of weight, temperature, and pulse. He failed, however, to acknowledge any of the psychological or social issues they raised, such as homesickness, complaints about institutional life, and the burdens imposed on patients and their families.

Flick responded angrily to any doubts about his methods. He rebuffed all suggestions that patients travel to other climates. Replying to a man who had requested more detailed information about his wife's condition, Flick wrote,

> I have explained the case fully to you, have told you frankly what I thought her chances of recovery were and I do not see how I can say any more to you on this score. I cannot expect to make an anatomist, physiologist and pathologist out of you and therefore cannot go into details as to where the injury in her lungs is located, how much lung is involved and what the pathological condition is . . . I am not willing to give you any further details than I have given nor am I willing to let you or anyone else dictate to me as to my methods of treating patients. You are willing to accept my services as they are or to leave them.[146]

Flick found "quite amusing" a husband who presumed to offer advice. "You seem to know so much about your wife and to be so glib with your advice as to what ought to be done for her that I do not know of anything better to do than to have you become her physician. You certainly have more confidence in yourself in regard to her treatment than I have in myself and I shall be very glad to resign in your favor."[147] He wrote to a mother who had expressed anxiety about her son's extended sanatorium stay, "Unless you feel entirely confident in my judgment and are willing to follow implicitly what I say without quibble, I would much prefer to have you place your son in the hands of someone else. It is impossible for me to explain every detail to you simply because you cannot understand the reasons and all I can say is that I am giving you my best judgment and honest advice. If you have any misgivings at all I would be glad to have you employ someone else."[148]

Flick also denied all requests to withhold information from patients. "I make it an absolute rule to decline to see patients who are to be kept ignorant of their condition," he wrote to the physician who feared his wife was too sensitive to bear a tuberculosis diagnosis.[149] Rather than attending to the details of individual lives, Flick relied on the formal application of supposedly neutral laws.

Flick did respond to some requests. He answered all questions about the treatment regime, no matter how trivial. He wrote to one woman, for example, "Your husband can have oysters occasionally in place of meat, but it is not worth while to waste time on poultry, as it is not sufficiently nourishing to answer the purpose. As a rule he should stick to the beefstek, roast beef and roast mutton."[150] Whether because Flick subscribed to the common belief that fear and discouragement retarded recovery or because he was overly confident in his methods, he also was sympathetic to requests for reassurance, seeking to rekindle hope whenever possible. In addition, Flick sometimes revised treatment plans. In response to complaints of nausea, he typically allowed patients to discontinue the special tonics and eggs (though not the milk). He also permitted a man to stay up later at night to play cards with his wife.[151]

Despite these concessions, Flick insisted on exerting control. Although his detailed replies to questions displayed some sensitivity to his correspondents' concerns, they also implied that nothing could be left to the caregivers' discretion. All challenges to Flick's authority met hostility. Most significantly, he attended selectively to the information he received. He acknowledged neither the practical problems caregivers and patients confronted nor the suffering they experienced.

In trying to assert authority over family caregivers, Flick closely resembled nineteenth-century physicians. As we saw in Chapter 3, they also touted the superiority of formal education, dismissed caregivers' judgment, and ignored the importance of social support. Several factors, however, distinguished Flick from his nineteenth-century predecessors. He enjoyed the enhanced prestige of the medical profession. He had new arguments for belittling the spiritual and emotional components of care—areas in which family members were the experts. His advice resonated with scientific authority. And because he had no aspirations to empathy, he was more easily able to distance himself emotionally from both patients and caregivers. In part, Flick's stance reflected his personality. A short-tempered man with few social graces, he wrote formally and brusquely even to close friends and family. But the tone of his letters to caregivers also expressed the increasingly impersonal orientation in medicine. Although many physicians continued to demonstrate genuine concern for their patients as individuals, the new optimism about medicine's technical prowess encouraged some doctors to define patients solely in terms of their disease.

～ ANTHROPOLOGIST Brigitte Jordan defines "authoritative knowledge" as that which is "important, relevant, and consequential for decision-making."[152] Both groups of letter writers examined in this chapter accepted expert advice as authoritative. Women wrote to the Children's Bureau because they viewed it as a repository of valuable child care information. Although some family members writing to Flick repudiated elements of his program, most respected his expertise.

Because of the nature of the two samples, the letters cannot tell us to what extent caregivers in general accepted medical authority in the early twentieth century. We heard nothing from the many women who either remained ignorant about the new child care advice or resented the intrusion of all experts into their lives. Family members who challenged the credibility of Flick's pronouncements were unlikely to consult him regularly about patient care.

Both groups of letter writers appear to have gained a sense of mastery and efficacy from following medical advice. To the extent that caregivers had their own reasons for deferring to expertise, we can view them as active agents, rather than as passive objects of medical control. Moreover, medical expertise continued to be contested even after establishing its preeminence. Some women writing to the Children's Bureau remained uneasily poised between traditional practices and expert teachings. It is possible that such women selectively appropriated those aspects of each that best served their purposes. Several correspondents to Flick made major treatment and life decisions independently. Some used Flick's authority to strengthen their own. And few accepted his rigid protocol without demur.

The two groups were able to retain critical distance from expertise for similar reasons. Medical ideology did not constitute a coherent set of beliefs in either case; different books and doctors offered conflicting child care advice, and doctors themselves were not a monolithic force. Doctors disagreed even about such emblems of scientific progress as vaccines and surgical procedures. Moreover, child care advice was constantly under revision. Within a decade after *Infant Care* first decreed that mothers should instill habits of regularity, some experts began to preach the new gospel of permissiveness. Some women appealed to the Children's Bureau as the final arbiter, asking the staff to decide where their children's best interest lay. But others viewed the agency primarily as an alternative source of medical knowledge, providing the information that would enable mothers to make their own decisions. Family members writing to Flick also heard advice that clashed with his dicta.

Above all, caregivers' empathic knowledge fostered skepticism. Even some mothers who valued the practical advice dispensed by professionals remained convinced that technical expertise did not invalidate their intimate understandings of their own children. Although Flick trusted only measurable information, his correspondents continued to convey the subjective experience of living with a serious chronic disease and to consider themselves experts on psychological issues. As a result, they remained very attentive to patient wishes despite Flick's injunction to focus primarily on surveillance and control.

~6

Negotiating Public Health Directives: Poor New Yorkers at the Turn of the Century

$\mathcal{I}$N 1918 the New York Charity Organization Society (COS), the city's most prominent charitable agency, engaged in an eight-month conflict with an Italian immigrant couple over the care of their twelve-year-old daughter.[1] The COS first visited the Germani household on January 25. The family consisted of a musician, his wife, and their six children. Mr. Germani was considered "a rather better class of Neapolitan man," but he lacked work, and the family could not make ends meet. Attention soon focused on the oldest child, Maria, who was ill.

At first, the Germanis did not object to the COS's plans for their daughter. They agreed to have Maria's sputum tested, and on March 7 a Department of Health physician diagnosed tuberculosis. The COS's next recommendation provoked more resistance. The COS learned that the doctor considered Maria "a hospital case" and believed that "the sooner she was rushed to the hospital, the better."

According to the report of the charity worker who came to take Maria to the hospital, the girl "cried and absolutely refused to go." On the morning of March 8, Mr. Germani told a charity worker that, rather than sending Maria to the hospital, he would take her to the home of his sister, who lived with her husband in an eight-room house on two acres of land in New Jersey. There Maria not only would be isolated from the other children but also would receive the fresh air and rich diet believed to have therapeutic value. Mr. Germani also said he had taken Maria to a Brooklyn doctor, who had confirmed the diagnosis but consented to the father's plan.

Mr. Germani's decision to send his daughter to New Jersey prompted the COS to report the case to the Society for the Prevention of Cruelty to Children (SPCC), requesting it to find a way to take Maria "by force" to the hospital. On March 29 the SPCC reported that it could take no action because Maria was leaving for her aunt's home in New Jersey. A COS charity worker who visited the girl in New Jersey confirmed that she was "getting along very well"; she had "gained weight" and had "plenty of fresh milk and eggs and good care." Nevertheless, the COS remained suspicious of the parents, warning them that the SPCC would be alerted if Maria returned to the city.

Maria did return. On July 9 a COS worker visiting the Germanis after the birth of a baby found Maria at home and her health still poor. She looked "pale and worn" and was dressed in "a heavy white sweater" despite the summer heat. Mrs. Germani insisted that her own doctor considered Maria "fine" and that she wore the sweater only because she had just returned from the park. The report for July 22 read,

> Maria was sitting in a large rocking chair, propped by a big pillow. Her mother said she had just come in from the park (which seemed very doubtful). Maria looks sick and weak and has a very loose cough. She coughs frequently. [The charity worker] asked if Maria might go with her to the doctor's the next time she called, or if the mother would prefer having the doctor call at the house. Mrs. Germani would much prefer the latter and wants an Italian doctor.

The COS informed the SPCC of Maria's return, but it again refused to intervene, noting that Maria was going back to New Jersey and that "the mother has promised to cooperate with the SPCC." The COS's own investigation confirmed that Maria received good care at her aunt's home. On August 15 a charity worker found Maria "sitting in the back yard under a grape arbor." The caseworker described the aunt as "a nice looking woman with a very kind, good face" who seemed "very fond of Maria and cannot do enough for her." Some New York relatives who were visiting were "nice refined people and all so interested in and concerned about Maria." The house was "out in the country where you can see the fields and woods for miles and miles. It is a very lovely spot for Maria if the air is dry enough." Although Maria refused the special foods prepared for her, the relatives promised to work harder at persuasion.

On September 23 the case took a dramatic turn. Maria was found at home and was hospitalized against her family's wishes. According to the charity worker's notes, Mrs. Cappetti, one of Mr. Germani's sisters living in New York,

> called at the office in a great state of excitement. She said that Maria and her mother had been to court this morning and the judge had ordered that Maria be placed in a hospital. She was taken to the Reception Hospital. The family feel very badly about this and fear the child will grieve herself to death because she is separated from her family. Mrs. Cappetti said her sister in [New Jersey] is willing to keep Maria and they feel that the child has been getting the proper care there and has shown improvement. Mrs. Cappetti takes her regularly to see [the doctor in Brooklyn]. Mrs. Cappetti explained that Maria had come into the city to go to see the doctor . . . The truant officer called and found Maria at home. Mrs. Germani probably was not able to explain fully to the officer that Maria was not living at home and he, seeing her there among so many children, no doubt thought the best place for her would be in a hospital. Mr. Germani is very much worried about it and asked Mrs. Cappetti to call and see if the COS could help get the child discharged from the hospital. Mrs. Cappetti was told that the Society would do what they could in the matter.

The Germani family faulted Maria's mother for the disaster. When the charity worker visited the Germani home the following morning, Mrs. Germani "implied that her husband and his family blamed her for Maria's commitment." Nevertheless, she had been powerless to prevent it. She had assumed that the officer who came to take her to court was from the school and wanted Maria examined. Her language difficulties had even more drastic consequences in court. The case file continued:

As [Mrs. Germani] cannot speak or understand the English language very well, she did not comprehend all that was going on in the court room. She tried to explain to the Judge that Maria did not live at home and that she was under a doctor's care, but no one seemed to pay any heed to her remarks. When they got into the automobile, she thought they were going to take Maria to the hospital for an examination, but when they arrived there she was told that the child would have to remain.

Maria was soon transferred to Metropolitan Hospital. Operated by the New York City Department of Public Welfare on the site of the old almshouse on Blackwell Island, this facility aroused more hostility among immigrants and the poor than any other city hospital. The COS was well aware of its deplorable conditions. In 1911 the organization issued a report castigating the city for the hospital's "disgraceful" overcrowding. Beds "regularly lined" the halls, and many patients were forced to sleep on mattresses on the floor.[2] Two years later, a patient who left the hospital "because he could not stand the place" vividly described his experiences in a letter to the COS. The bedding he received had been used by other patients without having been washed or even aired.[3] The COS staff were so impressed with this letter that they sent copies to numerous city officials, but conditions at the hospital remained unchanged.

Maria was miserable in the hospital and begged to be discharged. Her condition steadily deteriorated. In early October a charity worker found her "sitting on a rocking chair all bundled up in her sweater with the saddest and most forlorn look on her face." Mrs. Germani tried to obtain her daughter's release, pointing to Maria's special sensitivities, which made a hospital stay especially hard on her. Unlike her siblings, the girl never expressed her feelings directly but "all the time cries inside." Mrs. Germani feared Maria would die from homesickness if compelled to stay. The mother also expressed concern about her husband, who took many days off from his new job at a bakery and occasionally threatened suicide. In October, when the 1918 flu epidemic struck New York and city officials placed Metropolitan Hospital under quarantine, both parents became frantic with worry.

Charity workers tried to allay the Germanis' fears by contacting the hospital administrators to obtain information about Maria. In other ways, however, the COS remained impervious to the parents' concerns. Although various relatives beseeched the COS to work for Maria's release, the organization stonewalled. It repeatedly promised to appeal to influential people on Maria's behalf but then used interviews with those people to explain why Maria should remain in the hospital. As the family grew increasingly irate at the COS for its failure to act, charity workers turned the blame back on the parents, claiming that if they "had done as they promised to do and had not brought Maria home with them all this trouble would have been avoided." A hospital nurse similarly held the parents responsible, arguing that the girl might have recovered had the parents allowed her to enter the hospital sooner.

As the weeks passed, Maria's condition continued to worsen. By the middle of October she had stopped eating. "I think it is a sin to have a sick child suffer the way she is," wrote one of Maria's cousins on November 8. Maria died in the hospital eight days later, nearly two months after her admission.

Public Health Programs and Families

Like many of Dr. Lawrence Flick's correspondents described in the previous chapter, the Germanis sought to retain control of medical decision-making. For the Germanis, however, challenging medical advice had drastic consequences. Although Flick had considerable authority as a prominent physician, he could not wield official coercion. The Germanis confronted what David Arnold called, in another context, "a state centered system of scientific knowledge and power."[4] Public health programs not only derived authority from the ascendance of scientific medicine but also possessed formal powers of enforcement. When the Germanis persisted in pursuing their own course of treatment, they suffered serious sanctions that proved fatal to their child.

Barriers of culture and language undermined the Germanis' attempts to protect Maria. Although charity workers may have relied on a child or a neighbor to translate (as they often did in similar situations), we know from court and case records that Mrs. Germani had at least some difficulty communicating with the COS. When she tried to explain in court that Maria did not live at home and was under a doctor's care, "no one seemed to pay any heed to her remarks." Her limited English also led her to misconstrue several critical events leading to Maria's commitment.

The Germani's struggle with the COS and the Department of Health partly expressed a conflict about the meaning of Maria's life. To her parents, Maria was a uniquely precious child; they directed their attention to promoting her recovery, which they believed could occur only within her family. To charity workers and health officials, however, Maria was primarily a source of infection who should be segregated from both the family and the rest of society.

In framing their policy toward the Germanis, the COS and the Department of Health drew on widespread assumptions about the association of disease with poor people, especially immigrants and people of color. That perception had some empirical foundation. The health of the poor suffered greatly from the squalid conditions in which they lived and worked. Although tuberculosis affected the general population throughout the nineteenth century, after 1900 it was concentrated among low-income people.[5]

But the identification of disease with poor people could survive epidemiological falsification. Medical examinations at Ellis Island and other entry points found that the incidence of sexually transmitted diseases, for instance, was no higher than among the native-born population. Yet a professor of gynecology at the Johns Hopkins Medical School declared in 1910, "The tide of [venereal disease] has been raising owing to the inpouring of a large foreign population with lower ideals."[6] During the 1916 New York polio epidemic, health officials linked the disease to immigrants despite epidemiological reports showing that it affected affluent communities most severely.[7]

Moreover, poor people were viewed as agents of disease, not merely victims. We might have expected that greater knowledge of the pathogens responsible for specific ills and the routes of transmission would have dispelled some of the anxieties about the poor. But the germ theory did not easily or entirely eclipse older models. As Charles E. Rosenberg writes, the years between 1885 and 1920, which witnessed "the most enthusiastic and uncritical acceptance of the germ theory," were also the "period of most enthusiastic hereditarian thought."[8] Hermann Biggs, a New York City health official who eagerly embraced the new bacteriological knowledge, asserted that an inherited predisposition, as well as the spread of germs, explained the high rate of tuberculosis in certain families.[9]

Old attitudes about the association between dirt and disease also lingered. The conclusion of an 1893 *New York Times* article about street vendors on the Lower East Side illustrates both the nature of prevailing stereotypes and the persistent power of the filth theory of disease:

> This neighborhood, peopled almost entirely by the people who claim to have been driven from Poland and Russia, is the eyesore of New York and perhaps the filthiest place on the western continent. It is impossible for a Christian to live there because he will be driven out, either by blows or the dirt and stench. Cleanliness is an unknown quality to these people . . . If the cholera should ever get among these people, they would scatter its germs as a sower does grain.[10]

The germ theory bred fresh worries. A recurrent theme in the writings of health officials was the failure of germs to respect barriers of class and race. A tuberculosis nurse in Baltimore warned in 1905 that even the most scrupulous housekeeper could not guard the portals of her home against pollution. "Domestic servants, laundresses, dress makers, teachers and the like" spread infection "in ever-widening circles."[11] Moreover, fear of contagion coincided with deep social anxieties about the sexuality and revolutionary potential of the poor. By instilling discipline and exerting social control, it was argued, health officers could not only retard the spread of disease but also tame the sexual activity and reproduction of low-income people, create a docile workforce, and avert social disorder.[12]

Although all poor people were considered responsible for the spread of germs, caregivers were singled out for special blame. The previous chapter noted that the new confidence in medical science strengthened physicians' claims to superior knowledge and created a pretext for lavishing attention on maternal education. Poor women were especially likely to be perceived as ignorant. A 1913 study of 285 children at the Boston Dispensary Hospital concluded that 70 percent of the mothers needed education in child care, "general home hygiene and housekeeping," and the importance of professional medical treatment.[13] Education dominated both preventive and curative health programs directed toward the poor. To be sure, the prominent place of education on the public health agenda stemmed from various factors, including budgetary constraints and private physicians' hostility to free services. Client ignorance, however, was most frequently noted.[14]

Emotionalism was another trait attributed to caregivers in poor households. Whereas nineteenth-century cultural authorities encouraged caregivers to form close bonds with care recipients and respond sensitively to their sufferings, early-twentieth-century experts stressed the importance of maintaining emotional distance. Poor women were believed to be especially likely to indulge sick and disabled kin. In 1919, the annual report of the Out-Patient Department of the New York Society for the Relief of the Ruptured and Crippled cited the example of George, a "boy of 11 years [who] had been coming to clinic for some time with a tuberculous hip. As he was not improving, was referred for home investigation. The worker found boy to be an only child, very much spoiled by over-kindness." Improvement began, the report added, only after his mother agreed to make him drink the extra milk and cod-liver oil the society supplied.[15] An Italian father was blamed in a case reported by the Massachusetts Charitable Eye and Ear Infirmary: "His small daughter of three years [was] evidently a spoiled and petted child. The doctor thought the child could be treated safely at home, with three visits a week to the Infirmary. When several days had passed and the child did not return, a visit was made to the home. The father explained that the child had cried so much at the hospital and again cried so much each time an attempt was made to treat the eyes at home, that they had decided to do nothing."[16] Other indulgent parents loosened their crippled children's stays, allowed diabetic adolescents to depart from the recommended diet, and permitted cardiac patients to engage in vigorous physical exercise.

The affection inspiring such misguided solicitousness also came under attack. The director of social service work at Youngstown Hospital in Ohio explained why so many parents refused recommendations of hospital placement for their children this way: "Parents are prejudiced by their love for their child, and although it may be more of an animal love than human it must be recognized."[17] Open expressions of emotion repelled Anglo-American social workers and nurses accustomed to restraint. Visiting the home of a West Indian woman the day after her daughter died during surgery, a New York City charity worker wrote that the mother "had something very primitive about her grief over the child."[18]

If some poor women were described as caring too much about sick and disabled family members, others were criticized for caring too little. In a study of the reasons why children failed to return for follow-up visits to St. Louis Children's Hospital Dispensary, social service workers concluded that the fault lay with "indifferent" parents in eleven of fifty cases.[19] Many commentators located the source of indifference in the view that illness was unavoidable. One social worker argued that mothers refused to acknowledge the problems medical inspectors detected in schoolchildren because the mothers "are of the belief that the diseases of children are a necessary part of the life of the child."[20]

According to Josephine Baker, chief of the New York City Bureau of Child Hygiene, women normalized death as well as disease. Immigrant mothers "were just horribly fatalistic about [infant death]," she later wrote in her autobiography. "Babies always died in summer and there was no point in trying to do anything about it . . . I might as well have been trying to tell them to keep it from raining."[21] A public health nurse in Arizona described Gregoria, a twenty-two-year-old Hispanic mother, thus: "Five babies had been born to her in the seven years of her married life, but the good God had taken three of them. They had lived a few miserable months, and had then died. Gregoria sat huddled over her door-step and thought that nothing was of any use. The baby was always sick and some day the good God would take him as He had the others."[22] Nineteenth-century white caregivers had been praised for the strength of the religious conviction that enabled them to reconcile themselves to the inevitable, but privileged members of society had long viewed subordinate groups as fatalistic. Moreover, by the early twentieth century, optimism about science had become a central cultural value. No longer an important spiritual goal, acceptance of God's will was now portrayed as a sign of passivity, inadequate willpower, and failure to appreciate the benefits of modern medicine.

Although "discouraged" and "resigned" caregivers were assumed to hope for recovery, observers occasionally accused poor people of harboring the opposite wish. Richard Cabot, a Harvard professor and physician who established the first hospital social work department at Massachusetts General Hospital, wrote in a 1909 letter that one of the "two chief causes of infant mortality" was the "desire on the part of parents that the baby should die."[23]

Because charity workers, public health nurses, and health officials identified opposition to public health services with perceived negative attributes of the poor, it is important to understand the client perspective. The remainder of this chapter discusses how caregivers in destitute New York families at the turn of the century experienced that city's pioneering program of tuberculosis control. We will see that the Germanis were not the only caregivers who spurned some aspects of that program and incurred serious sanctions as a result.

Tuberculosis Control in New York City

We can glimpse the attitudes of poor New Yorkers through the case files of the New York Charity Organization Society. I examined all 119 files from the years 1894 through 1918 in which at least one family member had tuberculosis. The files included a standard intake form containing such basic information as the names, addresses, and ages of all family members and the occupations of those who were wage earners. On subsequent pages, COS staff recorded the results of interviews with neighbors, relatives, friends, employers, and clergy. Charity workers also made notes on every interaction with family members, whether at home or at the COS office. These entries both summarized conversations and recorded the investigators' impressions of the household. Few aspects of the clients' lives were too trivial or private to escape scrutiny. Copious notes described sleeping arrangements, the type of food served, the quality of the housekeeping, and the children's demeanor. In addition, several files contain correspondence, medical records, and reports from various institutions, including hospitals and sanatoriums.

The data from the files cannot be quantified, because some of these families had only brief interactions with the COS. Approximately one-third, however, remained on the caseload for years, and their voluminous records are especially enlightening. Because the philosophy of the COS changed significantly between 1894 and 1918, it is important to note that the records are concentrated in the later years. Most of the cases initiated during the 1890s continued into the first two decades of the twentieth century; the records in the later period thus include those that began a decade or more earlier.

Unfortunately, the records provide limited information about the health beliefs of caregivers. In interacting with COS staff, caregivers had to frame their appeals in language calculated to appeal to the organization. Because charity workers exhibited enormous faith in the germ theory, caregivers may have been reluctant to assert that they subscribed to an alternative explanation of disease causation.

If the records do not enable us to gauge the extent to which the health beliefs of clients coincided with those of charity workers and health officials, they do provide insight into the everyday context within which impoverished caregivers experienced public health measures. Recent studies demonstrate that life circumstances are the most important factor in explaining compliance with medical regimes.[24]

The late nineteenth and early twentieth centuries were, as Charles E. Rosenberg writes, the "heroic age of public health."[25] The New York City Department of Health was especially prominent in the field of tuberculosis control. It made tuberculosis a reportable disease, launched one of the first major health education campaigns, and provided free diagnosis and treatment. At a time when many cities had only fledgling health programs, New York boasted a remarkable array of services, offering curative medicine as well as prevention.[26]

Normative values infused the tuberculosis campaign. Although Hermann Biggs, the department's chief medical officer, claimed to be translating Koch's discovery of the tubercle bacillus into practice, the absence of a magic bullet left ample opportunity for ideological factors to shape health programs. Accepting the common belief that the habits of the poor predisposed them to contract and transmit tuberculosis, the department emphasized personal reform. Public health nurses visited clients in their homes and taught the values of thrift, sobriety, and restraint while providing instruction about hygiene, fresh air, and diet. A primary goal of the institutions established by the department was to refine and uplift their inmates.[27]

The New York Charity Organization Society collaborated closely with the Department of Health in many phases of its tuberculosis work. In its early years, the New York COS, like other charity organization societies in both the United States and Britain, initially attributed poverty to the moral failings of the poor, ignoring the social and economic forces that shaped individual behavior. One practice of the wealthy was also believed to undermine the character of the poor. By giving aid "indiscriminately," it was thought that affluent people encouraged "pauperism," or long-term dependence on handouts. COS charity workers visited the home of each applicant for relief, conducted a lengthy investigation, and then reported to a district committee, which decided whether the applicant was "worthy" of assistance and, if so, what form it should take. District committees originally gave no direct assistance themselves but, rather, coordinated the donations of other charitable groups.[28]

Founded during a period that venerated rationality, the organization labeled its approach "scientific." Josephine Shaw Lowell, the founder and "guiding spirit" of the New York COS, wrote that the "task of dealing with the poor and degraded has become a science, and has its well defined principles, recognized and conformed to, more or less closely, by all who really give time and thought to the subject."[29] Charity workers' relationships to their clients bolstered the claim to scientific authority. Although women held prominent positions in the COS, they sought to distinguish themselves from previous generations of female charity workers. Rather than viewing themselves as "sisters" to less fortunate women, COS staff cultivated the detachment considered proper for experts; emotion, sensitivity, and close personal connection, they asserted, had no place in scientific charity.[30] Such a stance enabled charity workers to argue that they, rather than family caregivers, could best discern the needs of the sick.

During the early twentieth century, district committees increasingly provided material assistance and acknowledged the social and economic causes of poverty. Nevertheless, the COS continued to distinguish between deserving and undeserving applicants. The most important criterion for assessing worthiness was willingness to work.[31]

It is important not to overstate the extent to which that criterion was gendered. Feminist historians often criticize turn-of-the-century charitable agencies for reinforcing the gender division of labor by demanding that married women remain out of the workforce, even when their husbands were too disabled to work.[32] For the COS, however, economic self-sufficiency took precedence over traditional gender relations. Two groups of women frequently asked for assistance so they could stay home and provide care—single mothers of sick or disabled young children and women who previously had relied on incomes of husbands or older children and suddenly found themselves without support when those breadwinners became incapacitated. The COS often refused to excuse either group from the duty to find paid employment.

The COS's preoccupation with work also shaped the organization's health-related programs. The delivery of health services expressed less a sense of connection and shared humanity with clients than a means of enhancing productivity and self-reliance. Charity workers frequently stated that their goal was to restore sick or disabled individuals to "wage earning power."

Ill health was one of the few causes of poverty the COS deemed acceptable; "able-bodied" adults without work constituted a high proportion of the unworthy. Nevertheless, the organization did not consider sick or disabled people entirely blameless. Illness, like poverty, was viewed as the result of personal failure. The COS abhorred weakness and dependence of any kind. When people lost vigor and could no longer engage in productive activities, they became "burdens"; family care consumed resources that could be better devoted to income-generating activities.

One way the COS assisted the Department of Health was by monitoring patients' behavior at home. In addition, the organization established the Committee on the Prevention of Tuberculosis (CPT), which published a handbook on tuberculosis prevention, established open-air classes for children with tuberculosis and a day camp for adults, organized an association to coordinate the activities of public and private tuberculosis clinics, and convinced the city government to increase its budget for tuberculosis control.[33]

Demographic information may help to introduce the COS clients. Although most Jews were referred to the United Hebrew Charities, other immigrant groups dominated the caseload. A 1916 study found that Italians represented 27.9 percent of the clients, Irish 14.6 percent, Germans 6.2 percent, and Austro-Hungarians 5.4 percent. Native-born Americans constituted 29.6 percent of the clientele. (The background of 16.3 percent of the clients was not specified.)[34] The study did not indicate what proportion of the clients were white; the case files suggest, however, that very few African Americans applied to the COS.

Almost all employed men were unskilled manual laborers; the majority earned between $12 and $14 a week. Most families lived in three-room apartments, paying between $8 and $12 a month in rent.[35]

The clients appear to have borne a very heavy burden of disease and disability. A 1910 study reported that 12 percent of the 5,387 families on the COS roster had at least one member with tuberculosis, and 75 percent had "another acute or chronic physical disability."[36] A high proportion of the women thus had at least one major caregiving responsibility. Because many clients lived in tenements without running water, electricity, or other modern conveniences, providing care at home must have been grueling.[37]

Outside employment often exacerbated the difficulties of caring for sick family members. According to a 1920 COS study, 42 percent of female clients held jobs. Of these, over half (54 percent) worked as janitors, office cleaners, laundresses, chambermaids, or domestic servants, 22 percent held factory jobs, 19 percent did home work, and 3 percent did clerical work.[38] Most earned very little. A 1916 COS study of the families of patients at a New York tuberculosis clinic examined several cases in which women entered the labor force in place of sick husbands. "In no instance," the study concluded, "are the earnings sufficient to maintain a decent standard of living unless supplemented by children's earnings or relief."[39] The practicalities of combining caregiving and paid employment proved daunting. Sick and disabled children were excluded from the few day nurseries that existed. Unlike healthy offspring, seriously ill patients could not easily be left with neighbors. And taking sick or disabled family members to work was rarely an option. Some employed women thus were forced to leave sick family members home unattended.[40]

Despite the COS's insistence that paid employment take precedence over caregiving responsibilities, household sickness drew some women back home. On January 20, 1904, the wife of a laborer suffering from tuberculosis applied for aid. Because her husband had been forced to quit work, the woman had supported the family for two years by cleaning offices. Six weeks prior to her application, however, her husband had become so ill that she had relinquished her job in order to tend him full-time. As a result, she could not afford to pay the rent or buy food, fuel, or clothing for the children.[41] In short, many women faced stark choices when illness visited their households. They could work, earn little, and leave sick family members alone, or they could decline work to provide care and suffer extreme poverty.

A few women sought to reconcile the antagonistic demands of work and care by finding jobs they could do at home, such as taking in board-ers, foundlings, laundry, or piecework. But home work paid extremely poorly and was not always available. As fears about germs spread, up-per-class people refrained from bringing washing or sewing to women whose family members suffered from communicable diseases. Work at home also consumed time needed for care. A dressmaker told the COS in 1897 that although she had a sewing machine at home, she could not keep it running while tending her bedridden husband.[42] Some women could not afford the soap and tubs required for washing or lacked the space needed to dry clothes. And women often undermined, rather than promoted, family health when they worked at home. Investigators in the early twentieth century attributed the high rate of lung infec-tions among home workers' children to the chemical fumes and fabric particles they inhaled. The use of sewing machines, hot irons, and boil-ing water led to injuries, burns, and scaldings. Work that involved chil-dren's participation deprived them of time for play and sleep.[43]

Although the COS frequently pressured tuberculosis sufferers di-rectly to comply with Department of Health advice, I focus on conflicts between charity workers and the wives, mothers, and daughters the or-ganization held responsible for the activities of sick family members. Given the pattern of male dominance prevailing in poor and immigrant households, it is hardly surprising that these women often told charity workers they were powerless to override male relatives' objections. Nevertheless, the organization blamed and penalized women when their family members failed to adhere to the prescribed medical regi-men.

We have seen that in cases involving children, the COS sometimes solicited the intervention of the SPCC.[44] An even more common coer-cive measure was withdrawal of relief. In situations of extreme need, the COS provided emergency supplies of groceries and fuel as soon as families applied. The organization then discontinued such help when-ever families demonstrated unworthiness, for instance, by rejecting medical advice. Some charity workers made the offer of assistance con-tingent on adherence to public health directives. When family mem-bers suffered from tuberculosis, the COS occasionally mobilized state power to compel compliance. In 1901 the New York City Department of Health instituted a policy of forcibly detaining tubercular patients; two years later, the department opened a special pavilion at Riverside Hospital to confine them.[45] Although charity workers frequently complained that the department failed to respond to requests for forcible detention, the threat of removal sometimes was enough to convince clients to comply.[46]

Advice for Tuberculosis Sufferers

A major responsibility the COS entrusted to caregivers was ensuring that tuberculosis sufferers obeyed Department of Health advice. Unwilling to take client accounts at face value, COS staff paid surprise visits to clients' homes to inspect beds, food, windows, and sputum cups. One charity worker made home visits before family members were awake in order to observe sleeping arrangements. Such examinations uncovered numerous tubercular people living in cramped, dark, and unsanitary quarters, sharing beds with the well, deviating from the prescribed diet, and allowing sputum cups to overflow.

The COS typically attributed noncompliance to ignorance but often failed to specify what it thought caregivers did not know. Some components of the tuberculosis program seemed to have as much to do with advancing the goal of assimilation as with controlling disease. Instructions about sleeping arrangements, for example, addressed moral, as well as medical, concerns. By advising tuberculosis patients to sleep alone, nurses and charity workers sought to control not just contagion but also promiscuity, which privileged members of society associated with overcrowding.[47] Because the discovery of the tubercle bacillus made disposal of the sputum an urgent issue, it is not surprising that educational circulars provided detailed instructions about hygiene. The concern with cleanliness, however, shaded easily into a focus on neatness and order. Both Department of Health nurses and COS staff supervising tubercular people noted whether beds were made, children's faces washed, and rooms kept tidy. Warnings about expectoration attempted to combat a practice the middle class considered not just dangerous but also socially abhorrent. In many cases, what charity workers interpreted as poor people's ignorance of the germ theory may have been refusal to adopt middle-class modes of behavior.

But even charity workers who were most inclined to blame clients for noncompliance acknowledged the constraints that material conditions imposed. "Nourishing food" and new beds were expensive, and many apartments were too small to accommodate additional beds. Many tenement rooms were windowless; windows that existed often opened onto air shafts rather than the street, thus providing neither the sunlight nor the ventilation that health officials considered essential. The dilapidated condition of buildings, the soot and ashes produced by coal-burning stoves and kerosene and gas lamps, and the serious overcrowding all made dirt unavoidable.[48]

To ameliorate some of these problems, both charity workers and health officials participated actively in the campaign for tenement house reform.[49] In addition, many clinics distributed eggs and milk to needy patients.[50] The COS Committee on the Prevention of Tuberculosis raised funds to furnish new beds, special foods, and sputum cups, and occasionally even helped move patients to sunnier and airier apartments. When clients lacked space for extra beds, the CPT provided folding cots to be used in the kitchen at night.[51]

Competing needs sometimes interfered with the intended use of this material assistance. A woman who received a new bed from the CPT saved it for her forthcoming confinement rather than giving it to her tubercular son to enable him to sleep alone.[52] Other assistance was inadequate. The number of eggs, for example, occasionally fell short of the amount doctors prescribed; a few people received money for moving expenses but no help with paying higher weekly rents. Moreover, some clients resented pressure to leave their apartments. Moving disrupted the patterns of social exchange on which poor people depended. Because janitors typically lived in damp and fetid basements, they were especially likely to be told to find new quarters. But such clients lost free rent as well as familiar surroundings when they moved.

Although charity workers sought to provide some of the resources that clients needed to follow the Department of Health's dictates, they were unwilling to relax their standards of hygiene, which often imposed exhausting burdens on poor women. Lacking indoor plumbing, many had to lug pails of water up several flights of stairs. As we have seen, some could eke out time for household chores only after long days in factories, laundries, or upper-class homes. Home work also consumed time while increasing dirt and congestion. Onerous childcare and nursing responsibilities further diminished women's abilities to meet charity workers' expectations. Dying patients created special problems. COS staff enjoined caregivers to observe "absolute cleanliness,"[53] but most poor women were virtually incapable of following such advice. People in the final stages of consumption coughed and vomited frequently, soiling themselves, their beds, and sometimes even the rooms around them.[54]

Outpatient Services

Clinic care was available to the tubercular poor both in the facilities established by the Department of Health and in a variety of hospital dispensaries. Most had very limited hours of operation, typically during the workweek.[55] Employed caregivers thus forfeited income when they accompanied family members to the clinic. According to the 1912 case records of the COS, one woman lost her job when she attended a hospital dispensary on her husband's behalf:

> Mrs. P. goes to the dispensary from time to time to get some medicine for Mr. P. Mrs. P. is a janitress and has been in present house for some three months. Last week she lost her position as janitress as while she went to the dispensary for the medicine a lady came to look for rooms, and Mr. P. not being able to walk the little boy took the lady upstairs and showed her the rooms. He was not able to tell her the price and could not explain that the mother would return soon and to have the lady wait. She made a complaint to the landlord that no one wanted to show her the rooms and that was the cause of [Mrs. P.] losing her position. At present they have either to pay $9.50 a month for these rooms or to leave. They have absolutely no money, no gas, no coal in the house.[56]

As we saw in Chapter 2, caregiving in the nineteenth century typically involved labor-intensive activities that clashed with women's domestic responsibilities. The conflict between work and care took new forms at the turn of the century, as the proportion of employed women grew and caregiving increasingly came to involve servicing work. Women now had to balance a wide variety of activities, each dominated by a different clock and located in a different site.

Inpatient Care

The sharpest conflicts between charity workers and caregivers focused on institutionalization. The major facility for the tubercular poor in New York was Metropolitan Hospital, which Maria Germani entered in 1918. A 1911 study by the CPT found 947 patients at that hospital on March 1. The special tuberculosis pavilion opened by the Department of Health at Riverside Hospital housed both people who were forcibly confined and those who entered voluntarily, a total of 238 on that same date. In addition, five private hospitals received subsidies from the Department of Public Charities to provide tubercular care for the poor; they accommodated a total of 918 people on March 1, 1911.[57] A few other private hospitals reserved free beds for tubercular patients.[58] Although the number of hospital beds for the tubercular poor tripled between 1897 and 1911,[59] all facilities remained oversubscribed; in 1911 the CPT estimated that half of the patients seeking hospitalization for tuberculosis had to wait for admission.[60]

In the late nineteenth and early twentieth century, poor New Yorkers had few opportunities for sanatorium care. They could try to find a free bed in a private institution or go to one of the boardinghouses that sprang up in communities surrounding sanatoriums. But few free beds were available, and boardinghouses charged high rates. One woman reported in 1906 that she was taking in extra washing to pay her son's board in Liberty, New York; in addition, his friends were "getting up a benefit for him."[61] Another woman noted in 1913 that her husband's sister in Norway had sent $50 to be used for his board in Liberty. Because the rate was $10 a week, "the $50 would not go far."[62] After the opening of the New York state sanatorium at Ray Brook in 1903 and the municipal sanatorium at Otisville in 1906, those facilities became major resources for COS clients. But both required applicants to wait several months for admission, and Otisville excluded noncitizens, a serious problem for many COS clients.

Because access to both hospitals and sanatoriums remained limited in the decades preceding World War I, some COS clients appealed for help in finding beds for family members. Many more caregivers, however, faced the opposite problem—staving off pressure to place their sick family members in institutions.

The COS insisted on the institutionalization of tuberculosis sufferers for many reasons. As we have seen, charity workers viewed tubercular people as menaces who should be segregated from their families and the rest of society. In addition, charity workers assumed that poor women were too emotional, ignorant, and fatalistic to deliver good care, and that the clients' living conditions were inadequate to foster recovery and protect family members from infection. And charity workers wanted to free women from responsibility for care to enable them to enter the workforce.

Caregivers had a variety of reasons for opposing the institutional placement recommended by COS workers. In some cases they felt that patients did not need institutional care. Although the Germanis agreed that Maria had tuberculosis, they contended that the girl was recovering satisfactorily at home. In another 1918 case, the mother disputed the diagnosis. At the COS's request, she had taken her eleven-year-old boy to the Manhattan Eye and Ear Hospital to have his sputum examined. Informed that her son was in the second stage of tuberculosis and should be hospitalized, the mother consulted her own physician, who stated that the boy had "weak lungs" but not tuberculosis. The mother noted that the hospital had examined the boy the previous October and found him in good health; she doubted that he "could have possibly developed tuberculosis in the second stage in such a short time." She also reminded the charity worker of a previous incident. When her six-year-old daughter was hospitalized for Saint Vitus' dance in 1916, the mother had overheard doctors saying that the girl had diphtheria and should be transferred to Willard Parker, the contagious disease hospital. The mother had brought the girl home and called her own doctor, who stated that the child was not seriously ill. Because the girl "immediately recovered," the mother had concluded that the hospital doctors had been "absolutely wrong in their diagnosis." In the absence of a definitive diagnosis of tuberculosis, she did not want her son exposed to contagious patients.[63]

Some women argued that they needed whatever income family members still were able to provide. As a COS committee wrote in 1906, "Even the scanty and occasional earnings of a consumptive are important to many a poor family, and frequent objection to hospital care is raised by father, mother, husband, or wife, even though the bread-winning power of the one needing such care has been reduced to the lowest point, if not, indeed, entirely taken away by sickness."[64]

Family members who could not obtain paid work occasionally provided other essential help. Some tubercular husbands, for example, cared for children during the day while their wives worked.

Institutionalization not only deprived women of critical assistance but also imposed new responsibilities and anxieties. One woman stated in 1911 that she "could not endure the thought of sending her husband to the hospital" because "the worry and strain" would be too great during her approaching confinement.[65] The difficulty of obtaining news of institutionalized patients intensified worries. Without access to telephones and often possessing only a weak command of English, women found communication with institutional staff extremely difficult. Many caregivers also suspected that institutions failed to provide accurate information or notify them promptly in emergencies.

Visiting institutionalized patients was often difficult and expensive. Whereas Martha Farnsworth had easy access to her niece in Topeka, New York City hospitals for the poor typically restricted visiting hours to two or three hours a week.[66] Employed caregivers often could not take advantage of those times. Carfare was another problem. One COS client removed her baby from a private hospital in 1902 because she could not afford to make regular trips to see the child.[67] Another woman refused to allow her husband to be transferred from Bellevue Hospital to Metropolitan in 1905 because the trip would be too far for her and the children; she wanted him to remain where they could visit him "every day or so."[68] The cost of transportation was especially great when family members were sent to sanatoriums outside the city. Few families could afford the train fare to Otisville, which was located seventy-five miles from New York City in the Catskill Mountains; in addition, travelers had to pay for at least one night's accommodation.[69] Because sanatoriums also involved the longest stays, many women desperately tried to prevent family members from being admitted.

Institutionalization could involve other expenses. The Department of Health sent patients admitted to Otisville a long list of outdoor clothing essential to withstand the cold; many individual items cost between $5 and $10, nearly a week's wages for most workers.[70] One woman told the COS in July 1912 that she had mortgaged her furniture to buy the outfit for her daughter. Six months later the woman was still unable to pay her debt.[71]

Caregivers continued to provide clothes and services after patients' departures. The wife of an Otisville inmate sent him a new pair of "arctics" costing $2.50 in February 1907 and a dollar to have his shoes repaired in April; in May she sent $1.50 for mending his clothes, $.50 for a new hat, $.50 for carfare, and $.25 for a haircut.[72] Another woman who visited her husband in 1904, three days after he entered a private hospital, was told, according to the case file, that "she would be compelled to do his laundry work and provide all necessary toilet articles, and would also have to get him a new suit of clothes, as the patients who were able to be about, must be neatly dressed. As it would be impossible for her to do all this, she brought the man home with her."[73]

Clients also defended their decisions against institutionalization by countering the COS assertion that they lacked the qualities necessary for rendering good care. One woman protested that she had been a hospital aide in Ireland.[74] Others sought to convince COS staff that they understood the special precautions the Department of Health recommended for the care of tubercular patients and were scrupulous about following them. In addition, several women claimed a type of knowledge that enabled them to provide better care than any institutional staff. Like many other groups of caregivers we have studied in this book, these women asserted that they alone understood family members' unique qualities and could best respond to their individual needs.

Rather than accepting criticism of their living conditions as a justification for institutionalization, moreover, some women argued that the responsibility of the COS was to improve conditions, not to remove the sick. The women also complained about the poor quality of care at institutions. Caregivers frequently argued that hospitals and sanatoriums endangered, rather than promoted, health; many were convinced that family members would die soon after admission. Women who had previously lost family members in institutions vowed never again to surrender their kin.

Visits to institutionalized family members and letters from them convinced many women to seek early discharge. One woman noted that although her tubercular daughter had seemed to be "getting along nicely" when she first went to a private hospital, she recently had written "begging" to be brought home. The girl had developed pleurisy and neuralgia, which she attributed to the rain that came through an open window onto her bed.[75]

We can see that, according to charity workers' reports, the caregivers in client families generally remained within the interpretive grid imposed by the COS. Rather than rooting their criticisms of institutional care in an alternative system of medical knowledge, the caregivers relied on biomedical concepts to buttress their stance. Like the COS staff, women stressed the importance of cleanliness and the dangers of exposure to germs. Many also sought to portray themselves as delivering the type of care the COS valued, providing fresh air and ample food to tubercular patients and making them sleep alone. Some asked for the resources they needed to follow the recommended treatment plan. Moreover, although they pointed to factors very different from those disturbing charity workers, the caregivers focused on the burdens and stresses that encumbered their lives.

In one crucial respect, however, the caregivers departed from COS frameworks. Whereas charity workers elevated the virtues of self-reliance and rationality, caregivers appear to have spoken the language of emotion and intimacy. Caregiving was not just a set of exhausting tasks and demands to them but also a profound human experience that conferred meaning on their lives. Certain losses seemed overwhelmingly painful. Under pressure to hospitalize her husband with advanced tuberculosis, one woman said that she "never had been separated from him and could not bear to let him go now that he is so ill."[76] Women stressed not just their own grief but also that of their sick family members. When the COS urged a fourteen-year-old girl to enter a city hospital six months after leaving Otisville in 1912, the mother argued that the girl's extreme loneliness at the sanatorium showed that another separation from home would hasten her death.[77] Many parents sought to retrieve homesick children.

The COS responded to caregivers' arguments in various ways. Just as charity workers facilitated compliance with medical advice at home by providing special foods, so they tried to mute some objections to institutional care by occasionally paying the cost of transportation for family visits, providing outfits for people admitted to Otisville, obtaining information about institutionalized patients, and requesting transfers of patients in upstate New York to city facilities closer to their families. We have seen that the organization also urged the city to improve conditions in the hospitals it administered.

Nevertheless, charity workers disparaged most client complaints about the quality of institutional care. Although the COS was clearly aware of the terrible conditions at Metropolitan Hospital when Maria Germani entered that facility in 1918, charity workers tried to convince the parents that the girl was well treated there. The focus by caregivers on the strength of their personal ties also met criticism. Where women claimed to provide special attentiveness to family members' individual needs, charity workers and visiting nurses reproached them for overindulgence. Just as many caregivers who corresponded with Dr. Lawrence Flick sought to make him aware of patients' particularities, so Mrs. Germani stressed her daughter's special sensitivities, which made hospitalization intolerable to her. Although the COS did not comment on Mrs. Germani's assertion, the organization's unwillingness to intervene suggests that it considered Maria's personality irrelevant to her care. In a similar case seven years earlier, a COS charity worker complained about Italian immigrant parents who "absolutely refused" to compel their tubercular daughter to enter a sanatorium. "The child is very obstinate," the worker wrote, "and her family honor all her whims."[78]

There were exceptions to these patterns. I have noted that some women asked the COS for help in finding institutional placements for family members. In addition, some caregivers readily acceded to recommendations for institutionalization. Because caregiving is embedded in personal relationships, the quality of those relationships has always influenced the amount and type of care women are willing to provide. Clients who had the greatest conflict with sick family members were the most receptive to requests for institutionalization; in fact, a few women appear to have viewed institutional placement as a means of gaining protection from abusive husbands. Moreover, women's interpretations of their children's needs occasionally changed. Some who had adamantly refused to consider institutionalization when their children were very young dropped their opposition when those children grew older. The COS occasionally softened its demand that women find paid jobs when breadwinners were incapacitated. In a few cases, the organization provided small pensions to compensate for the lost incomes of institutionalized earners, thus enabling women to remain outside the labor force. In addition, the organization continued aiding a few families who rejected recommendations for institutionalization. Families accorded either type of special treatment tended to be considered unusually deserving.

Protecting Children

Some facilities sought to prevent tuberculosis rather than cure it. In 1909 Alfred Hess, a New York City pediatrician, established a "preventorium" for poorly nourished children who had been exposed to infection at home.[79] The facility accommodated 150 children between the ages of four and fourteen, who stayed an average of three months.[80] "The plan of treatment is simple," Hess wrote. "Plenty of good food, a twenty-four-hour-day in the open air, an intimate acquaintanceship with the fields and woods, and a practical lesson in cleanliness and hygiene."[81] The Department of Health assumed responsibility for selecting children.[82] Department of Health doctors also often recommended that children at high risk of tuberculosis be sent to boarding homes in the country for a few weeks; the COS made the arrangements for children in client families and raised money to pay for the trips.

Although Hess argued that parents willingly relinquished even very young children,[83] the COS case files suggest otherwise. The difficulty of visiting children may have sharpened parental opposition. Hess wrote that he wanted his facility to be "far enough from the city for the items of expenditure of time and money to act as a deterrent to frequent visits on the part of mothers."[84] Parents who could afford trips to the country sometimes were denied permission to see their children.

Parents also may have been reluctant to subject their children to the scrutiny of people who considered themselves socially superior. One boarding home owner complained that two boys sent by the COS "have no nightclothes nor proper underwear," were "inclined to be somewhat wild," and were "not very cleanly in person." Although the owner subsequently reported that the boys were "improving in manners," the parents may have been less pleased with the change.[85] Another boarding home owner expelled a boy after finding lice in his hair; the boy was accused of infecting the owner's wife and child.[86] Because moral uplift was central to Hess's program, preventorium staff, too, may have harshly judged the children in their charge.

Parents had their own fears and suspicions. Pressed to send her daughter to the country, one woman demanded assurances that the boarding home "is a good respectable place and that those who control it have a good reputation."[87] Just as a boarding home owner refused to tolerate a boy with verminous hair, so a mother was described as "very worried" by the discovery of nits in her daughter's hair after she returned from the country.[88] One man who was able to visit his son and daughter in a country house was "not pleased with the appearance of the place." The food was "poor" and did not include milk and eggs. His wife found bedbugs on the children's clothes after they returned. In addition, the girl had stomach cramps, which the mother attributed to the crab apples the child had been permitted to eat.[89]

⌒ A MAJOR THEME of Part Two of this volume is the impact of the expanding formal health care system on family caregiving. Lacking access to most private services, poor caregivers in New York City at the turn of the century relied on those established by the Department of Health. Not only were public health programs oversubscribed and underfunded, but they also encoded prevailing social anxieties about the poor and implicated caregivers in various state-centered forms of regulation. Although Dr. Lawrence Flick invoked the authority of medical expertise, he could not penalize caregivers who failed to comply with his instructions. Charity workers, however, were able to use the enforcement powers of the state to remove Maria Germani from her parents' custody when they disregarded doctor's orders.

Caregivers were hardly passive recipients of the advice they received. They sought out second opinions, allowed patients to miss clinic appointments and share beds with others, refused to heed advice about diet and cleanliness, and repeatedly rejected recommendations for placement in hospitals, sanatoriums, and preventoriums.

We should be cautious, however, about romanticizing resistance to public health authority. Social theorists currently emphasize resistance in order to describe the patterns of dominant groups without casting subordinate groups solely as victims. But our desire to restore agency to poor caregivers should not blind us to the fact that the advice they disregarded often addressed real needs. Caregivers who refused to clean sputum cups adequately, segregate tuberculosis sufferers at home, or enroll them in institutions endangered other family members. Although we no longer place faith in the therapeutic value of rich food for tuberculosis patients, contemporaries had reason to believe that any deviation from the prescribed diet brought serious risks.

Nevertheless, caregivers' responses to the tuberculosis program often made sense when viewed from their perspective. The prescribed standards of hygiene imposed overwhelming burdens on women without plumbing facilities. We saw in Chapter 4 that the growth of the formal service sector not only relieved family caregivers but also imposed new obligations on them. The task of mediating between sick people and formal services was especially onerous for poor women. Many could not afford to provide the outfits sanatoriums required or to visit institutionalized family members. In an era without personal leave days or job security, the many women who worked for pay risked dismissal when they took sick patients to clinic appointments or visited them in hospitals. Interactions with formal service providers also exposed caregivers to harsh assessment. They were faulted when their homes were considered too disorderly, their children too ill mannered, and their tubercular husbands too undisciplined. Above all, caregivers' emotionalism received condemnation. Many caregivers were proud of the special love and attention they bestowed on very sick people. To both health officials and charity workers, however, women's desires to nurse sick family members at home represented yet another indulgence of the poor.

~7

Caregiving during the Great Depression: Mothers Seeking Children's Health Care and American Indians Encountering Public Health Nurses

*T*HE STOCK MARKET crash of 1929, which plunged millions of Americans into poverty, drastically reduced access to formal health care services and, thus, dramatically altered the context of informal care. Lacking health insurance, most people paid out of pocket for medical care, but its cost had risen rapidly in the first decades of the twentieth century.[1] Although some doctors provided free services, a government committee estimated in 1938 that even the most basic health care was beyond the reach of a third to a half of all Americans; the cost of medical care for serious illness and long-term disability was prohibitive for the great majority.[2]

Few public services were available. Most large cities operated municipal hospitals, but many people lived in areas without such facilities. Moreover, shortages of beds, staff, and equipment seriously undermined the quality of care delivered in all public hospitals.[3] The three Depression-era programs that helped to fill some of the gaps in public services were grossly inadequate. As early as 1930, local relief offices began to provide special payments to cover the cost of medical care.[4] In 1937 the Farm Security Administration created a medical care program for poor farmers, sharecroppers, and migrant workers.[5] Crippled Children's Services, established under the Social Security Act of 1935, also expanded care, but eligibility varied widely because the act allowed state governments to define "crippled."

The lack of access to health care was felt especially acutely because the economic crisis coincided with heightened confidence in medicine. By the 1930s, such fearsome diseases as cholera, typhoid fever, and smallpox, which had reached epidemic proportions just decades earlier, were virtually eliminated, and other common killers, including rickets, syphilis, and dysentery, had lost much of their menace. Although historians now debate the extent to which medical advances contributed to the decline in infectious diseases, many people gave credit to science alone.[6] The growing efficacy of health care added a sense of urgency to the task of spreading its benefits to all sectors of society.

But public sentiment was hardly unanimous. Opposition to a national health program came not only from organized medicine but also from the many lay people convinced that health care should be distributed solely on the basis of market principles. Thus, although the Social Security Act greatly expanded social protection and made some provision for maternal and child health care, most health benefits remained part of public assistance, and typical welfare criteria continued to guide client selection.

Access to hospitals continued to be almost completely denied to people of color. Many Americans interpreted Darwinian theory as implying that both African Americans and American Indians were inherently inferior mentally and physically and thus, were doomed to extinction; neither education nor health care in this view could prevent the fulfillment of this biological destiny.[7] Throughout the South, most African Americans could gain admittance only to segregated wards, located in the basements of city hospitals.[8] Although people of color benefited when the control of public health programs was shifted from the states to Washington during the 1930s, discrimination continued. A 1940 study reported that only 2 percent of crippled African American children in rural Georgia received hospital care, compared to 40 percent of crippled white children.[9] Because most municipal hospitals refused to admit American Indians, they could receive care only in special institutions operated by the Office of Indian Affairs (OIA). The number of OIA hospitals rose during the 1930s, but most had too little equipment to provide even rudimentary treatment. Many American Indians had no access to any hospital.[10]

Not surprisingly, different groups of caregivers responded very differently to access problems. In this chapter we hear first from mothers who were anxious to receive the benefits of modern medicine for ailing children. We then examine American Indian caregivers on reservations. Some rejected the few services that public health nurses sought to impose, while others accepted them on their own terms.

"One God Is over All": Appealing for Children's Health Care

The emergence of the welfare state in the early twentieth century inaugurated a new stage in family caregiving. "Servicing work" expanded to include not just taking patients to medical appointments and visiting them in hospitals but also pressing claims on behalf of family members and negotiating with government bureaucrats. This section examines a collection of 258 letters mothers wrote to either Eleanor and Franklin D. Roosevelt or the Children's Bureau between 1929 and 1940. This collection, now located in the Children's Bureau Records in the National Archives,[11] also contains reports of investigations conducted by caseworkers and public health officials. During the 1930s, the Children's Bureau routinely referred letters to state and local agencies with a request that they follow up. In 56 cases, the agencies sent reports back to the Bureau. After the election of 1932, thousands of people also wrote to Eleanor and Franklin D. Roosevelt. Although the Roosevelts or their staffs answered many letters themselves, many others were routed to relevant government agencies. The Children's Bureau was the destination for correspondence about children's health.

The letters in this collection were written by a variety of relatives; even a few children wrote on their own behalf. The overwhelming majority of correspondents, however, were mothers, and I therefore refer to the letter writers collectively as such. In the 1930s, as today, women had primary responsibility for preventing illness among family members, caring for them in times of sickness, and getting help from outside services.[12] Because of the way the letters were collected, we cannot be sure how representative they are. Nevertheless, nearly a third of the women provided some demographic information about themselves. That information enables us to sketch a portrait of the letter writers.

The Depression frayed marital bonds, and single women were particularly vulnerable to economic distress.[13] It is thus not surprising that more than 25 percent of these women were either unmarried or separated from their husbands. Married women also reported serious economic problems when husbands either could not work, were unemployed, or held only part-time or irregular jobs. Although other husbands worked full-time, their earnings were still insufficient to pay for medical care.

Many correspondents indicated that they were just getting by. Although they could pay for the routine necessities of life, they had nothing left for emergencies. Relatively few letter writers, however, appear to have come from the ranks of the most impoverished. Although one correspondent was living in a migrant workers' camp and another was sleeping in a car, writing letters was not likely to be a high priority for the great majority of those engaged in the most desperate struggles for survival. The only correspondents identified as people of color were African Americans.

The medical conditions discussed in these letters are heavily biased toward chronic illnesses and disabilities, perhaps because mothers were unlikely to embark on the lengthy process of soliciting help from the federal government for problems that could be resolved relatively quickly. The health complaints most frequently noted in the letters were eye problems (77), tonsils and adenoids (30), asthma (25), ear problems (25), heart problems (23), tuberculosis (22), dental problems (17), orthopedic problems (16), diabetes (13), and skin problems (10).

Although most correspondents lacked access to the health care system, some complained about the quality of services available. They wanted private medical care, which they assumed was superior to public care. Others had already seen private providers but were dissatisfied with the results. Convinced that elite practitioners could provide a cure, they wanted the government to send their children to such eminent institutions as Johns Hopkins Hospital, or the Mayo Clinic, or to "a great doctor" or "the best authority in the field."

Women typically wrote to the Children's Bureau or the White House only after exhausting other avenues of help. Many mothers reported that repeated rebuffs had made them "desperate." They recited a litany of complaints about the private health care system. Although some women sought help paying medical bills, many complained that health care providers had refused to furnish treatment without payment. One mother asked Franklin D. Roosevelt to find help for her sixteen-month-old daughter stricken with spinal meningitis. A private hospital had admitted the child but then withheld treatment while waiting for the mother to pay.[14] An Arkansas mother wrote about her experience with local doctors: "I call the Dr. he says Mrs. B. . . . you owe me and I cant come. All I can Say is yes I owe you some but I Cant help it and then on the other hand you look at it [his fees] are so high, it would tax a rich man to have them. I lost my little girl with pnemonia and membras croup because the Dr. Just Set Down and would not come Back. Now I had a man out the other Day Saying you are going to Pay the Dr. or you Cant get one we have a medicine bord to that Effect."[15]

Other women recounted their difficulties gaining access to public programs and services. Some learned that they had not lived in a particular county long enough to qualify for help. A rural Michigan woman wrote Eleanor Roosevelt in January 1939:

Before thanksgiving Robert my 14 year old son was sent home from school and ordered to have a chest exray he had it and the Dr. said he has T.B. Have all your children exrayed I did and all 5 had T.B. They put them all out of school and said they would send the children to a T.B. Hospital Now it is two months they are fighting between counties to see who will do it the oldest boy is getting worse when he coughs he raises blood. Now I lived in Berriam Co. Niles town ship about 3 years and I moved to Cass Co. Howard town ship last July the 9 . . . What county is supposed to take the children? I have done every thing I can do and all I was told to do and the house I live in is to cold for animals let alone sick children.[16]

Other parents discovered that the conditions from which their children suffered fell outside the scope of public programs. The father of a twelve-year-old boy with asthma in West Virginia wrote, "My heart has been full of good faith that sure I was going to get some kind help for my boy when Mrs. Carr [of the State Department of Public Assistance] from Princeton W. Va. come to investigate my case. But today my dreams have disappear because she said they can't do anything for my boy that is chronic case."[17]

Although some letter writers pointed to restrictive regulations disqualifying them from public programs, most correspondents interpreted their rejections as the result of individuals' decisions. The claimants assumed that local officials exercised broad discretion and had denied their requests out of callousness or indifference.

It has become almost commonplace to argue that state welfare programs historically have served to forestall social unrest by placating the poor and defusing their hostility.[18] But the letters in this study suggest that these programs could heighten, as well as dampen, resentment. Several parents expressed anger at their sense of powerlessness. They could not make authorities listen to them or acknowledge the urgency of their requests. Another West Virginia father, who had sought help for his daughter, wrote, "I have apeald to our County Welfare to help me have her treated and the[y] Seem to not Pay me eny mind."[19] The frustration of not being able to communicate with public officials is also evident in the following letter from a rural Minnesota woman who had unsuccessfully sought both medical and dental care for her five children. "I believe that you are doing all you [can]," she wrote to Franklin D. Roosevelt, "but there's those who hold offices who don't believe a poor person what they say to them. It's hard for me to explain to you too."[20]

Respecting medical expertise, many parents were shocked to realize that relief officers would disregard requests for services that doctors had ordered. "Here is my problem," wrote a mother in New York City in 1939. "I am now on Home Relief. I have two children, one of whom is a heart case . . . This boy who is ill needs special food as he is 11 years of age and much under weight (63 lbs.) This child must have digitalis, (3 a day) and I don't seem to be able to obtain such from my investigator. For some reason she does not think it necessary."[21] A Louisiana woman wrote to Eleanor Roosevelt,

> I have been at the Welfare Office to ask them to give me a help to take care of my sick boy. He has Masthoid. There are a month that he hasn't been treated for I haven't any money to take him to the Hospital he was suppose to see the doctor every week. My husband is working on the W.P.A. and he only get $29.92 a month. And Mrs. Kathleen Troxler the Parish Welfare Director want me to use that money to take care of the child. Now Mrs. Roosevelt if I use this little salary to take care of the sick child, What will the rest do. I have to support 3 boys going to school what will I give them to eat?[22]

Many parents interpreted the denial of essential services as evidence that officials had no regard for their children's basic worth and humanity. An African American grandmother requesting assistance from Franklin D. Roosevelt reminded him of the religious injunction to regard every human life as precious. "Plese dont throw this letter in the Wast Basket and let that settle it," she wrote. Her grandson was "a Colored boy But he is Human and one God is over all."[23] Several mothers described particularly blatant forms of humiliation. One wrote on behalf of her sixteen-year-old diabetic son. "Please let me know who to go to so I can get help," she implored Franklin D. Roosevelt. "They say at the relief office that there is no way to help him and one man said to me when I ask him (quote) 'O he is your boy no one cares if he dies it is only one kid out [of] the way.' Now I dont like that kind of an answer."[24]

Some women sought monetary assistance to purchase care from private health providers, while others turned to services delivered directly by the public sector. But these, too, drew criticism. Mothers were well aware that public hospitals frequently offered inferior care. A typical comment came from a woman in California, who described herself as "almost worried to death" about her three-year-old son, who had both a rupture and an undescended testicle. She had tried to save money to pay for a private doctor, but her income was too meager. "Perhaps you will ask 'Why dont I take him to the County Hospital?'" she wrote to Eleanor Roosevelt. "I will answer honestly. I haven't any confidence in them. I have had him out there before. Please try to under stand. He is my boy and I love him. I want him under a good doctor."[25]

The letter writers framed their requests in two ways. The majority of women who wrote to either Eleanor or Franklin D. Roosevelt appealed to them as individuals. A typical letter to Eleanor Roosevelt began this way: "Mrs. Roosevelt, since you are both a Mother and a Grandmother, you can readily understand the anxiety we are feeling about our little baby's health."[26] Several correspondents addressed Eleanor Roosevelt as "Dear Friend" or "Kind Lady." Others expressed the belief that the New Deal reflected Franklin D. Roosevelt's essential goodness. Giving him sole credit for the new programs, the letter writers distinguished him from the local officials who had ignored their children's needs and denied them dignity. The Roosevelts' charitable acts also impressed some letter writers. "I have heard how good and kind you both are, and of the kind deeds you have done or the many people who have needed them," wrote a Chicago mother. "Couldn't I be another of these people?"[27] Some expected Eleanor or Franklin D. Roosevelt not only to single them out for special attention but also to intervene personally on their behalf. One woman, for example, asked Franklin D. Roosevelt to lend her the money to buy a cow.[28]

Other letter writers put their faith in the development of national programs rather than individual acts of compassion. Numerous observers have noted that the expansion of welfare programs often increases citizens' sense of entitlement.[29] The passage of the New Deal legislation had enlarged the felt needs of many correspondents and given them courage to articulate new grievances and make further demands on the state for social protection. Assuming that health care was a right they could claim as citizens, they were shocked to discover how little was available. "Isn't there some fund?" women repeatedly asked, to pay for the various services their children needed. Pointing out that many of Franklin D. Roosevelt's charitable deeds focused narrowly on the victims of infantile paralysis, they urged him to extend the range of his beneficence.

Regardless of whether they presented their cases in terms of personal benevolence or social justice, the letter writers sought to demonstrate their moral worth. Numerous correspondents claimed the classic traits of the deserving poor: they were thrifty, hardworking, sober, and self-reliant. "We are not lazy people," wrote a mother in Horseshoe Bend, Idaho, seeking money for her son's tonsillectomy. "Hard luck has just come our way."[30] Several stressed that neither they nor their children should be blamed for illnesses. Many supplied references to buttress their claims that they were upstanding citizens.

The women also sought to compose acceptable portraits of the men in their families. Letter after letter noted that husbands had been in the military; some also included the information that the men had received honorable discharges or had been wounded in battle. Women also expressed pride in their husbands' occupational histories. The mother of a boy with rickets wrote of her husband, "He is known as a sober, honest and reliable man where ever he has worked."[31]

Women presented themselves as fulfilling the cultural definition of good mothers. They wrote that they had devotedly nursed sick children, searched tirelessly for appropriate services, and denied themselves all luxuries. Five noted that they had not purchased new clothes for themselves in over a year.

In addition, mothers frequently pointed to the unique characteristics of their children. Several women enclosed snapshots of their offspring in particularly charming poses. One woman asked permission to bring her mute sister to visit Eleanor Roosevelt, adding, "I am sure you would try to help if you could only see her because she is such a sweet child and is a picture of health and well being"; friends of the family already had agreed to pay the fare.[32] Other women wrote that their children learned quickly, earned good grades in school, had high occupational aspirations, or demonstrated unusual artistic or musical abilities. A woman whose eleven-year-old daughter had multiple physical problems remarked, "She's smart enough she's in 5th grade and her marks are good, that's why I can't see why she can't be helped."[33]

Finally, some letter writers sought to demonstrate their worthiness by noting that they were white, native-born Christians. A few claimed what they considered especially distinguished lineages. A woman who alerted the authorities to the health problems of her sister's children commented, "These people are natives of the State of Tennessee as far back as 8 generations their families had paid taxes there so I believe you will agree with me that they deserve help if anyone does."[34]

How can we understand the effort to demonstrate personal worth? In many cases it may have been a rhetorical strategy. Because health care remained part of the welfare system, women seeking benefits from the federal government, like clients of charitable organizations, had to display individual merit. But it is likely that the mothers also were exhibiting the parochialism too often associated with caregiving. Preoccupation with the problems of particular children often obscured the needs of more distant ones.[35] I write throughout this book about the empathic knowledge that caregivers frequently counterpose to professional knowledge. Here mothers were using their deep and intimate understanding of their own children to advocate for them alone. In addition, many letter writers may have shared the cultural assumptions that were current at the time. In Chapter 2 we saw several examples of white, middle-class women in the nineteenth century who used their shared vulnerability to suffering to forge close bonds of interdependence. But we also saw that mutuality rarely crossed lines of class and race. Most employers, for example, felt little responsibility for servants who fell ill. In the 1930s, as well, social prejudices narrowed the range of concern. Letter writers from relatively privileged backgrounds believed that their children had special entitlement to meager government resources.

Although the Children's Bureau answered every letter, its replies became shorter and less personal as the agency grew more bureaucratic during the 1930s.[36] The increasingly standard response informed correspondents that the federal government could not offer the assistance they sought and that the letter would be referred to the relevant agencies at either the state or local level. Of the 258 letters in this collection, the Children's Bureau referred 135 elsewhere. A few were sent to voluntary agencies, such as children's aid societies; the great majority were sent to public entities. Although some letters went directly to local agencies, most were addressed to state authorities, such as health or welfare departments, with a request that they refer the letters to the appropriate agencies at the local level. Several letters went to the very officials about whom the mothers had complained.

The Children's Bureau typically did not ask for or receive reports on its referrals. Many of the replies merely acknowledged receipt of the letters. There is, therefore, no way of determining how often authorities actually followed up. In 56 cases, however, the authorities enclosed reports of investigations and provided some indication of the actions taken in response to the mothers' requests.

Children occasionally received at least some of the medical care their parents had requested.[37] When a Missouri woman learned that a county clinic would provide both her daughter and granddaughter with the antisyphilitic treatment she had sought, she expressed her joy in a letter to the State Board of Health. "I believe heaven fell in my arms," she wrote. "When Dr. T. L. Waddle of State Health District No. 2 of Dexter Mo. sent his Nurse to see me last week . . . I was so Happy. That was the first time I ever was that close to H. on Earth."[38]

The state and local authorities most likely to fulfill the mothers' requests were those who interpreted their jurisdictions broadly, drawing on private, as well as public, resources. In one case, a state official directed a county health officer to work harder to galvanize voluntary aid. The county health officer of Laurens County, South Carolina, had reported to R. W. Ball, the director of maternal and child health of the

State Board of Health, that a young girl with syphilis could obtain treatment at a local clinic but that she had no means of getting there.[39] Ball wrote back, urging the health officer to "contact the various service groups, churches, civic groups, etc., as the case may be, with transportation as your objective."[40] A month later Ball was able to inform the Children's Bureau that arrangements had been made for the girl's transportation and that she was undergoing treatment.[41]

Few cases ended so happily. Most authorities had to explain to the Children's Bureau why they could not fulfill the mothers' requests. Just as letter writers strove to compose acceptable portraits of themselves, so state and local authorities hoped their replies to the Bureau would reflect well on themselves. Many health care programs they administered received federal funding, and some, such as Crippled Children's Services, were under the direct control of the Children's Bureau. Especially in the South, state and local authorities frequently resented federal interference, but all had an interest in creating a favorable impression.

Government officials justified their denials of assistance in several ways. Some pointed to restrictive eligibility criteria in various programs and services. Children with heart problems or hearing difficulties fell outside the scope of Crippled Children's Services in several states. The residency requirements of welfare departments and public hospitals excluded many other claimants.

Segregation provided another rationale for inaction. The city health officer of Asheville, North Carolina, explained her inability to satisfy one mother's request this way: "Our hospital facilities in Asheville for colored people are very limited, there being only fifteen beds available for them. During the winter months these beds are filled with sick patients and it is only during warm weather that we can use them for a tonsillectomy."[42]

Officials also pointed out that no publicly funded program could reach more than a tiny fraction of needy children. The staff of some public agencies acknowledged that they had been compelled to ration services on the basis of cost. The director of the Wilson County Department of Public Health in Tennessee wrote that although insulin was necessary to keep a thirteen-year-old girl alive, her supply had been discontinued because of the expense.[43]

Officials also excused themselves from extending assistance in some cases by pointing to the enormous misery surrounding them. Several authorities wrote that they were inundated by requests for help. Another common justification for inaction was mothers' erroneous description of children's health status. All reports included results of medical examinations conducted by either the investigators themselves or local physicians. On this basis, some reports accused letter writers of fabricating their stories of illness. Others asserted that the prognosis was more hopeless than mothers had indicated and that treatment would therefore be futile. Investigators drew on the mystique of medical science to establish their accounts as authoritative; many reports gave precise numbers and diagnoses to counter the mothers' vague terminology.

Because health benefits remained part of public assistance, social and economic factors were as important as medical diagnoses in determining eligibility. The investigators followed the standard procedures for evaluating applicants, making home visits and conducting interviews with employers, neighbors, schoolteachers, welfare officers, and the staff of various social service agencies. Home visits were especially intrusive. Like the charity workers examined in the previous chapter, investigators arrived unannounced to observe the cleanliness of the home, the range and quality of household possessions, and the nature of family relationships.

In a few cases, investigators concluded that the letter writers had lied about their inability to pay for medical care. They reported that some women who claimed to have been deserted had husbands living at home, some who asserted that their husbands were unemployed were relying on their husbands' weekly paychecks, and some who stated that their husbands were too ill to work had husbands who were perfectly able bodied.

Letter writers and investigators also clashed about the amount of money needed to support a family. A widow in West Virginia, for example, had written that her six children were "awful sick" and that she was "in need very much." She had needed to destroy all her bedding following the death of her husband from tuberculosis and received only $28 a month from Aid to Dependent Children (ADC).[44] The county health officer, however, believed her income was adequate. "This woman," he concluded, "is apparently of a very shiftless sort, and expects some one else to assume all her responsibilities."[45]

Another recurrent charge was that women spent too much on unnecessary purchases. Complaints about "poor management" were common. As noted, a preeminent concern of the letter writers was to demonstrate that they were willing to sacrifice all but the most basic goods. But what was a necessity to a correspondent was often a luxury to an investigator.[46] One woman protested her caseworker's demand that she relinquish her radio, thus saving the cost of its monthly rental charge. "The lady from Child Welfare said that I cant have no Radio," the mother wrote to the Children's Bureau. "So I tell her I am allways home. I just go to Church. That's my only pleasure I have."[47] The investigators whose reports are included in this chapter viewed a wide range of possessions as dispensable. They pointed to cars, telephones, refrigerators, "a power washing machine," and a "modern cook stove" as evidence that parents had disposable income and, therefore, could purchase medical care without government assistance.

Investigators also focused on the letter writers' qualities as parents. As Winifred Bell showed in her classic study, a key requirement of income maintenance programs in the early twentieth century was that recipients be "fit parents" and maintain "suitable homes."[48] These concepts were central to client selection for the mothers' pensions enacted in individual states after 1911 and then in the federal Aid to Dependent Children (ADC) program, which followed in 1935. Because health benefits were viewed as part of income protection, it is not surprising that these criteria guided investigators reporting to the Children's Bureau.[49] None questioned the appropriateness of denying aid to children because their parents were deemed incapable of rearing them properly.

Failure to uphold high moral standards was held against many letter writers. Like countless charity workers and relief officers, investigators routinely interpreted children's illegitimacy, the presence of boarders in the home, and crowded sleeping arrangements as signs of depravity. Investigators also found repeated examples of poor housekeeping skills. Several nurses who made home visits reported that the housekeeping was "atrocious" or "deplorable." Children's misbehavior also could be grounds for denying them help. When children "roamed the streets" during school hours or received poor grades in school, they showed that their parents were ill equipped to exercise custodial responsibilities.

Some of the harshest criticism was reserved for those who refused to defer to their social superiors. Despite the pressure on letter writers to present themselves as worthy of aid, a few failed to display approved behaviors and attitudes. Several mothers also maintained distance from professional authority. Because they were seeking health services, all correspondents had at least some faith in medical expertise, but some had consulted chiropractors or other alternative medical practitioners, failed to keep medical appointments for their children, or refused to comply with recommendations for institutionalization. Those who avoided public hospitals and clinics were especially likely to incur the wrath of investigators. I have noted that many women expressed anxiety about the quality of care provided in municipal facilities, but to investigators, this was no excuse for spurning such services. A representative of the Fayette County Children's Bureau in Kentucky criticized a mother who had "gone ahead taking her children to private doctors, building up drug bills in drug stores because as she said, she could not bear to go to the public clinic with her children."[50]

The complaints of an African American woman in Missouri about the treatment rendered in segregated facilities also elicited little sympathy. The woman's grandson suffered from a serious skin condition, and she had sought help from Franklin D. Roosevelt. Although the boy had received care in the city hospital, the grandmother wrote that "they never did any good," and she asked Roosevelt to pay the fee of a private physician who had promised a cure. The Children's Bureau referred the letter to the state health department, which in turn sent it to Mayme Penn, the social service worker in the Kansas City Colored Hospital. Penn reported that the grandmother had frequently missed appointments at the hospital for the boy. Ignoring the grandmother's complaint about the quality of care the boy had received and her desire to obtain private medical care for him, Penn explained why she could dismiss the case: "I know you will see by the information given that the family has received treatment and the real cause for not receiving any further treatment on all occasions is their non-cooperative attitude."[51]

If investigators rebuked some claimants for their lack of confidence in public services, they reproached others for their extravagant faith in medical science. One South Dakota father had described a particularly harrowing plight. Two of his children had died of diabetes. Four of the remaining eight suffered from the same disease; two were blind, and another was rapidly losing his eyesight. The father requested that his ailing children be sent to the illustrious Mayo Clinic. But the field-worker for the Department of Social Security who investigated the case concluded that the real problem was the father's inability to reconcile himself to his losses. "It is our impression," the field-worker wrote, "that the family can be aided further only by helping them to better understand their problems and the part they must play in coping with all the difficulties in which they find themselves."[52]

Parents also were faulted for failing to accept the limitations of local agencies. Many state and local authorities expressed anger at parents' efforts to seek recourse from the federal government. Charges of discrimination provoked particular outrage. The medical director of the Department of Institutions and Agencies in New Jersey answered one mother's complaint this way: "When I think of the terrific load which Atlantic City and Atlantic County carry for the negro group, I get impatient at their attitude that they are discriminated against because they are negroes."[53]

As noted, many women appealed to Washington after having exhausted every other channel of help. Some mothers spoke with pride of their persistence, which they presented as a sign of maternal devotion. To investigators, however, mothers who wrote to high government officials were "complainers." They showed a lack of appreciation for the benefits they had received and an inability to adjust to the inevitable.

The evaluation process left ample leeway for cultural, racial, and other biases. All investigators presented themselves as neutral and impartial, but the prejudices pervading their reports are readily apparent to present-day readers. The director of the Marshall County Health Department in Mississippi, for example, wrote of a mother whose case he had investigated, "I think she is typical of the ignorant and superstitious class we find among our poor people."[54]

Because most investigators in these cases did not identify the race of letter writers, it is difficult to determine the extent to which racial prejudices skewed judgments. Other researchers, however, report that the "fit parent" and "suitable home" requirements of the mothers' pension and ADC programs routinely served to exclude African Americans from benefits.[55] It is likely that many investigators reporting to the Children's Bureau also were prone to dismiss African Americans as unworthy.

The concept of deservedness also incorporated the prevailing gender assumptions of the time. Although investigators expected women to justify their failure to get a job before they could be considered for public programs, the employment histories of men received far more intense scrutiny than those of women. Mothers alone, however, were judged on their ability to manage scarce household resources and minister to the needs of chronically ill or disabled children.

Despite the biases evident in these reports, they invariably were accepted as objective and neutral. In no case did the state or local officials who had commissioned the investigations question the findings. When reports contradicted letter writers' assertions, officials invariably assumed that investigators had uncovered the truth. I have noted that the Children's Bureau rarely asked to be informed of the results of investigations. The agency also typically refrained from commenting on reports that were sent, even when they revealed that authorities had bestowed only the most cursory attention on the letter writers' problems.

American Indians on Reservations

The economic situation of American Indians during the Depression was even more desperate than that of most mothers who wrote to Washington about their children's health problems. By the 1930s, American Indian people had undergone two centuries of catastrophic upheaval. Encroachment by white entrepreneurs, farmers, and soldiers, as well as years of warfare, had left many people dependent on rations from the federal government. The Depression caused new devastation, further increasing reliance on government resources.[56]

In order to survive, American Indians had long made many accommodations, such as sending children to boarding schools, using the agricultural and ranching methods taught by government agents, and moving into log houses. Contrary to the assimilationist credo, these changes neither reflected nor produced wholesale repudiation of traditional values and beliefs. By selectively appropriating white practices, American Indians were able to transform their cultures without destroying them. In this section I argue that caregivers on reservations adopted a similar strategy in their encounters with public health nurses. The nurses viewed caregivers as passive recipients of white knowledge and predefined services. The caregivers, however, retained their own beliefs and practices, while picking and choosing among the types of care the nurses offered.[57]

Most American Indian people had a health care system based on the interrelationship between people and the environment. Because health was considered the result of harmony and balance, disease was thought to stem from some form of disequilibrium. American Indians drew a distinction between diseases that originated in environmental disruptions, which could be cured by healers trained in natural remedies, and those that resulted from spiritual forces and required the intervention of spiritual healers.[58]

Various assaults had seriously weakened this system by 1930. Much traditional knowledge was lost during epidemics because large numbers of healers died before they could transmit healing lore to the members of younger generations. The consolidation of reservations in the early twentieth century reduced access to the plants from which traditional remedies were derived. And Europeans introduced lethal infectious diseases that were unfamiliar to indigenous healers. Although many American Indian people assumed that white practitioners were best equipped to provide some services, they did not embrace white medicine as a substitute for the declining American Indian health care system.[59]

Nurses hired by the Office of Indian Affairs (OIA) were responsible for dispensing most of the government health services provided on reservations in the 1930s.[60] Dubbed "field nurses" to differentiate them from nurses employed by the Public Health Service, most were white, native-born women from middle-class backgrounds. They typically arrived on reservations knowing little or nothing about the people they were expected to serve. Although some sought opportunities to learn about American Indian cultures, others saw no reason to do so; few tried to learn an American Indian language.[61]

The field nurses dismissed American Indian health beliefs as arbitrary and bizarre. Most nurses believed that American Indians were capable of reason but had to be taught how to exercise it. Subscribing to a notion of reason transcending historical and social conditions, the nurses denied the possibility that American Indians could be active participants in the construction of meaning and knowledge. They assumed that American Indians would follow a linear progression from understanding the principles of health to the eradication of all traditional practices. That model left no room for ambiguity or syncretism.

This section relies on two different types of sources. We first examine the accounts of the field nurses, including their letters, memoirs, and, above all, their monthly and annual reports to Washington.[62] These reports consisted of a two-page statistical section, in which the nurses enumerated the services they had rendered, and a longer narrative section, in which they delineated their goals, chronicled their activities, and discussed individual cases. Because the nurses had little direct supervision, these reports were the principal means of monitoring their performance. Thus, the nurses had an obvious interest in presenting their work in the best possible light and expressing attitudes that mirrored those of officials. Nevertheless, the reports provide some insight into the nurses' assumptions and their work.

I also draw on oral histories of the field nurses' clients. In-depth, semistructured interviews were conducted with residents of two Sioux reservations in South Dakota in August 1993. The twenty-three respondents included seventeen women and six men. All were at least seventy years old and, thus, old enough to have interacted with the field nurses in the 1930s.[63]

Again, caveats are necessary. First, because there are significant differences among the Sioux people, I may draw questionable generalizations from the respondents. Second, although I rely on the reports of field nurses throughout the country, I have interviews from members of only one tribe; nurses who worked in more than one region occasionally remarked that different tribes responded differently to their work. In addition, the interviews rely on the ability to recall events occurring more than half a century earlier; we can assume that the intervening years affected many memories. The respondents were children when they had contact with the field nurses and were asked in the interviews to discuss actions taken by parents on their behalf. Although the respondents could identify fundamental family values and beliefs, they may have misconstrued some of their parents' actions. Because of these limitations, we cannot assume that the interviews offer a more objective account than do the field nurses' reports. Nevertheless, the respondents powerfully challenge the nurses' interpretation of their interactions with American Indian people.

Although the field nurses insisted that health education was their primary focus, they engaged in a broad range of activities, including screening for such conditions as trachoma, tuberculosis, and sexually transmitted diseases, providing immunizations, delivering home care, and placing clients in institutions for sickness and childbirth. A recurrent theme in the nurses' reports was opposition by caregivers to their services. Like the destitute New Yorkers discussed in Chapter 6, some caregivers sought to hide family illnesses from outsiders. One mother took particularly aggressive steps to avoid detection. Seeing a nurse arrive, she "threw a blanket over the child." When the nurse "rashly . . . picked up the edge of the blanket to look under," the mother snatched it away and threatened the nurse with a knife.[64] The day after Nettie Johnston Story attended a home birth, she learned that a family living in a back room of the house had remained hidden because their baby was gravely ill with pneumonia.[65] Other parents reassured nurses that children were "all right," "fine," or "getting better" when, in fact, death was imminent.

Even caregivers who welcomed the nurses into their homes often rejected the nurses' claims to special expertise. Denied permission to take a child with a nasal hemorrhage to the hospital, M. Gertrude Sturges packed the nose herself. Returning to the home a few hours later, she found that "they had removed the packing." Although Sturges repacked the nose and applied ice, she could not convince the family of the merits of her treatment. At sundown "the medicine man arrived and we were forced to give up and go away. Their comment was, 'the nurse was no good, nose packing was no good, I should have been able to give medicine to have stopped the bleeding.'"[66]

The greatest resistance was to institutionalization. Report after report describes confrontations with parents who refused to send their sick children to hospitals or sanatoriums. "In some ways, this has been a very difficult month," wrote Ruth I. Peffley, explaining that a one-year-old child had developed bronchial pneumonia. "It was diagnosed at the very onset by the government doctor and urged to go to hospital. The family refused and three days later drove the babe fifty miles to an off the reservation doctor only to receive the same advice . . . Finally after much maneuvering and running about by the family, they were again approached concerning the hospital with the same negative reply. At the end of the eight days the babe died. A deliberate sacrifice to false beliefs."[67]

Resistance continued after institutionalization. Margaret Mary Schorn, a Washington nurse, wrote, "A very trying situation confronts us in that the parents of tubercular children take the patients out of the sanatorium against advice. The little tots go back into the contaminative, unhygienic homes and peculiar habits, some descript and some nondescript and the splended work of the sanatoria is completely obliterated."[68]

Because the field nurses' reports provide no insight into the reasons why American Indians rejected or accepted specific services, it is necessary to turn to other sources. Our interviews suggest that although the nurses expected American Indians to abjure all traditional practices, most people accepted white medical care to supplement their own healing system, not to supplant it. Caregivers thus agreed to institutionalization only when their own efforts no longer seemed adequate. Examining the conflicts that arose over the care of children with tuberculosis helps to illuminate the two competing perspectives.

In the words of the Merriam Report, written at the request of the secretary of the interior in 1928, tuberculosis was "without a doubt the most serious disease among Indians."[69] The tuberculosis death rate was seven times that of the rest of the population.[70] According to Sarah Smith, the disease was present "in almost every home" in Pine Ridge.[71]

Despite official statements of concern about the prevalence of tuberculosis, the government never committed the funds necessary to mount an effective campaign of control. In 1934 the OIA operated fifteen sanatoriums, containing 1,315 beds.[72] Occupancy rates were extremely high. Many field nurses convinced clients to enroll in institutions only to discover that vacancies did not exist. "No room at the inn," wrote Anna A. Perry, a Wisconsin nurse. "I wish I had a good stable somewhere for T.B. children of pre-school age."[73] The few places available were often hundreds of miles away. Zelma Butcher reported driving three days to take Pine Ridge patients to a sanatorium in Albuquerque.[74] The poor quality of the roads, coupled with bad weather conditions, made such journeys perilous. After noting that tubercular patients in Washington and Oregon had to travel two days by "day coach" before embarking on a long car trip to reach a Nevada sanatorium, the Merriam Report commented, "Obviously such a trip is beyond all reason for a case of active tuberculosis."[75] Many of the government cars the nurses drove were open;[76] those that were closed lacked heat.[77] All were in poor condition and frequently broke down.

The sanatoriums operated by the OIA were seriously deficient. The 1935 annual report of the Phoenix Indian Sanatorium stated, "The crying need of the entire institution . . . is an increase in the operating allotment. For the past fiscal year, the per diem cost per patient was less than $1.50." The majority of buildings were "in a most deplorable condition"; the equipment was "woefully inadequate."[78] Carrie Brilstra, a nurse at the sanatorium in Dulce, New Mexico, later wrote that she was shocked to discover that the institution had only four thermometers for eighty patients and that X-ray films frequently were "unreadable."[79]

Just as the New York Charity Organization Society viewed the Germanis' refusal to place Maria in an overcrowded and underfunded hospital as evidence of their personal failings, so the nurses focused on the shortcomings of American Indian caregivers when explaining their resistance to sanatorium placement. Because they were "superstitious," "backward," and "prejudiced," nurses claimed, American Indian caregivers clung to traditional practices and believed even outrageous rumors about sanatoriums. Such labels permitted the nurses to disregard the motives of caregivers, treating them as obstacles on the path to progress. The nurses could thus construct accounts in which all initiative came from them. Institutionalization occurred, in the nurses' view, because they "educated" caregivers, "sold" them on the benefits of sanatoriums, and "persuaded" them to enter. Margaret Mary Schorn wrote, "In many instances I made five to six trips to some families selling them the idea of hospitalization. All their prejudices, misinformation, suspicion etc. was very hard to overcome. However, we won to the extent that we gained consent from every parent who had a tuberculous child . . . I count this as a decided victory for the medical workers in the field."[80] Assuming that American Indian parents could not be trusted to determine the best interests of their children, Schorn depicted herself as engaged in a campaign to wrest consent from the parents. Each child's entry into the sanatorium thus represented a personal triumph.

We interviewed three Sioux women who had suffered from tuberculosis as children; their comments help to restore agency to the field nurses' clients. All three believed that their parents and grandparents had not opposed sanatorium placement in all circumstances but had viewed institutionalization as an option to be considered only when home care proved inadequate. A woman who had lived with her grandmother said, "One time I was about 17 years old I was really sick. At that time the people really have TB. And I had it too, at that time. So those tell me I should go to the government sanatorium. I didn't go, I stayed home. And I'd get up early in the morning to go outside and go for a walk and then come back. And I was all right. Miss Butcher [the field nurse], she was there. She give me clothes or stuff that I drink in the morning." Despite the nurse's insistence on sanatorium placement, "Grandma didn't want me to go so I didn't. Stayed home." This girl had been relatively isolated from other family members and appeared to be in no immediate danger; the grandmother considered herself qualified to give care. Unable to institutionalize the girl, the nurse assisted the grandmother, providing clothes and special food.

The comments of the two other respondents suggest that even parents who complied with recommendations for institutionalization did so on their own terms. One recalled,

> At that time, you know, TB was going through the reservation. My mom was a good nurse. She kept me clean. There was a whole bundle of bandages there. Denver mud. That's what they treated me with. Part of the time I stayed at home. But there was a time that my dad took me to Rapid City on the train and left me over there. I really cried so bad . . . There was another girl that was with me at that time. And she didn't go and she's dead. So my dad thought you better go for that so I went. And I survived.

This woman had been able to remain at home for a period because her mother was a "good nurse" who knew how to care for her.

The third woman reported yet another experience:

> My mother . . . died. And then, after that . . . it just seemed like I didn't feel good at all. And that was when Mrs. Hemm, the field nurse, took me into the clinic in Rosebud and they run a series of tests on me and they said I had TB. So what did they do, they sent me to Iowa. It's on the Sac and Fox reservation. And the reason I was sent there was when my dad was in Carlisle [a boarding school] he befriended a man from there and became blood brothers, more binding than birth brothers. So anyway there he knew that he and his wife would give me good attention because he wrote him a letter explaining that my mother had died. So then I was in the hospital in there.

Circumstances, not conversion to white medicine, explained this father's acceptance of institutional care. Unlike the caregivers in the first two cases, he did not have the resources to tend his daughter at home. Because his wife had died and he had a full-time job at the subagency, he concluded that the best way to care for his daughter was to send her away. Nevertheless, he was determined to remain in charge of his daughter's care. Although patients from Rosebud and Pine Ridge did not normally go to the sanatorium at Sac and Fox, he insisted that his daughter be close to a man he trusted to look after her. When the father concluded that his friend was not fulfilling his responsibility adequately, he brought the girl home.

～ THE TASK of mediating between ailing family members and formal service providers was very different for the two groups of caregivers examined in this chapter. Sharing the widespread faith in medical science, those who wrote to the Roosevelts or the Children's Bureau sought its benefits for their children. Some had already engaged in lengthy campaigns to obtain surgery, hospitalization, drugs, or physicians' services. Those who criticized the care their children had received believed that a better doctor or more eminent clinic could solve the problem. The letter writers also seem to have viewed the government positively. Many assumed that public officials wanted to establish a truly humane social policy. Although some complained about the actions of local government agencies, all looked to Washington for redress. Few could have imagined that their letters would be referred to the very officials against whom they had lodged complaints. American Indian caregivers on reservations were far less trusting of the federal government and far more skeptical about the value of white medicine. Many rejected the services public health nurses offered; the rest accepted them selectively and strategically.

Both groups of caregivers had to contend with agents of the state who refused to honor the basic humanity of their sick family members. One letter writer reported that a relief officer told her that "no one cares" if her son died. Rejecting the alleged weakness of American Indians, the field nurses assumed that access to health care was essential, and many endured enormous personal sacrifices to deliver services themselves. But many nurses revealed their contempt for American Indians by accepting the grossly substandard institutions serving that population.

Both groups of caregivers demanded respect for their kin. One letter writer reminded Franklin D. Roosevelt of the significance of every human life. Although her grandson was "a Colored boy," he was "Human and one God is over all." Recognizing the need to curry favor with government officials, most correspondents used prevailing notions of deservedness to construct their accounts. Nevertheless, they challenged narrow definitions of human worth by asserting the fundamental value of their children. Although we did not hear directly from American Indian caregivers, we can assume that their objections to sanatorium placement were based in part on the belief that their children were precious family and community members who deserved the most sensitive and attentive care.

Both groups of caregivers were subject to official scrutiny. Health and welfare officers investigating the letter writers' appeals found "atrocious" housekeeping, poor economic management, and lax child rearing. One field nurse wrote that American Indian children with tuberculosis died outside sanatoriums because their homes were "contaminative" and "unhygienic." The death of a baby with bronchial pneumonia represented "a deliberate sacrifice to false beliefs," according to another nurse.

Caregivers who fought back risked confirming the harsh judgments directed toward them. Although many letter writers were proud of their persistence in fighting for their children's needs, investigators labeled such mothers "complainers." When an African American woman failed to bring her grandson back to a segregated clinic where she believed he had received poor care, she was faulted for having a "noncooperative attitude." The refusal of American Indian mothers and grandmothers to surrender tubercular children reinforced the nurses' belief that all Indians were "backward," "superstitious," and "prejudiced."

Ironically, American Indian caregivers appear to have achieved greater success than Depression-era mothers seeking health care for children. Although American Indians depended far more heavily on the federal government for survival than did most of the correspondents, it was much easier to reject medical services than to obtain them. Some American Indian caregivers were able to resist, or at least delay, institutional placement of tubercular children. Letter writers trying to extract welfare benefits from a parsimonious government, however, met overwhelming defeat.

~8

"Very Dear to My Heart": Confronting Labels of Feeblemindedness and Epilepsy

𝓜RS. CARTER, an Illinois woman married to a railroad laborer, wrote to the Children's Bureau in July 1914, requesting its new pamphlet about babies, as well as advice about caring for Charles, her ten-year-old son, who was doing poorly in school.[1] The Bureau chief, Julia Lathrop, replied a few days later, noting that *Infant Care* would be available the following month and discussing various special education classes and institutions for mentally defective children. Mrs. Carter waited impatiently for the publication and was delighted when she received *Prenatal Care* as well as *Infant Care*. In subsequent letters she noted that she benefited from both publications. Although she had given birth to six children, she wrote, "I have read the book 'Prenatal Care,' I learned several things that did me good."[2] Lathrop's advice about Charles, however, appalled the mother. Writing to thank Lathrop for the material, she rejected out of hand the suggestion that she place him in an institution. "I believe my boy would worry his self sick if sent away to school," she remarked.[3] Nor did she want him labeled "imbecile" or "part-witted."

Mrs. Carter questioned the counsel of other professionals as well. She refused, for example, to accept the school's assessment of her son. From her perspective, the problem was not his failure to learn designated skills but the way his teachers damaged his self-esteem. Instead of helping him realize his full potential, they undermined his sense of worth. She used her intimate understanding as a mother to challenge the teachers' assessment of his capabilities. They considered him "backward," but "at home he is more dependable and uses better knowledge than all the rest of the children."[4] Her landlord, a farmer who occasionally spent days with Mrs. Carter's boys, concurred. He, too, she wrote, found that "this boy uses better judgement in any *work* he is put at than other boys of his age [and is] more careful and [uses] better judgement than his 12 year old brother or 8 year old brother, who are getting along so well at school."[5] Mrs. Carter reiterated that although her son fell behind in his schoolwork, he did "not seem dull at work or chores."[6]

She had no greater confidence in doctors. Charles's teachers had urged her to seek a medical diagnosis of his disability. The first doctor found a nonexistent problem on the boy's nose and advised a senseless operation to correct it. "I could not help feeling like he was after the money," she wrote.[7] The second did not merit the dollar he charged, and she adamantly refused his recommendation that they return for another visit.

Previous chapters have demonstrated that women caring for family members with physical ailments distanced themselves from doctors' authority by relying on their own empathic knowledge. This chapter explores the extent to which women continued to rely on that knowledge when children were diagnosed as "feebleminded" or epileptic. Experts argued that many of the traits mothers valued in such children actually expressed mental problems. A label of feeblemindedness or epilepsy thus had the potential to change maternal feelings and alter the way mothers viewed their children's behavior. Nevertheless, I argue that many mothers continued to use their intimate knowledge of offspring to resist the advice of an array of professionals.

Two sections of this chapter explore mothers' attitudes toward children living at home. The first discusses the responses of indigent New Yorkers to recommendations that they place offspring in institutions, focusing on the years from 1895 to 1910, a period of extreme contempt for, and suspicion of, people labeled as epileptic or feebleminded. The second section examines the types of assistance mothers sought during the 1930s. Although some of the hostility directed at those with epilepsy or feeblemindedness had faded by that decade, institutionalization remained the primary recommendation. The third section of this chapter examines the experiences of mothers who tried to sustain contact with institutionalized children and influence their care.

I follow several recent historians in using words like "feebleminded," "backward," and "mental defect." Although considered offensive today, such usage avoids the problem of imposing late-twentieth-century meanings on early-twentieth-century phenomena. Feebleminded and epileptic children differed greatly from each other, but I discuss them together because they aroused similar social anxieties at the time; moreover, it was widely believed that epilepsy led to feeblemindedness.[8]

Once again, it is important not to glorify women's rejection of expert advice. We will see that many experts were overready to label some groups of children mentally defective; however, it may also be true that some mothers were unwilling to acknowledge even unambiguous symptoms. Rather than attempt to evaluate the competing claims of professional and empathic knowledge, I examine the extent to which mothers relied on their own understandings of children to challenge expert authority.

Mothers and Charity Workers, 1895–1910

The files of the New York Charity Organization Society (COS) include five cases containing extensive discussions of feebleminded or epileptic children between 1895 and 1910. During that period, the growing eugenics movement transformed the cultural and social climate surrounding feeblemindedness and epilepsy. Much of the sympathy formerly extended to parents of such children evaporated as attention focused on the role of heredity in mental disabilities. The New York Association for the Improvement of the Condition of the Poor (AICP), which worked closely with the COS, proclaimed in 1912: "The strongest factor for producing feeble-mindedness is heredity. The affliction of one parent is likely to result in feeble-mindedness of one or more of the children. All children will probably be feeble-minded if both parents are afflicted."[9] Thus, parents whose own mental capabilities escaped suspicion were faulted for transmitting inferior genes.

The popular rhetoric about these conditions became especially negative. As Joan Gittens writes, "The early word for all handicapped people had been 'afflicted,' with its connotations of randomness, innocence, and the mysterious actions of Providence . . . By the late nineteenth century, the retarded, as well as the epileptic, were called defective, no longer the personification of an inscrutable message from God to man, but merely lacking in the necessary qualifications for full humanity—not a product of a mysterious Providence but of the inexorable dictates of heredity."[10] In their 1892 annual report, the Board of Directors of the Illinois State Institution for the Feeble-minded referred to their inmates as "the waste products of humanity."[11]

The word "menace" increasingly was applied to both epileptic and feebleminded people.[12] The menace was perceived to take two forms. First, sexual offenses, crime, pauperism, homelessness, and drunkenness were attributed to feeblemindedness and epilepsy. An 1890 article in the *American Journal of Insanity* pronounced that "the history of epilepsy is the history of violence, of crime, of homicide."[13] The AICP warned, "Feeble-minded women are sources of debauchery and licentiousness, which pollute the minds of boys and youths of the community, disseminate disease and bring young children into the world destined to repeat their history."[14] Adolescent boys considered feebleminded were believed to be prone to other forms of antisocial behavior. In 1914 a charity worker discussing a seventeen-year-old boy, who had been labeled a "cretin," wrote, "Although the object of tender solicitude, his parents realize that he is a dangerous element in the family life. His moods are variable and often violent. The younger children may not be left with him a moment. The spark of intelligence which might, under proper treatment and training be developed for usefulness, is now only a menace."[15] The second perceived threat was that feebleminded and epileptic people were oversexed and, thus, reproduced at abnormal rates. Permanent institutionalization was the most popular solution for both problems.[16]

The native-born middle class saw mental impairments as overrepresented among immigrants. H. H. Goddard, the preeminent researcher of mental abilities in this period, appeared to confirm that impression. In 1917 he concluded that 40 to 50 percent of immigrants arriving at Ellis Island were feebleminded.[17] Although some contemporary critics disputed his findings, these numbers strongly influenced public opinion and policy.[18] Serving a predominantly immigrant population, Charity Organization Society workers were thus predisposed to discover mental defects among their clients.[19]

The COS also pressed vigorously for the institutionalization of children labeled feebleminded or epileptic. In two of the five cases I examine, parents successfully resisted this pressure. The case of the Penucci family—an Italian immigrant candy factory worker, his wife, and five children—was opened in 1907 at the request of a school principal.[20] Mrs. Penucci rebuffed financial assistance but thought the COS might help her twelve-year-old son, John, whose "unruly" behavior she blamed on his teacher's leniency. The school principal reported that she knew "all about" the boy, who attended the "defective class" in her school and lived close by. According to her, "his teacher has had a continued struggle to keep him from using the vilest language in class and as yet has not entirely succeeded. He seems to absorb all the evil of the street and he brings it into the school." Furthermore, he physically tormented weaker classmates. The principal concluded that the boy was "in a fair way to become a menace to the community" and should be institutionalized.

Whereas the principal pigeonholed the boy, emphasizing the danger he posed, the mother stressed his potential and her attachment to him. Informed of the principal's recommendation on January 26, Mrs. Penucci "resented very much the idea of the boy being somewhat defective," arguing that he had "always been perfectly well both physically and mentally." Although she "finally admitted" having come to the United States partly to find a better environment for John, she rejected institutionalization because she "hated to think of parting with the boy." Nevertheless, she promised to discuss the matter with her husband. On February 2 Mrs. Penucci reported that she and her husband had decided to keep John out of an institution. In an interview two days later, she pointed out that in his one year in the United States, his schoolwork and conduct had improved as he learned more English. The case closed shortly thereafter.

Why was the charity worker so willing to drop the issue of institutionalization? Two possible explanations come to mind. First, the parents agreed to exercise greater control over the boy, and the principal soon reported improved behavior. Second, because the parents did not need financial assistance, the COS had no leverage to compel compliance with their treatment plan. As we will see, the COS's most common coercive measure was withdrawing relief.

The struggle over institutional placement was far more protracted in the second case.[21] In March 1907 a Department of Health nurse alerted the COS to the "distressing circumstances" of the Marafinos, an Italian immigrant family with four children. Attention soon focused on the oldest son, Charles, who had suffered from "epileptic fits" for four years. Because he was eighteen when the case began, the COS pressured him directly. Nevertheless, it interacted primarily with his mother, whom it held at least partly responsible for his care.

The charity worker recommended that Charles "be placed in the ward for epileptics at Bellevue [Hospital] for observation, with a view of sending him to Craig Colony for Epileptics." Established in 1896, Craig Colony was a public institution in upstate New York providing long-term care for epileptic people.[22] Charles's physician supported that advice, noting that at Craig Colony "his living would be best suited to his needs." A home visit in June gave the charity worker additional evidence of the need for institutionalization. "The family have insufficient food and his condition is aggravated by this." She witnessed "Charles [having] a fit and it was evident that the entire family are under a nervous strain." Two younger Marafino children "especially seemed to be affected by Charles' suffering." In drawing that conclusion, the charity worker reflected the common belief that epileptics imposed overwhelming stress on their families.[23]

The first problem the charity worker encountered was the family's alienage. Despite widespread alarm about the high rate of feeblemindedness and epilepsy among immigrants, Craig Colony refused admission to noncitizens. The charity worker next recommended a farm colony on Staten Island. Although Charles and his mother do not appear to have explicitly rejected that advice, they delayed applying until the deadline had passed.

When Charles's health seemed to improve, the charity worker devoted her energy to increasing his economic contribution to the family. Because epileptics faced employment discrimination, the charity worker assumed a job search would be futile. Nevertheless, she encouraged him to earn some money by learning to play the mandolin.

His condition deteriorated the following year, and the COS resumed its campaign for institutionalization. Once again the charity worker attributed the strains of the household entirely to his seizures. Charles spent some time in the hospital in 1909, but he still had not entered a long-term care institution when the case closed in April 1912.

In the other three cases I examine here, the COS eventually did obtain parental consent for institutional placement. The first case began in June 1892.[24] The initial investigation described Mrs. Williams as "a bad character: lazy, intemperate, bad tempered, and quarrelsome." She had three children, each by a different man. Although she claimed to have left her current husband, the charity worker thought otherwise: "Rather think he has left her."

The scathing assessment of Mrs. Williams helped to justify demands for the removal of her youngest daughter—first to a hospital, then to an institution for feebleminded children, and finally to Craig Colony. Jessie Williams was paralyzed on one side and had difficulty speaking; several physicians consulted by the COS urged hospitalization. Mrs. Williams resisted, declaring that her "heart will break" were she forced to surrender the girl. But a woman who once had assisted Mrs. Williams financially wrote the COS that the mother was a "wicked woman" who was "too lazy for work" and kept Jessie "with her to excite the sympathy of strangers." The girl "swears dreadfully" and should be taken from the "degrading moral influence" of her mother and put in an institution where she "would be brought up properly." The COS soon had further evidence of maternal incompetence in the form of a charge of physical abuse. In September 1892 Mrs. Williams finally agreed to Jessie's removal, and the charity worker escorted the girl to the hospital. On the way, Jessie expressed her eagerness to leave her mother, who she said "used to *lick* me too much." Jessie remained in the hospital for three months, during which time the COS lost contact with Mrs. Williams.

The case reopened on August 18, 1896, when Mrs. Williams appeared at the COS office, stating that she and Jessie were homeless and needed $3 for a furnished room. Although the COS did not explain its refusal in the case file, the desire to force Mrs. Williams to relinquish the girl may have been a factor. On August 25 Jessie entered the city's major institution for mentally deficient children, established on Randall's Island in 1866.[25] In the subsequent weeks, Mrs. Williams continued to object, asserting "that Jessie was not properly cared for" and would be removed as soon as suitable accommodation was available.

Because the case file remained closed for the next four years, we do not know whether Mrs. Williams indeed tried to regain custody of her daughter. The file indicates, however, that Jessie was still on Randall's

Island in November 1900, when Mrs. Williams next applied for assistance. She now faced pressure to allow Jessie to go to Craig Colony. Although Mrs. Williams protested that the distance was too great, Jessie was transferred there some time during the next year and a half. Mrs. Williams accompanied her daughter to upstate New York, living and working nearby for four months. She returned to the city upon learning that regulations prevented her becoming an attendant in the colony.

The mother in the next case, Mrs. Lazarre, applied to the COS in April 1904 because her husband "had been idle four weeks owing to a strike," and she could not afford to care for her three children, who had "considerable sickness."[26] The condition of two-year-old Thomas, the middle boy, was especially serious. The next month he had convulsions, and in June he contracted spinal meningitis. When the COS next contacted the mother in January 1906, the charity worker wrote that Thomas had "arrested mental development." He could not "reason at all and either chews his clothing or a block constantly; he slavers and drools all the time; his body seems to be somewhat humped." Because the boy "cannot walk when he is on the street," his mother "does not know what to do with the other children, as she has to carry him." A wealthy woman who had aided the family complained to the COS that the mother kept the children inside too much and "always asked for something," recently a carriage "large enough to hold Thomas and the baby."

Thomas's physician advised placement in "the hospital for mentally deficient children on Randall's Island" because "the mother has neither the time nor the ability to develop his intellect, and the only chance that I see of doing the child much good is to place him in an institution where his mind can be trained in accordance with scientific methods." Whereas the physician appealed to scientific authority, Mrs. Lazarre spoke in terms of emotion and intimacy. Thomas's extreme vulnerability appears to have created a special attachment. She stated that "she loves him more than all her other children and that it would nearly kill her and she thinks it would kill him to be separated from her." The charity worker tried to "reason" with Mrs. Lazarre and "show her the great necessity of giving the child a chance to receive the proper treatment now while he was young." The use of the word "reason" reminds us of the belief that emotional connection undermined rationality; the charity worker appears to have believed herself better able to understand the boy's needs because she was emotionally disengaged.

The COS took Thomas to two doctors at Cornell University, who concurred with the recommendation that he be sent to Randall's Island. But medical opinion was not unanimous. The COS recorded that Dr. Fielder of Bellevue Hospital, whom it also consulted, "hesitates very much about having the boy go to Randall's Island because he feels he will not have the individual attention which he really requires; that in all public institutions where a child shows itself at all unruly, it is likely to receive pretty rough treatment; he fully realizes how devoted the mother is to him and that she is really wearing herself out in caring for him, but at the present he sees nothing else but to have him remain with his mother." Mrs. Lazarre took advantage of this fissure in medical opinion. The record continued, "As Dr. Fielder has advised her about Randall's Island and as she has heard so many bad reports from there, she will not under any circumstances, permit Thomas to go."

Dr. Fielder suggested that Thomas go to a private facility in Morristown, New Jersey. The COS made financial arrangements, and in early February Thomas was admitted. Two days later, however, Mrs. Lazarre was informed that he was "too troublesome" to stay.

With that option eliminated, the COS redoubled its efforts to send Thomas to Randall's Island. The organization tried to persuade Dr. Fielder to drop his objection and warned Mrs. Lazarre that financial assistance would cease until she consented to Thomas's institutionalization.

A series of events that spring began to erode her resistance. Thomas's health deteriorated further. The report for May 7 read, "Found Mrs. Lazarre with remains of black eye, which she stated had been given her by Thomas during one of his fits, his head striking her in the eye and knocking her senseless; when she recovered she found Thomas walking around the room covered with blood. At the time of these fits he falls striking his head and face and injuring himself very badly." Mrs. Lazarre may have had more difficulty managing Thomas because her own health had declined; in September she would be diagnosed with tuberculosis. Moreover, a new strike loomed at her husband's factory, threatening the family's income and, thus, increasing their dependence on the COS. On June 2 Mrs. Lazarre announced that she had "put in an application to Randall's Island on May 26." The charity worker wrote on June 22, "Mrs. Lazarre called, stated that Thomas was sent to Randall's Island on the fifteenth; that she has visited him and he seems to be improving; has not had any of his attacks since he has been there; is sorry that she did not put him away long ago; he is quite contented and does not cry at all." Mrs. Lazarre's apparent acceptance of Thomas's situation may have expressed genuine conviction about the benefits of institutional care coupled with immense, if unexpected, relief after the responsibility had been lifted from her. But her comments also may have reflected a desire to demonstrate gratitude to the COS for its help. Had she continued to argue that Thomas would be better off at home, she would not have appeared properly appreciative.

Thomas's commitment failed, however, to resolve the controversy about his care. Because Dr. Fielder described the problem as epilepsy, Randall's Island sought to transfer him to Craig Colony. According to the case file, "Mrs. Lazarre objects very much to his going so far away from home; that she was going to see Dr. Fielder this afternoon and ask him if he could not change his statement somewhat about the child being epileptic, so that he would be kept on Randall's Island." In the absence of tests yielding a definitive diagnosis, Mrs. Lazarre appears to have hoped that social factors could influence the process of medical diagnosis. It is unclear whether Thomas eventually went to Craig Colony.

The final case began in January 1906 when a school nurse reported that a widow named Mrs. Martin and her two children, ages fourteen and eleven, had "nothing to live on."[27] A home visit revealed that the younger child, Evelyn, "has some mental difficulty, about which the woman is most indefinite. Child is unable to speak intelligently and has falling attacks which the woman insists is only due to a weakness of the limbs." The girl often accompanied the mother when she did "day's work," which was "a great hindrance to her." The physician consulted by the COS concluded that Evelyn "should be placed in the Deaf and Dumb Asylum." Evelyn's school principal concurred, arguing that the girl would "respond quickly to scientific treatment." The mother repeatedly agreed verbally to the recommendation but took no steps to carry it out. In March the COS withdrew financial assistance and asked the school authorities to bring all "possible pressure to bear to have the child placed in the proper institution." The principal reported that the mother so feared the COS's influence that she kept the girl home. Concluding that Mrs. Martin was "unwilling to act on the advice given," the COS closed the case in early June.

When Mrs. Martin next applied for assistance, on July 12, she was informed that "further aid would not be considered until the child should be placed in the proper institution." The next day she returned

> to say she has reconsidered the matter of placing Evelyn in an institution . . . ; said she would act honorably in the matter and would surely let her go if she promised to do so; has been obliged to take Evelyn with her to work, many times had no carfare and obliged to walk and drag the child with her; thinks it would be a rest and change for the child and would also enable woman to get on her feet; thinks probably she has not done right by Evelyn in not giving her all the chance for an education possible.

Mrs. Martin's initial opposition turned out to be only the first hurdle. On July 21 the New York Institute for Instruction of Deaf Mutes decided that Evelyn "was not a proper subject for the institution." The COS then sought to convince Mrs. Martin to take Evelyn to a doctor who would recommend an appropriate placement. In September the charity worker interviewed Mrs. Martin's sister-in-law, Mrs. McGrady, "who feels that woman is inclined to put obstacles in the way of Evelyn's welfare by her short-sighted affection for the child; will use her influence to induce her to consent to any plan that may seem wise." "Short-sighted affection" may have been Mrs. McGrady's phrase, but it clearly expressed the COS perspective.

On October 17 the charity worker gave the mother "a card of introduction to Dr. Bryant," a "specialist in speech instruction." When Mrs. Martin requested aid on December 6, she had "no satisfactory excuse for not having called on Dr. Bryant." A week later, however, she allowed Evelyn to go to the doctor with the charity worker, who wrote that he "thinks that the child was simply undeveloped as shown by her speech, her general lack of intelligence and the hesitating character of her movements; says she is in the mental condition of a child of about three and was not a candidate for a deaf mute asylum . . . ; thinks that the best place for her is a home for feeble minded."

Once again an economic crisis forced compliance. Early on January

7, 1907, Mrs. Martin was evicted from her home and sought emergency assistance. That afternoon she agreed to send Evelyn to Randall's Island. Learning that Mrs. Martin was planning to remove the girl a few weeks later, the COS threatened to alert the Society for the Prevention of Cruelty to Children (SPCC), as it did in the case of Maria Germani, discussed in Chapter 6. In May the charity worker wrote, "Evelyn is doing very well, is gaining in weight, and is having good care. Woman does not seem as determined as formerly to have her at home again."

⌒ THE FIVE WOMEN whose cases we have examined were hardly alone in insisting that children labeled feebleminded belonged at home. The Social Service Department of the Massachusetts General Hospital described a typical case involving a "little feeble-minded girl" in 1918: "The doctor asks us if we will have a talk with the mother and persuade her to send her child to a school for the feeble-minded. She may willingly fill out the application paper; but on the other hand she may have many reasons for not doing so, which it may take us months to eradicate."[28] Testifying before a New York State commission on services for the feebleminded, Elisabeth Irwin complained of the difficulty of convincing New York City parents to institutionalize children between the ages of twelve and sixteen. Only 20 of 100 families eventually agreed to institutional placement, and 18 of those 20 families removed the children within a year.[29]

The COS cases help us understand parental resistance. Because women often tried to avoid direct confrontations, the files do not always reveal how the mothers framed their objections. Nevertheless, the few comments that are available suggest that mothers rejected widespread conceptions about their children. Mirroring dominant social attitudes, the COS assumed that epilepsy and mental retardation diminished children's worth and humanity. The mothers, however, spoke of their children in relational terms; because the children were intimately bound to the entire family, their lives had special value and meaning.

To overcome client opposition, the COS often deployed the language of benevolence, arguing that institutional placement would promote the well-being of not just the disabled child but also the whole family. The mothers contended that the grief of separation would dwarf any benefits of institutionalization.

The COS responded in two ways to clients' focus on the strength of their personal ties. In one case, charity workers charged a mother with indifference, and even hostility, to the child she purported to love. But charity workers who credited women's emotions were equally disapproving. While mothers claimed that empathic knowledge enabled them to be especially attentive to the children's needs, the charity workers implied that close bonds distorted maternal perceptions. One charity worker quoted a relative's complaint about a mother's "short-sighted affection." Another worker described trying to "reason" with a mother who invoked her strong attachment as justification for keeping her son at home.

Circumstances help to explain why mothers sometimes acceded to demands for institutionalization. Poverty greatly exacerbated the problems of caring for disabled children. One mother had to "drag" her daughter along when she went out to do "day's work." Another lacked the financial resources to purchase the prescribed food for her epileptic son. Another could not afford a carriage to transport her disabled son. And another had no place for her son to play except the street, where he got into trouble and was under the surveillance of his school principal.

Poverty also subordinated the mothers to the COS, which employed various strategies to produce acquiescence. The COS gave no help to alleviate the burdens of home care. It discontinued monetary relief when mothers refused institutionalization. In one case, it threatened to notify the SPCC if the mother withdrew her consent to her child's placement in an institution.

Still, the COS's power was hardly limitless. Charity workers often could not find vacancies in appropriate institutions. At least one physician to whom charity workers appealed refused to endorse the COS's recommendation. And clients themselves were not totally powerless. Two mothers effectively blocked institutionalization; the other three delayed it for substantial periods. Charity workers finally prevailed in those three cases only when new financial emergencies increased the mothers' reliance on the COS and weakened their ability to disregard expert opinion.

Responding to Experts in the 1930s

By the 1930s, the rhetoric surrounding feebleminded and epileptic people had grown somewhat less virulent. Experiments in the 1920s with discharging and "paroling" the feebleminded and other disabled people from institutions had demonstrated that many former inmates could manage successfully in the community. The advent of new drugs to control epileptic seizures helped to win new tolerance from the rest of society.[30] And a better understanding of genetics and the etiology of various forms of mental retardation had begun to undermine eugenic beliefs.[31]

Nevertheless, institutional placement remained the principal recommendation for feebleminded and epileptic children.[32] When an Ohio mother wrote to the Children's Bureau that she hesitated to put her eleven-year-old "Mongolian type" boy in an institution, Agnes K. Hanna, the director of the Bureau's social service division, responded,

> Although we appreciate how difficult it is for you to reconcile yourself to do so, we believe that since the recommendation has been made by competent doctors, that it would be best to place your son in an institution while he is young enough to make a happy adjustment easily. After the first strangeness wears off, he would be happy in the companionship of other boys of his age and capacity, would be taught to be as useful as possible, and he would not be made unhappy by trying to compete with children better equipped than he is.[33]

Professionals continued to contrast the reasonableness of institutionalization with the emotionality of maternal resistance. Asked to investigate a two-year-old child whose mother had consulted the Children's Bureau, a Florida doctor wrote that if the parents attempt to care for her at home "it will be at the expense of what the Other Members of the family, particularly the Children, should enjoy. In my opinion there is no justifiable reason for giving this attention to a child who absolutely can not appreciate what is being done for Her." To this doctor, a mentally disabled child was simply a burden, exhausting family resources yet unable to benefit from personal care. He acknowledged that "of course a mother feels much differently towards her own child than some one who is removed from the environment would feel." But he was confident that professional expertise would prevail. "I believe the mother can be brought to see the problem from our standpoint."[34]

This section relies on 122 letters from parents of feebleminded children and 21 letters from parents of epileptic children, written between 1929 and 1940. Like the correspondence discussed in Chapter 7, these letters were addressed either to the Children's Bureau or to Eleanor and Franklin D. Roosevelt.

The correspondents differed from the COS clients examined in the previous section in two significant ways. First, a large percentage were native-born women in small towns throughout the United States; only a small fraction were immigrants. Second, although many letter writers cited severe economic hardships, few appeared utterly destitute.

A key concern expressed in some letters was to preserve the family's social status. James W. Trent writes, "To have a defective in the family was to be associated with vice, immorality, failure, bad blood, and stupidity. To place that defective in a public facility was to be associated with the lower classes."[35] Several letter writers sought to distance themselves from the taint of heredity by blaming their children's deficiencies on injuries or on diseases like encephalitis or spinal meningitis, which had no genetic component. In addition, correspondents stressed that other children in the family were healthy and "normal," developing satisfactorily and doing well in school.

Some parents also sought to avoid the stigma of state institutions. Private facilities proliferated during the early twentieth century, but the Great Depression put them beyond the reach of many parents. "I am from one of the oldest families in Hillsboro," wrote an Illinois woman, the mother of a fifteen-year-old, in 1935. "We lost our money during the depression . . . We have tried to find some backward school for Peter, but the ones we can send him to are private schools and they cost to much." One reason she cited for refusing to consider the state institution at Lincoln was that the boy "has been brought up in a good religious home."[36] Special education classes were equally abhorrent to some correspondents. A Pennsylvania woman explained why she recoiled from the suggestion that her son enroll in the class she visited near their home: "[The] special class was a disgrace to a township as rich as Montgomery Co. A dismal room with colored boys and girls, 3 feeble minded from 1 family, a place to send a child in order to be relieved from their care."[37]

The overriding problem for many letter writers, however, was gaining access to public services, not avoiding them. Special education classes reached only a fraction of needy children in the 1930s. "We are sorry to say," wrote Hanna to a New Jersey father in 1939, "that many communities throughout the United States do not have financial resources for the special educational needs of many physically or mentally handicapped children. Special classes for educable children unable to adapt themselves to regular school courses and home teaching for children who are unable to attend school are provided in some, but by no means all, of our large cities and such resources are not available in a large proportion of our smaller communities."[38]

Although the number of public institutions had multiplied since 1900, access problems intensified during the Depression, as state legislatures froze or cut funding. Waiting lists contained hundreds, and sometimes thousands, of names.[39] Some groups were ineligible. Two African American letter writers who had been told there were no institutions in their states later learned that such institutions existed but admitted only whites.[40]

As demand for institutional places increased, criticism of mothers occasionally took a new turn. Many now were reproached, not for their reluctance to relinquish their children, but for attempting to shirk responsibility for them. In response to a mother's statement that poor health prevented her from caring for her severely disabled twelve-year-old son in addition to three other children, a caseworker wrote that the boy's "needs are simple and do not require facilities that you do not have."[41] The caseworker told the Children's Bureau that the mother "can give her son adequate care if she so desires."[42]

Assumptions about women's caregiving obligations pervaded the reports of other investigators as well. A North Carolina mother had written two letters to the Children's Bureau asking the staff to institutionalize her son. But the superintendent of public welfare of Sampson County, to whom the Bureau referred the letter, concluded that the problem was not the boy but the mother, who "resents having to wait on the child." The superintendent disregarded the mother's comments about the burdens of care. "This child is not completely helpless," he wrote. "It is able to get about but clearly is a mental case which requires a lot of watch-care and supervision. We have other families with mentally deficient children who are in considerably worse condition in every way than this family." The superintendent decided that the boy should remain at home because the parents were "strong and able bodied."[43]

A major reason for writing to Washington was to obtain information about children's problems. Several mothers were just beginning to suspect that something was amiss; others had recently received specific diagnoses and wanted to know more about prognosis and treatment. One mother wrote, "I have a 7 year old son who is the picture of health in every way yet about three weeks ago I began to notice that at times he would grow rigid and not know anything for a second. I took him to the doctor and he says he has epilepsy. They tell me there is no known cure. But to watch his diet. Can you give me any help? Is there a cure for this trouble? Will you, please send me any and all information you can on how to treat him?"[44] Another woman had just been told by a physician that her eight-month-old daughter was a "Mongolian idiocy type." "Now what I am writing you for," the mother explained, "is I want to know just what he means by 'Mongolian idiocy' and what you would suggest me doing in regard to her care etc. and if there is any literature you have on babies of this type I would greatly appreciate your sending it to me."[45] A third woman sought information about what to expect in the future: "My baby is a Mongolian child. I have heard my child is phisically strong but mentally weak. He will not be smart, and maybe not attend school. Naturally I feel grieved . . . Can you help me about what does a Mongolian child amount to in this world. Is he useless."[46]

Whereas other women argued that their children's personalities transcended their diagnoses, these mothers were trying to understand their children as a generality or "type." By offering an interpretive framework, the labels also shaped mothers' perceptions of their children. These letters thus remind us of the difficulty of disentangling expert and empathic knowledge.

Most letter writers fell into one of two categories.[47] Women in the first pleaded for institutional places to relieve the stress of caring for severely disabled children. Because their letters focused on the enormous burdens of time, energy, and emotion that the children imposed on them, I refer to members of this group as "overwhelmed mothers." Many complained that feeding, carrying, and toileting was difficult and unremitting work. One wrote to Eleanor Roosevelt, "The baby keeps me in so much that our home is nothing but a prison to me. It's not right for a normal healthy person to be cooped up inside always. Don't you agree?"[48]

Many of these letter writers reported multiple, competing caregiving obligations. A Missouri mother, for example, had seven children in addition to a twelve-year-old girl "with an undeveloped brain."[49] Caregiving also conflicted with economic responsibilities. The mother of a seven-year-old epileptic boy wrote, "I am a widow woman with no support, only the labor of my hands. I don't mind work. But with the care it takes for him there is no time for other work—A farm woman, and you can imagine my round of duties."[50] Two employed mothers could not provide the supervision their children needed. One locked two feebleminded daughters in the apartment during the day.[51] The other reported that her son wandered into town during her absence; on two occasions the elevator at a nearby mill had nearly crushed him to death.[52]

Several women expressed concern about other children in the household. A few mothers feared that their retarded children posed physical threats to younger siblings. Others shared the widespread belief that all children suffered emotional harm from the presence of feebleminded or epileptic siblings. Neighbors' reactions heightened the anxiety of one mother of a mentally retarded girl: "So many of the neighbors make the remark that it is a shame to raise a child like her in a home where there are other normal healthy children, but under the circumstances I am unable to do anything about it."[53]

Although a few "overwhelmed mothers" sought places for babies, most had tended their children for years. The experiences of these letter writers support the conclusion reached by other studies that parents typically saw institutionalization as a last resort.[54] A New Mexico mother explained that she needed institutional care because her new husband was cruel to her mentally retarded daughter.[55] Several cited the recent deterioration of their own health. Aging mothers worried about who would provide care when they were gone.

The maturation of offspring also prompted the search for institutional placement. Adolescents were more likely to engage in disruptive behavior, and many could no longer be physically restrained at home.

Mothers of mentally retarded girls expressed concerns about increased sexual vulnerability.

Many letter writers related the need for institutionalization to the Depression. One mother wrote, "I have a son of twenty four with the mentality of an eight year old. Due to lack of money we are forced to move into very small quarters. My sister has been providing a home for us but my boy is too much for her nervous system as she works very hard and must have an atmosphere of quiet when she is home that is impossible with my boy. There seems no alternative but to send him to a state institution."[56] Others would have remained home to provide care had the Depression not forced them to contribute to the household income by working. As the Georgia Department of Public Welfare wrote in 1931, "Many families who in ordinary times are able to care for their own unfortunate children, find it impossible to do so now."[57]

By emphasizing their burdens, "overwhelmed mothers" separated their offspring from the family's affective life, thus denying the emotional bonds that are the precondition of empathic knowledge. By contrast, another group of women, whom I call "challengers," relied heavily on their own intimate understanding of their children to frame their accounts. Some resisted labeling; a few criticized the process used to identify feeblemindedness. By 1913 intelligence tests were used to examine 72 percent of those eligible for special education in the United States.[58] But one woman asserted that her son's teacher had neglected his poor eyesight when interpreting the results.[59] Another protested that her son's teacher had "mentally retarded" him by using the wrong age to calculate his score; when the mother gave the boy a test from *Parents' Magazine* he "stood up to the normal mark."[60] In addition, several parents blamed physical problems for the slowness that doctors characterized as feeblemindedness. And some attributed poor school performance to insensitive teachers who had wounded the children's self-confidence.

More commonly, the "challengers" acknowledged their children's disabilities but disputed the meaning assigned to them. Rita Charon writes that "medical case histories conceptually enclose narration, constrain signs to mean only one thing, and tie utterances down to unalterable meanings, whereas patients' narratives improvise, recombine dissimilar elements, go someplace without knowing where they are going, and open possibilities."[61] Many letters in this group resemble patients' narratives in important respects. For several women, epilepsy or feeblemindedness did not encapsulate their children's identities. "I have a little girl of eight years old who is mentally retarded," wrote one mother. "The child isn't foolish by any means. She eats plays and sleeps just like any other."[62] The mother of a seven-year-old boy recently diagnosed with epilepsy wrote, "Except for the second that these spells are on him I never saw a more perfect specimen of childhood."[63]

I have noted that both epileptic and feebleminded people were seen as prone to antisocial behavior. The letter writers, however, frequently depicted their children as loving and well behaved. "He is good," wrote a mother of a "backward" fourteen-year-old boy. "He does every thing he can to help me and as good and better than most boys."[64] The mother of another fourteen-year-old boy wrote, "Marvin has a very nice personality, much nicer than his brothers. He is kind and very affectionate. He has sympathy and consideration for others. He loves animals and has brought home many a stray dog and cat. I'm sure if I would except them I wouldnt have room in my home to live."[65]

Like the patients in illness narratives, "challengers" sometimes described their children in contradictory terms. One mother wrote about her five-year-old son, "The child's brain at birth was injured, which has retarded his development, in that he does not talk or walk very well. He is not defective. In fact he is very alert."[66] Others noted that their offspring were "bright" and "intelligent," even if "subnormal mentally," "backward," or "deficient."

Mothers created possibilities by emphasizing their children's developmental capacity. One hallmark of expert knowledge is its claim to predict and control behavior.[67] This helps to explain the popularity of I.Q. tests. Paula S. Fass writes, "In the United States, [Alfred] Binet's tests were greeted with an enthusiasm that they failed to arouse anywhere else, including his native France, precisely because Binet's tests, as distinct from Binet's views, offered the possibility of measuring innate ability and unchanging potential."[68] But while testers emphasized the static quality of mental capacities, mothers focused on their children's progress. After summarizing her son's achievements, one mother commented, "Considering the baby I had at 1 year and the boy I have at 9 God has been quite good to me."[69] Some also argued that their children's abilities transcended the testers' metric. The mother of a thirteen-year-old boy wrote, "He likes to build things and seems to use his hands very well. He goes most any place he wants to—crosses the streets where traffic is a plenty . . . I know he can learn because he took piano lessons and could play some."[70]

It has become common to argue that experts seek dominance by relying on objective, quantifiable data to supplant subjective lay judgments.[71] These mothers, however, implicitly claimed knowledge that was unavailable to detached observers. They had experienced the children's capacity for intimacy, which many professionals denied. Close contact, the mothers claimed, allowed them to discern capabilities that eluded the measurement process. Whereas testers observed the children at one moment in time, mothers had a long-term perspective. Familiarity also enabled them to communicate with children whose language was opaque to others. Noting that her daughter "doesn't talk plain," a mother remarked, "One has to be used to her to understand her."[72]

A Pennsylvania mother not only asserted the superiority of her own knowledge but also questioned the legitimacy of outsiders to predict her son's performance. Officials had excluded the boy from school based on a psychologist's test. "They were heartless in their remarks," the mother wrote. "Said I wouldn't raise him, the state don't bother about an individual . . . My whole heart is centered on my boy and why should they be able to prophesies his future?"[73]

Whereas "overwhelmed mothers" presented themselves as burdened by difficult children, "challengers" portrayed themselves as embattled by a hostile society. The hurts their children experienced wounded them also. "My boy is very dear to my heart," wrote a woman whose son had been deemed ineligible to attend the local public school. "It hurts so much to see him growing up with no education."[74] An Alabama mother of a fourteen-year-old boy wrote, "People tease him and have fun with him, not realizing how it breaks my heart."[75] In addition, many women had experienced stigma and discrimination firsthand when seeking services for their children.

Some "challengers" refused to consider publicly funded institutions, citing their poor conditions. A Tennessee mother wrote that the state institution was so overcrowded that children slept two to a bed.[76] A Pennsylvania woman had removed her mentally retarded son from a state hospital after receiving reports of abuse and vowed never to send him back.[77] A New Jersey mother wanted the government to pay her son's tuition at a private institution. A series of tragedies had visited the family. The only other child, a "very bright" ten-year-old boy, had died suddenly of pneumonia. The father, a real estate salesman, had lost his money in the Depression and then suffered a paralyzing stroke. "We have been so plunged in despair with the last cross we have been called upon to bear," the mother wrote. "I am heart broken to even think of parting with my baby, particularly after losing my other boy. I do pray when he leaves my arms, I can feel he will be tenderly cared for."[78]

Several women also asserted that the unique needs of their children would not be served by public institutions. Three mothers maintained that although mental handicaps prevented their children from attending local schools, they were too bright for state institutions. One wrote, "Vermont has a State school for Feeble Minded but it would be a crime to send Mark there . . . All I have seen of this school isn't what Mark needs and the associations would prove detrimental I am sure. If he were Feeble Minded in full sense of the word he probably wouldn't know the difference. But he isn't. He needs a chance."[79]

Like COS clients at the turn of the century, some letter writers in the 1930s also argued that the welfare of the family was inseparable from that of the child and that institutionalization would destroy the family rather than save it. Distance aggravated such concerns. A New York City woman had removed her eight-year-old son from Craig Colony—the facility that had aroused fierce resistance from COS clients—because she had been able to see him just twice during his twenty-one months there. "It will break my heart and his if he goes back where he was," the mother wrote. "So please try to understand my feelings."[80]

"Challengers" who sought institutional placement stressed the benefits to the children rather than to themselves. Some insisted that the children could be cured or restored to normality. Others emphasized the need for training to enable their offspring to support themselves. One mother, for example, explained why she wanted to find an appropriate institution for her son, whose "mental processes have been retarded" as a result of epilepsy. The doctor she consulted was optimistic "that under proper training and care this boy will not have to spend his life as a public charge."[81] The mother of a thirteen-year-old feeble-minded son wanted him institutionalized because "he needs schooling and discipline to make a useful citizen out of him."[82]

It is important not to exaggerate the extent to which these women rejected the prevailing social definition of mentally disabled children. Faye D. Ginsburg and Rayna Rapp note that "people cannot develop oppositional positions independent of the categories of the dominant culture, even as they attempt to destabilize them."[83] By stressing their children's productive potential, the letter writers challenged contemporary assumptions about feebleminded and epileptic children. However, they also drew on reigning notions of human worth, which tended to stigmatize such children.

The women's use of the language of entitlement also contained a contradiction. The Social Security Act of 1935 provided assistance to both crippled children and blind people of all ages. Several mothers invoked that legislation to argue that mentally disabled children were a government responsibility. A typical comment came from an Oklahoma woman: "It seems to me much is being done for blind, deaf and crippled children—for which I am happy—but there are many children who are handicapped by other afflictions who are just as badly in need of opportunity to develop to the limit of their capacity as are these."[84] In making rights claims, the mothers asserted the worth of children others devalued. But we have seen that these women also highlighted the traits differentiating their offspring from other feebleminded or epileptic children. Appealing to Washington on the basis of their children's unique qualities, the mothers relied on the same distinction between the deserving and undeserving that the larger society used to justify the exclusion of all mentally disabled children from social protection.

How can we account for the contrast between these two groups of letters? One explanation lies in differences in the degree of disability. Most "overwhelmed mothers" had offspring with severe disabilities that, to a large extent, defined the children's interactions with the world. The many "challengers" whose children had more moderate limitations found it easier to focus on other aspects of their personalities. But it is also possible that some women's responses reflected changing circumstances. Many "overwhelmed mothers" indicated that they had been better able to bear the stresses of care before the Depression devastated their lives. Because we have only a single letter from most mothers, we cannot trace changes in attitudes. Recent accounts by Helen Featherstone and others suggest that most parents vacillate between viewing mentally disabled children as intolerable burdens and cherished family members.[85] We can assume that the attitudes of many women writing to Washington during the 1930s also wavered throughout the course of caregiving.

⌒ MOTHERS OF FEEBLEMINDED or epileptic children writing to the Children's Bureau or to the Roosevelts in the 1930s related to expert advice in diverse ways. Those struggling to accept their children's impairments hoped that expert knowledge would increase their own understanding. Mothers pleading for relief from caregiving responsibilities drew on the same concepts as professionals. Like many charity workers and public officials, those women portrayed mentally defective children primarily as burdens. Other mothers, however, treasured their children despite, or even because of, their disabilities. Some drew on their empathic knowledge to cast doubt on experts' diagnoses.

A much larger group of women accepted the categorization but not its implications. Although labels may have shaped these mothers' understanding of their children, the labels did not obliterate that understanding. Like the mothers of children with physical health problems discussed in previous chapters, these letter writers negotiated different modes of knowing.

Various circumstances help to explain why many letter writers sought institutional care. Just as indigent COS clients were most likely to relinquish children during personal crises, so many women writing to Washington in the 1930s accepted institutionalization only when the Depression magnified the burdens of caregiving. Mothers often consented to institutional placement because they needed to take an outside job or "double up" in apartments. The Depression also forced families to draw on the productive potential of every member. When funding cutbacks compelled school boards to disband special education programs or delay the establishment of new ones, mothers turned to institutional care. Experts encouraged mothers in the belief that institutions offered useful training. We will see, however, that a primary concern of institutional superintendents after admission was to convince mothers to lower their expectations.

So far, we have explored the attitudes of mothers whose feebleminded or epileptic children were living at home. Once children entered institutions, experts had even more powerful ways of discrediting maternal knowledge. The following section explores the extent to which mothers of institutionalized children were able to use such knowledge to sustain relationships with their offspring and influence their care.

After Institutionalization

It is easy to understand why mothers may have wanted to distance themselves from children after their admission to institutions. Some mothers had exhausted their physical, emotional, and financial resources before commitment. Those feeling the stigma of having borne mentally defective children may have hoped that total disengagement would help to hide the stain on the family's reputation. And still others may have been able to endure the anguish of loss only by severing all ties.

External factors also can shed light on why some mothers withdrew. In the late nineteenth and early twentieth centuries, the bucolic setting of the country was widely believed to have healing powers, especially for mentally defective people. A 1920 report of the South Carolina state institution for the feebleminded called it "the ideal situation for a school, as it is composed of woodland, cultivated fields, hills and valley."[86] Although most facilities were in rural areas, the great majority of families of institutionalized children lived in cities. Visits to inmates were thus often difficult, if not impossible, for many parents. In 1902 the $14 round-trip train fare between New York City and Craig Colony for Epileptics, located 360 miles upstate, exceeded the weekly income of many poor families.[87] Chicago parents had to take a 3:00 A.M. train to the Illinois state institution for mentally defective people in Lincoln.[88] Regulations also deterred visitors; some institutions prohibited visits on Sunday, the one day many working people were free to travel.[89]

Attempts to bring children home, either temporarily or permanently, forced parents to confront their loss of control. Recalling his term as a psychologist at the Southbury Training School, Connecticut's state institution for the feebleminded, Seymour B. Sarason wrote, "The state assumed the role of legal guardian. And legal guardianship meant that we at Southbury determined when and under what conditions a child could go home for visits, extended stays, or a work placement. In principle as well as in practice, it was similar to being sent to prison, that is, the state was in charge of your future."[90]

Craig Colony required parents to apply in writing for permission to bring children home for visits. The few parents whose requests were approved had to personally chaperone their children both ways, expending twice the train fare and time. Parents who found other escorts or asked that their children travel alone had to sign forms absolving the colony of responsibility.[91] The maximum length of home stays was thirty days; inmates who stayed away longer were involuntarily discharged.[92]

I have noted that many states established parole and discharge programs during the 1920s, reversing their previous emphasis on warehousing feebleminded and epileptic people. But home investigations frequently convinced superintendents that parents, especially poor immigrants and people of color, were unfit to control their children. Most requests for the release of adolescent girls and young women were also rejected. Although the rapid growth of sterilization programs during the 1930s allayed some fears about the propagation of the "unfit," superintendents continued to argue that women should remain in institutions during their reproductive years. In 1940 a mother wrote to the Children's Bureau that she missed her daughter, a resident in the New Hampshire state school for the feebleminded, and wanted her home. The Bureau forwarded the letter to the superintendent, who replied,

> Looking at it from the trained gaze of the social agencies and of this institution A. Y. is unquestionably a subnormal individual, call it feebleminded or what one may. She . . . is young, simple-minded and highly emotional and judging from past experiences in many similar instances she would be exposed to the possibility and perhaps even the probability of becoming the mother of an illegitimate child, which child would be possessed of poor mental equipment, and to the family and community this would be a social and economic burden.
>
> The family is emotional and affectionate but as such families are employed, if they can find employment, and as such families seldom can maintain social supervision it has been deemed wise, at State expense, to care for the girl at this institution.
>
> New Hampshire has a legal sterilizing law which is sometimes

applied; it is not always desirable however in those of such low mental and social ability as to be unable to protect themselves to some extent.[93]

The very conditions that made poor families vulnerable to losing children made it difficult for the parents to retrieve their children after commitment. In a phrase redolent of Foucault, this superintendent's "trained gaze" trumped the mother's emotional bond.

An exchange of letters between a New York City woman and the Children's Bureau in 1935 reveals the extralegal pressures on parents to disengage from their sons and daughters after they had been committed. Mrs. Gray first wrote to the Bureau on April 12, shortly after a Bellevue Hospital doctor had diagnosed her young son as a "mongolian type" and recommended his admission to the children's institution on Randall's Island. "I have been miserable ever since I have been advised that because this baby is very dear to me," she wrote. "He is such a very very good little chap in every respect, and [I] have no trouble at all with him. I just can't make up my mind what is best for the child."[94] Ella Oppenheimer, a pediatrician employed by the Bureau, responded by urging Mrs. Gray to heed the doctor's opinion.[95]

Mrs. Gray's next letter was dated May 21. After noting that she had institutionalized her son the previous day, his second birthday, she asked Oppenheimer to write the medical superintendent regarding his care. She explained her concern: "As far as the institution is concerned, my baby is just another case. If I were only sure that my little fellow was being taken care of properly, I would feel so much better." She was certain that a letter from the Bureau "would help so much."[96] Oppenheimer replied on June 15, "I am glad to write to you that I have had a letter from the hospital where your little son is being cared for. The doctor tells me that I may assure you that [the boy] is receiving all the care and attention he needs."[97]

But on her first visit to her son in October, Mrs. Gray was horrified, and she again solicited Oppenheimer's assistance:

Instead of improving, he is getting worse and worse. At home, I had sun-ray [lamp] treatments given him, 3 times a week, and thought that they would give him that at the institution, as he has a terrible case of rickets, but he does not even get the sun outside.

All they do at the institution is keep him nice and clean and give him his food, but as far as medical aid to help his case, they have not the facilities.

Is Mongolian type children a case of just letting the child exist until he passes away? Is there no help at all for these children? Please, Dr. Oppenheimer, let me know what I can do? He has been losing weight steadily since he is there and has been sick all along.

Is there no hospital in the U.S. that would really aid these children physically and mentally?[98]

Oppenheimer preached acquiescence: "I feel that I must tell you that there is very little that can be done for children like [yours]. Had it been possible to do something for your child, your doctor would not have recommended that he be sent to the institution. Dr. McGaffin (the Superintendent of the Hospital) seemed friendly and sympathetic in his letter, and I believe you can rest assured that your little son is having the care he needs."[99]

Mothers who appealed directly to administrators were similarly encouraged to accept their children's new identities as institutional inmates. Letters to and from relatives, preserved in the patient files of several institutions, illuminate the clash between administrators and family members.[100] The remainder of this section draws primarily on the correspondence of superintendents at Craig Colony, although I also incorporate a few letters to administrators of other institutions.[101] Because mothers wrote the majority of letters, I again refer to the letter writers collectively as "mothers"; however, I occasionally rely on the correspondence of other relatives that supports the mothers' accounts.

Not all letter writers wanted to sustain relationships with their institutionalized children. In response to her son's request to go home for a visit, one mother wrote to the Craig Colony superintendent, "I would much rather he would *not* come for a while yet—and wish you would talk to him and tell him it would not be best for him to go. Work has been very poor for me this winter and I really do not feel able to take care of him just now."[102] Most mothers, however, sought to maintain connections. Several requested information. Many residents were incapable of writing; even when they sent letters, mothers often tried to verify their accounts. Notices of illness frequently elicited requests for details. After learning that her fifteen-year-old son had a contagious skin disease, one mother wrote, "The pain and anxiety caused me by my not being able to be near my son when he needs me, will be much lessened, if without hiding from me as to the condition of my son, you will be kind enough to let me know all about him."[103]

Other letter writers wanted to be able to imagine their children's daily lives. An Oklahoma father wrote to the superintendent of an Illinois institution, "We hope to have a letter from you any day now, telling us how our little one is getting on in her new home. The little details, such of them as you can give, will be appreciated. The crumbs, even, will feed graciously our hungry hearts."[104] Mothers who wrote to the Craig Colony asked about their children's emotional well-being and how they spent their time.

Some letters seem to have accompanied presents; a few requested that administrators investigate gifts gone astray. Some presents may have expressed guilt for having committed children or having failed to stay in touch, but presents also softened the rigors of institutional life. When one mother learned that her son had tuberculosis, she dispatched beef, fruit, iron tablets, wine, and cognac.[105] Clothing from home enabled children to reject institutional outfits and thus retain at least some semblance of individuality. Some mothers sent cameras in order to get snapshots of the children they missed. And a few mothers sent gifts to attendants, hoping to secure special consideration for their offspring.

Mothers also suggested ways to improve the quality of care. Some requested the comforts of religion for their children, especially at the end of life. A few asked administrators to summon priests when death seemed imminent. Informed that her son was seriously ill, one mother urged his attendant to read aloud the psalms that had soothed him at home.[106]

Although religion was peripheral to superintendents' domain of expertise, they also received advice that encroached on their authority. A vast array of treatments for epilepsy was available in the early twentieth century.[107] One mother wrote after her son's visit, "The last week John was at home, we got a bottle of Dr. Khier's Epileptic Remedy, and gave it to John, and while he was taking it, he took no seizures . . . Would it be against the rules for him to take it while up there. If he would be allowed to take it, I would buy it and send it up."[108] Although parents lost control over most aspects of their institutionalized children's lives, major medical procedures still needed parental consent. The high rate of refusals testifies to parental skepticism about superintendents' judgment.

Other letters protested the lack of academic instruction. I have noted that mothers often consented to institutional care in the hope that it would promote their children's productivity and self-sufficiency. Some were shocked to discover that their children received no training of any kind. Expectations of cure were also disappointed. Seven years after her son's admission to Craig Colony, one mother wrote, "I should think there should be some improvement with all those years up there, if he is getting any treatment or att[ent]ion at all."[109] Another woman wrote thirteen years after her sister entered the facility, "Our main reason for committing her to your care was to cure her taste for drink which caused her Epileptic spells. She has been away much longer than the time said to cure such cases."[110]

Women had other grievances. One complained about her son's unkempt appearance: "He was Very Dirty went I was thear to see Him. For I Done Like to see hime in Long Pant that Done Fit him at all and Shoes to Big for his Feet he has 2 suit of Cloth there and 2 Pair of shoes and I Done See Why he Cant Wear them."[111] A second complained that her son was "encouraged to chew and is furnished tobacco; this is not right. When my daughter visited him five years ago, at which time he was just fourteen years of age, his teeth were completely ruined from chewing tobacco, and such practice would certainly have ill effect on his health as well as moral."[112] A mother whose son had resided in the same cottage for nine years wrote that he "should be transferred to a more cheerful house where his mind would have an opportunity to develop. Constant company of bad boys for so many years cannot possibly improve him."[113] When transfers occurred, women often criticized the new quarters.

Like sanatoriums, institutions for mentally defective people relied on the labor of higher-functioning inmates. Mothers often charged that these work assignments damaged their children's health. Harsh discipline further distressed correspondents. Some argued that their children's offenses were too trivial for severe punishments.[114] One mother implied that responsibility for her son's transgression lay with the institution rather than with him: "You mention that he stays out after nine o'clock from his cottage and this I do not understand because I believe you regulate the mode of living for all patients and I do not understand how he can disregard the rules."[115]

One unusual mother accepted the Craig Colony superintendent's interpretation of an assault on her son. Informed that he was in the hospital because his jaw had been broken by another patient, she wrote,

> I regret, very much, to learn this, feeling that Robert is, perhaps, not controling his temper as he should.
>
> I also received your letter of earlier date stating Robert had received a burn on the top of his foot. As a rule when things happen, he writes and tells us, but the burn was never mentioned. The two mishaps, convince me more than ever, he is not trying to do his part.
>
> I shall write him very sharply, and wonder if a good talking to by you, or someone, would calm him down.[116]

Most relatives, however, held superintendents responsible for protecting the residents from harm and became incensed when injury, or worse, befell them while they were in the institution's care. The sister of a Craig Colony resident received this stunning news:

> I regret to advise you that [Samuel] was drowned on April 6th. Yesterday morning Jewish Services were held at the Colony and your brother in company with several other patients started for Church. It would seem that while on his way to Church he became disturbed, left the rest of the boys and wandered away. Shortly after this he was reported missing and men were sent out looking for him. A diligent search was made but no trace of him was found until 4:30 in the afternoon when a local freight crew of the Pennsylvania Railroad Company while passing through the Colony on a train saw the body of a man lying in the water of the Kishaqua Creek. They stopped the train and took the body from the water. Word was immediately sent to the Colony and men were sent to the site of the drowning and identified the remains as that of Samuel.[117]

In her reply, the sister charged the institution with abuse and neglect:

> You have often stated in your letters that he was carefully watched
> and guarded, if so how was it possible that he wandered away and
> no one seen him do so. I don't think he was taken care of, wich
> people of his condition should, for such foule play would befolen
> him.
>
> No doubt you have seen him before his body was shiped home,
> and have noticed all those bruises on the side of his forhead, nose
> and eare . . .
>
> We were very much disappointed in the care he received. For
> each guard knows how many pupils is in his charge and should be
> able to manage them as not to disappiar under his eye.[118]

The final reason for writing to superintendents was to seek permission for residents to leave, temporarily or permanently. Poor health or
work obligations prevented many mothers from traveling. Moreover,
children who came home could participate in family life, attending
weddings and birthdays, sitting by the beds of dying siblings, and seeing visiting grandparents. Although a desire for help with housework
or for another wage earner may have prompted some requests for discharge, many letter writers expressed a genuine longing for reunion. A
woman who had been informed of her brother's serious illness wrote,
"It brakes our hart to have our dear Brother out thair and if he is to die
i would wish if forehand to bring him home first of carse it would be
very hard as we have not the money to hire help, but i can not bare to
think of my poor brother ding out thair a way from us."[119] Another
woman explained why she wanted her fifty-six-year-old sister-in-law
home: "I wrote you about two years ago asking her release and you advised me to wait a while longer. We are all growing older and dont feel
its wise to be so far separated, sickness or death [may come] and we
should like to be together at that time *if possible.*"[120]

In their replies, superintendents agreed to distribute presents to the
residents and trace lost parcels. However, they prohibited attendants
from accepting gifts, opposed home visits and parole, refused to change
cottage and work assignments, rejected mothers' medical recommendations, and countered all complaints.

Although in many cases Craig Colony superintendents gave no explanations for their decisions, those who did advanced three major arguments. First, mothers were too parochial. In 1912 a doctor forwarded a mother's request that her son be allowed greater freedom. The superintendent replied that the mother "did not seem to realize the necessity of having [the boy] kept under close supervision. From her attitude it would seem to me that she is rather selfish in her view, considering [her son] and not the Institution and its patients."[121] Employing the terminology of feminist moral philosophers today, we could say that the superintendent relied on an ethic of justice, the mother on an ethic of care.[122] The superintendent had an obligation to treat all inmates equally; the mother focused on the needs of her particular child.

Second, administrators discredited mothers' knowledge claims. I have argued that mothers based those claims on personal experiences and intimate relationships with their children. Superintendents asserted that the passage of time eroded the value of such knowledge and that residents transferred their affections from home to the institution.

The third argument rested on prevailing understandings of epilepsy. Superintendents denied the possibility of intimate knowledge of inmates because the disease was believed to erase personal characteristics.[123] Replying to mothers who had called attention to the special needs of their particular children, superintendents discussed epileptics in general, often referring to "them" or "these people." The most common rationale for refusing requests for discharge was that epileptics required institutional structure and discipline. Superintendents countered demands for training by asserting that many epileptics became too feebleminded to learn. Residents' complaints were dismissed as symptoms of their disease. In response to a woman who asked that her niece be transferred from the infirmary, which she detested, the superintendent wrote, "It is quite characteristic of patients suffering from epilepsy that their disposition becomes more irritable and fault finding as time goes on and this is true of Jenny's case."[124]

The form, as well as the content, of the administrators' replies served to rebuff attempts to influence care. In contrast to the mothers' warm and engaged epistolary style, superintendents adopted what Kathryn Montgomery Hunter calls the "clinical tone"—"objective, detached, impersonal, unemotional about death and loss and limitation."[125] Their answers were couched in medical terminology. Mothers who begged for minutiae about their children's lives received only terse, summary replies. Although superintendents answered the specific questions posed to them, they supplied no extraneous details. The deep emotions the mothers expressed met silence.

The archives suggest that most mothers wrote to administrators only once or twice. The few who wrote regularly after their children's admission either sent fewer letters as time went on or stopped altogether. Trent argues that letters to institutions for the feebleminded became less frequent because parents "came to terms" with their children as institutional inmates,[126] but there may have been other reasons. Most mothers were unaccustomed to writing letters, especially to their social superiors. Some expressed a fear of incurring the superintendents' displeasure; as we have seen, superintendents did nothing to allay such concerns. As years passed, some mothers died, and others became too frail to write. And residents who had left home as young children outgrew the traits their mothers most treasured.

Moreover, it seems that most appeals to superintendents were fruitless. The mother of an eighteen-year-old boy who had been in Craig Colony for nine years explained the recent break in her correspondence thus: "I am forever thinking about him, yet I do not write often as I always get the same sad news."[127] Thwarted by the superintendents, parents sometimes sought the intercession of other officials. The files of the Children's Bureau contain numerous letters from parents complaining about deplorable conditions at institutions. When an Illinois father found his son severely burned in 1915, he contacted his state representative, who launched an investigation.[128] Rather than repeatedly petitioning unyielding superintendents, some parents asked federal or state officials to reverse denials of parole or discharge.[129] And a few took direct action, kidnapping children whom superintendents refused to release.[130]

If we can only speculate about why mothers stopped writing, we know more about the attitudes of those who continued. Very few of those who persisted in writing to Craig Colony accepted the superintendents' accounts of their children. One set of letters provides a particularly striking example of a mother's continued faith in her own understanding, despite a superintendent's repeated denigration.[131] Mrs. Stein was a Jewish New York City woman whose son, Milton, entered Craig Colony at the age of eight in November 1910. She wrote every few months, sending books, food, and clothing, inquiring about his health, and seeking his return for visits. Because poor health prevented her from traveling, she could see Milton only at home. The superintendent repeatedly replied that Milton's frequent and severe seizures required him to remain in the colony.

Mrs. Stein initially deferred to the superintendent's judgment. "Dear sir," she wrote in September 1914, "as my son is 4 years at the Colony can you advise me if I can take him home, for you know if he is better or not." She was unwilling, however, to accept the superintendent's assessment of Milton's mental capacity. When the superintendent proclaimed the boy "extremely feebleminded" in 1916, Mrs. Stein expressed incredulity, "for at home, he was never feeble-minded; and was an apt scholar at school." She also noted that she found his letters "thoughtful."

Mrs. Stein finally visited the colony in August 1918, eight years after Milton's admission. "When I departed," she wrote, "he had a seizure but was not unconscious for during the attack, he clung to me and kept crying, 'Mother do not leave me.' How I wished then that I would remain and mother my boy. But it is impossible." Three months later, the superintendent informed her that Milton's condition had seriously deteriorated. She replied,

> You wrote that he is failing mentally, but I simply cannot grasp it. When I went up to see him, Dr. Shanahan, he related things that happened ten and twelve years ago. He introduced me to the boys telling me their names and where they lived. He begged so hard to go home. So we went to see the Doctor who had taken your place and Milton asked the Doctor to transfer him to Randall's Island if he cant send him home. The doctor asked my boy why he wished to be transferred and Milton answered, "My folks will be able to see me more often than they would here, because it costs a great deal of money to come up to the Colony." Dr. Shanahan in all his letters he writes, "mother I would love to be near you I cannot bear to be so far away." And I think Dr. Shanahan that this thought drives everything out of his mind and he simply forgets everything else.

The superintendent responded, "We will again repeat to you that Milton Stein is failing mentally and is undergoing a progressive deterioration. You must realize, of course that the endowments of Milton were always more or less deficient and that the size and shape of his head, his gait and his general appearance would indicate that there is a serious defect of the central nervous system. From such a condition there could not be expected any great improvement."

Mrs. Stein remained unconvinced. In February 1920 she asked, "Do you think if he were at home near his mother and those very dear to him, that it would be better for him." As usual, the response was pessimistic: "We can give you no hope for any improvement in Milton's condition." Nevertheless, Mrs. Stein brought Milton home for a few weeks in the spring of 1921. After his return to Craig Colony, her letters became more sporadic. Although she stopped pleading for his release, she never completely relinquished hope for some kind of recovery. In June 1928 she wrote, "I hope Dr. Shanahan the kind God has worked some of his miracles as only He can do." Milton died of meningitis in March 1930, twenty years after entering the colony.

Although Mrs. Stein may have been deluded about her son's capabilities, she was not alone in clinging to hope in the face of constant discouragement. One woman wrote to the superintendent of a private Illinois institution where her son resided, "Sometimes I still have hope for him although I know it is useless."[132] A mother writing to Craig Colony reproached the superintendent for failing to understand the importance of hope in alleviating suffering. Asked whether her fifteen-year-old son had any "remembrance of home" after four years at the colony, the superintendent replied, "His mentality is quite poor and he seems to take little notice of his surroundings. I hardly think he has any memory of his home life." The mother responded, "Your letters regarding my son have almost taken away from me that great comforter of the unfortunate 'Hope.' Is it really true, doctor, that I must regard my poor boy as lost both to me and to the world forever? Will life have no more meaning to him any more?"[133] Such women appear to have remained hopeful, not because they denied the superintendents' prognoses, but because they refused to accept those prognoses as the only reality. Information about disease processes did not extinguish the mothers' belief in their children's wholeness.

⁓ THE SUPERINTENDENTS of institutions employed various methods to sever the connections between mothers and their feebleminded or epileptic children. They restricted visits, rejected requests for parole and discharge, concealed information, deflected complaints, and subtly, or not so subtly, denied mothers' knowledge claims. Many mothers may have withdrawn as a result; some may have had other reasons for distancing themselves. Nevertheless, at least some women continued to view their children as integral members of their families and fought to preserve affective ties. In response to superintendents who treated the residents as an undifferentiated mass, mothers stressed their children's distinctive characteristics and asserted their basic worth. Some refused to abandon hope despite grim prognoses, thus rejecting the reductionism of institutional reports and challenging the scientific outlook that bolstered the superintendents' authority.

Conclusion

Today the "bad mother" is typically portrayed as indifferent to her children and unwilling to assume caregiving obligations. In the early twentieth century, charity workers, superintendents of institutions, government officials, and physicians occasionally issued a similar indictment of mothers of feebleminded and epileptic children. The accusation of neglect leveled at one COS client helped to justify the campaign to institutionalize her daughter. When the Depression forced institutions to reject new applicants, public officials reproached mothers for seeking to evade their responsibilities to provide care. Far more often, however, mothers were derided for being overly attached to their children. Rather than seeking to strengthen family ties, professionals sought to rupture them, and some ridiculed the deep bonds that prevented women from surrendering their children.

Conflicts between professionals and mothers frequently were embedded in broader systems of power. We have seen that professionals were predisposed to diagnose cases of epilepsy and feeblemindedness among families of the poor, immigrants, and racial minorities. In addition, many professionals viewed socially marginalized mothers as unfit to supervise their own children. Both charity workers and welfare officials made monetary relief conditional on children's removal from the home. After institutional placement, superintendents invoked legal authority to enforce their definition of children's problems.

Nevertheless, mothers were not entirely powerless. Despite overwhelming pressure to defer to expert authority, many continued to trust their own understanding of their children. Some kept children home much longer than charity workers, public officials, and doctors recommended. Some consented to institutionalization only when outside circumstances made it impossible for them to continue providing care. And some persisted in their belief that institutionalized children remained unique individuals who deserved the best care. Although the labels of feeblemindedness and epilepsy carried the luster of science, their ability to shape maternal feelings and knowledge was sharply limited.[134]

～9

"Like Ordinary Hearing Children": Raising Offspring according to Oralist Dictates

$\mathcal{E}$ARLY-TWENTIETH-CENTURY mothers of deaf children escaped much of the blame and moral censure faced by mothers of fee-bleminded or epileptic children. The role entrusted to them was also very different. Rather than permanently exiling their offspring to institutions, mothers of deaf children were supposed to prepare them for integration into the broader society. Nevertheless, these women also operated within a set of assumptions that disparaged their attachment to handicapped children and diminished the children's essential worth.

Most nineteenth-century educators of deaf children had been "manualists," emphasizing instruction in sign language and establishing residential schools that fostered the creation of a distinct deaf community. At the end of the century, however, "oralism" became the dominant discourse. Like charity workers and public health nurses encountering immigrants and people of color, oralists preached the virtues of assimilation. Those who founded residential schools taught lipreading and speech exclusively, and discouraged the formation of separate deaf cultures. Some advocated boarding school placement only when appropriate day schools were unavailable.[1]

Douglas C. Baynton links the triumph of oralism to the increasing importance of the concept of normality. "Oralists argued that 'the best principles of work with other children are best also for the deaf,' that they were 'trying to make our children like ordinary hearing children,' and would therefore try anything that came 'nearer to making them like hearing people.'"[2] Appearance was almost as important as performance. Even when "normal" functioning was impossible, deaf people were expected to imitate the hearing and thus appear less obviously different.

Once again we are examining a practice considered scientific in the late nineteenth and early twentieth centuries but now widely discredited. Oralist reformers were often educators rather than physicians, but they spoke with the absolute conviction and authority of medical science. Recent research suggests that the suppression of sign language disastrously affected several generations of deaf people. Although deaf children often learned to sign eventually, the denial of language during their formative years seriously retarded their ability to learn.[3] Oliver Sacks cites a 1972 study which concluded that the average deaf eighteen-year-old high school graduate could read only at the fourth grade level.[4] Today many educators of the deaf provide instruction in the use of sign language along with lipreading and speech.[5]

Growing numbers of deaf people now regard themselves as members of a distinct linguistic and cultural minority,[6] but in this chapter I consider deaf children a disabled group because both the experts and caregivers I examine viewed them as such. Whereas several previous chapters discussed the extent to which caregivers conformed with expert advice, I focus here on the costs of compliance to caregivers.

This chapter draws from articles appearing in the *Volta Review* in the 1930s, as well as from mothers' letters published by the journal. The *Volta Review* was established in 1899 as the *Association Review* of the American Association to Promote the Teaching of Speech to the Deaf, the leading oralist organization.[7] The association's first president was the inventor Alexander Graham Bell, who had deafness in the family and advocated integrating deaf people into society to prevent the "formation of a deaf variety of the human race."[8] In 1910 the name of the association was changed to the Volta Bureau, and the name of the journal to the *Volta Review*.[9] The journal published numerous articles by teachers and other experts offering advice for mothers of deaf children. In the early 1930s, the Bureau established correspondence clubs for mothers. Club members communicated with one another by means of a "roundabout letter," portions of which appeared in the journal each month. Women who felt profoundly alone raising deaf children in a hearing world looked to the clubs for suggestions, inspiration, and support.

Experts writing in the *Volta Review* shared the dominant cultural belief that mothers could assume virtually unlimited responsibilities for their children. "All parenthood means sacrifice," an article proclaimed, "but the parents of deaf children are called upon far more than the normal amount because of the extraordinary means that must be used in overcoming the handicap of a missing major sense."[10] Another article noted that mothers had to take the lead because fathers "may become discouraged, some of them even a bit estranged, from the children who require so much and respond so slowly."[11]

A central obligation of mothers was teaching their children to speak and read lips. Although schools for the deaf undertook this work, most accepted students beginning at the age of six or seven, long after training was supposed to commence; oralist doctrine held that even infants could, and should, be given special sensory training.[12] Mothers of day school students were supposed to supplement classroom instruction at home in the afternoons and evenings. Those whose children attended residential schools needed to provide extra training during vacations and holidays to prevent laxness and carelessness.

During the intervals between formal lessons, mothers were expected to exert constant vigilance over their children, preventing them from acquiring any of the "telltale" habits of the deaf, such as gesturing or pantomiming. The emphasis on social acceptability also meant that mothers were admonished to pay particular attention to discipline. Deaf children were believed to be especially prone to temper tantrums. One of the hallmarks of the good mother was the ability to control such undesirable displays of frustration and rage.

Mothers also were exhorted to control their own emotions. Baynton argues that late-nineteenth-century oralist leaders tended to sentimentalize the mother-child relationship, which their methods were intended to foster. Rather than surrendering children to the alien culture of deaf schools, mothers could keep their offspring home, teaching them "the satisfying, comforting language of kith and kin."[13] We have seen, however, that mother love lost favor among childcare experts during the 1920s and 1930s. Maternal affection was assumed to be especially dangerous for deaf children. Indulgent mothers responded to gestures, ignored misbehavior, allowed children to play rather than study, and, in general, failed to prepare them for the hostile world awaiting them.

It was especially important for mothers to be wise and intelligent as school age approached. Late-nineteenth-century oralists had envisioned replacing residential schools for the deaf with day schools. Largely as a result of the efforts of oralist leaders, many large public school systems established special schools for the deaf in the late nineteenth and early twentieth centuries. Boarding schools, however, remained the only option for the great majority of deaf students living in small towns and rural areas.[14] Ironically, many oralists now advocated sending deaf children to separate schools in the name of integration. Unlike the earlier boarding schools that oralists had long opposed, these new institutions taught speech and lipreading as the only forms of communication, and most prohibited students from signing even outside the classroom. The real tragedy, according to oralist experts of the 1930s, was not the child banished to an impersonal and foreign institution but rather the one "who is kept at home because his parents could not bear to part with him."[15]

Maternal sorrow over a diagnosis of deafness was also deemed self-indulgent and unacceptable. Today it is generally agreed that the discovery of a child's disability precipitates a period of grief, as parents mourn the "perfect" child they had expected. Like people experiencing the death of loved ones, such parents pass through various stages: "denial," "bargaining," "anger," and "acceptance."[16] But experts writing in the *Volta Review* expected mothers to bypass that process entirely, converting adversity into challenge.

Article after article reminded women of the "cheery courage," "invincible spirit," and "endless patience" expected of them. In his study of polio patients and their families in the 1950s, Fred Davis writes that "the paralytic polio treatment procedure is of the quintessence of the Protestant ideology of achievement in America—namely, slow, patient, and regularly applied effort in pursuit of a long-range goal."[17] Like the physical therapy regime imposed on recovering polio sufferers, the job of teaching deaf children to communicate orally in the 1930s was exceedingly arduous, painstaking, and frustrating, involving endless repetition and often producing imperceptible results. One observer compared the effort by profoundly deaf children to master oral communication to that of English speakers attempting to learn Japanese in soundproof glass enclosures.[18] Nevertheless, the *Volta Review* assumed that all mothers could prevail, given sufficient determination, will-power, and optimism.

Extenuating circumstances were rarely noted in *Volta Review* accounts. Inspirational stories about students' achievements typically failed to mention the level and onset of the hearing loss, although both profoundly affect the ability to master speech. At a time when conditions in state schools for the deaf were deteriorating, as the Depression forced state legislatures to cut budgets, *Volta Review* authors minimized the differences between public and private schools. The experts also occasionally implied that more women could afford private school tuitions if they were more creative, thrifty, or self-sacrificing. Limited income, like deafness, was simply an obstacle any suitably motivated individual could successfully overcome.

The mothers' roundabout letters provide a window into the way women negotiated the messages directed at them. Like the authors of many other letters analyzed in this book, the *Volta Review* correspondence club members were overwhelmingly white and middle class. Although oralists claimed that their model was culturally neutral, it has traditionally been associated with social privilege; indeed, one of the attractions of oralism was its promise to keep children apart from the stigmatized deaf community.[19] The children displayed in photographs accompanying the letters typically were impeccably dressed and posed in large yards or affluent houses. Even in the depths of the Depression, most letter writers remained out of the workforce. Many were able to afford private school tuitions or hire special tutors. None identified herself as deaf. These letters must be read with even greater care than those we have previously examined from manuscript collections. Just a few of the mothers' contributions to the roundabout letters were published, and rather than including each contribution in its entirety, the editors selected certain portions.[20]

Not surprisingly, the mothers' writings echoed themes found in the journal articles. Many women portrayed themselves in heroic terms, harnessing extraordinary willpower and determination to the task of teaching their children to act like the hearing. Several employed the language of war. A West Virginia mother wrote, "After a period of heartache and despondency we brushed away the tears and bravely began the battle of preparing her for life."[21]

The letter writers also asserted that they cheerfully sacrificed friend-ships, time alone, and even other household responsibilities to devote themselves to their children. A Texas woman explained how she made time for her son's lessons: "From the very beginning Charles and I have kept regular hours, and have allowed nothing to interfere. My friends have cooperated beautifully. They never telephone me in the mornings, and after the first month or so stopped inviting me to lun-cheons."[22] When one mother noted that she had just begun transport-ing her son to day school, another responded,

> I am glad you are getting Richard off to school and that you don't mind the half hour's drive. It will take two hours of your day five times a week, but it will be the best ten hours you ever spent. I know because I spend an hour traveling each day to get Billy, and an hour traveling home with him. But I love it, because I know I am helping him in the best way I can. When I call for him and he proudly produces a paper out of the inside pocket of his first suit, I feel that life is grand.[23]

No difficulty was insurmountable. Because appropriate schooling was unavailable locally, two women moved, one to a town with a special public school for the deaf, another to Northampton, Massachusetts, the location of the Clarke School, a well-known private institution.[24] Although one woman feared she would be unable to afford private tui-tion, she "did manage . . . by undertaking great economies at home."[25] After a flood forced a Harrisburg, Pennsylvania, woman to flee her home, she reported, "Things have been so topsy-turvy for awhile that I have done little else but clean, and get furniture to rights. Yet I've man-aged somehow to keep on talking to Nancy as much as ever."[26] External hardships occasionally became blessings in disguise. A woman who originally resented having to do her own housework in addition to training her two deaf sons gradually realized that her onerous workload "teaches the children to be helpful, gives me no time to spoil them and affords many opportunities to teach the homely—and homelike—things of life."[27]

The progress women witnessed confirmed their faith in the virtues of hard work. The following quotations are typical:

We can see much improvement in Frank this year, especially in his desire to talk. When we have a guest, he comes and asks the name.[28]

Lately I have noticed [Richard] uses any number of colloqualisms, which make his speech more natural.[29]

We feel that Priscilla is gaining in her ability to read our lips. It is seldom that she fails to get our meaning about things when we try to tell her.[30]

I am just now beginning to appreciate fully the miracle of oral training and we are all getting so much pleasure out of talking to Barbara and asking her about things, just enjoying how much she has learned.[31]

As spoken language improved, children became more tractable. A woman living in Mexico reported, "In the past we had quite a lot of temper tantrums and crying to combat and we are glad that, with her increased power of making us understand and our power to make her understand us, she seems to be an entirely changed child. Her disposition has improved so much, and she is such a happy, lovable child now."[32]

Mothers were proud when their children could pass as hearing. A California mother wrote, "I am sometimes amused at the look of utter bewilderment on the faces of sympathetic strangers and acquaintances (whom I've told, 'I have a little deaf girl') when she barges in with that give-no-quarter-and-expect-none air, and all full of smiles and interest. She usually shakes hands and then drags out candy . . . and passes it— sometimes specifying 'One' if the supply is low!"[33] Another mother wrote, "I take my child everywhere I go, parties and just everywhere . . . You cannot tell in any way by his actions that he is deaf. He never seems to be puzzled by not understanding what I say."[34] Other women delighted in the friendships their children developed with hearing children. "It is the most wonderful thing in the world to me to learn that children of all ages really like my little deaf boys and want to be with them," wrote an Iowa woman.[35]

Women also took pride in their own sense of mastery. Many letter writers portrayed themselves as accomplished individuals who had learned a set of technical skills and now had valuable experiences and specialized knowledge to share. Women filled their letters with suggestions for others. "I should like to tell you of a little experiment that is working out beautifully for all of us," wrote a mother who made a doll to take speech exercises with her five-year-old son and make him more comfortable with his lessons.[36] Other women described strategies they had perfected for enforcing discipline, engaging babies' attention, and communicating with residential school students who were too young to read letters from home.

Nevertheless, compliance with oralist dictates was often imperfect, even among members of the *Volta Review* correspondence clubs. Some women lacked the material advantages the journal took for granted. "I know I do not devote enough time to Margie," one mother wrote, "but in addition to all the usual work of a housewife I run a filling station, take care of a large yard and do a lot of my own sewing. We live in back of the station and about the time Margie and I get a lesson started someone is sure to stop and want gasoline, so we are usually interrupted."[37] Another wrote, "I believe I am much behind you other mothers with my teaching. I did not start until Eddie was almost 4 years old. You might ask 'Where were you the rest of the time?' Well, you see, I have eleven other children besides Eddie—one younger—so I had no time."[38] Whereas one letter writer extolled the benefits of driving children to school, another noted that she lacked access to a car. The credo that all difficulties could be overcome must have had a hollow ring to many women.

A few letter writers admitted that they departed from key oralist recommendations. "I have a confession to make," a North Carolina mother wrote. "I do use quite a few signs."[39] Another woman unabashedly wrote, "My boys all speak well, and they also use the sign language and the manual alphabet. I think this opens up a world they could never enter by lip reading alone."[40]

Opposition to boarding school placement was common. A mother who lived outside the catchment area of the closest public day school for the deaf wrote, "Peter is a splendid boy, but has his peculiarities. At table he never eats very much, but I try to find things he likes. Another thing, he occasionally has involuntaries [bed wetting] at night, and he would have them oftener if I did not get up with him every night. These are just two of the many things I do for him, and who would understand him and do such things for him if I send him away?"[41] After other mothers tried to extinguish her fears, she decided she was "mistaken" and made plans to visit the state residential school. Nevertheless, she remained ambivalent:

> If I could be sure that in an hour or so he would cease crying, and not carry on until he is exhausted, if I were sure that his pillow would not be soaked with uncontrollable weeping, I could stand it. It is only for the dear child that I feel. I wonder if leaving a deaf child so completely alone and miserable doesn't cause a severe nervous shock, even if it doesn't destroy his confidence in mother, whom he always trusted, and who has never before failed him? I went for two years to a boarding school far from my home, and although I was sixteen I was so homesick I was ill.[42]

A New Jersey mother wrote,

> I visited a residential school and almost decided to send my little girl there as a resident from Mondays through Fridays. But when I came home I had such terrible dreams about her lying in one of those little white beds calling and calling for me, and I couldn't go through with it. I know she probably would not take it nearly so hard as I, but I still can't bring myself around to sending her away from home. She is very sensitive, and to send her off to where she knows no one and has no one to love and comfort her, especially at night, would have an effect on her personality and character for life. It seems to me it would be like sending one of us to jail.

Although she realized that schools conferred important benefits, she concluded that "a little girl needs the love and association of her parents."[43] Oralist discourse implied that women's empathic knowledge was irrelevant because children were predictable and malleable, and could be relied on to respond to standardized training. These mothers, however, continued to trust their own understandings of the characteristics and needs of their offspring.

Some fears transcended children's individual personalities. Reports of cruelty at state schools frightened mothers who could not afford private tuitions. Although women expressed confidence in the private schools they selected, these facilities often accepted students as young as three years old, when children were still closely bound to their mothers and had no way of comprehending their banishment. Moreover, private boarding schools frequently were located hundreds of miles from home.

After children departed, many women continued to express ambivalence, interlacing descriptions of the stunning grief that assailed them with assertions of the advantages of residential schooling. One mother wrote,

> I have just been through the trying circumstances of leaving my little three year old daughter, Joyce, in school. We placed her in Central Institute, St. Louis. It was a three days' drive from our home to St. Louis . . . She cried a great deal and it was all I could do to restrain myself; but I did not let her see the agony it cost me . . . We have heard from the school every week, since our return home, and the reports from her teacher . . . have been most encouraging. I miss her more every day. Joyce seems essential to my life. Even her pony comes and hangs his head over the fence, and her dog sits before the door and whines. Her little sister, Helen Ruth, runs all over the house crying, 'Oyce, Oyce!' You see, it isn't easy to have her gone, but we feel we are doing the best that can be done for her.[44]

Four months later she wrote, "My deepest fear is that I may have lost something I'll never regain."[45]

Another mother justified her decision to send her young son away to school thus: "He is so strong willed that I feel a residential school is the place for him until he learns there are certain rules which must be obeyed. He is an only child, so the school offers the additional advantage of the companionship of the other children." Nevertheless, leaving him "was one of the hardest things I have ever had to do. There were no tears until we were safely out of sight, but then there was a regular flood."[46] A New York woman recalled that her son's first years as a weekly boarder at the Lexington School were

> terribly hard for both of us. He cried every Sunday when it came time to take him back to school, and when he used to say, "I don't want to learn how to talk or write, I want to stay home with Mama," it just broke my heart. I had to grit my teeth to see that he

arrived at school on Sunday evening. I realized that he had his own way to make in the world, and I wanted to do everything in my power to help make him a good citizen. I used to keep the door of his room closed all week while he was away, for it seemed to me sometimes as if he had died; but I have got over that foolish idea.[47]

Some mothers never reconciled themselves to the loss. At the end of a school holiday, one mother wrote that her daughter "seems to like school better every year. For a week, she kept counting the days, and when we took her back to school she was the first one out of the car and ready to go in. Naturally, this makes us happy at the thought of leaving her where she is so contented and satisfied; but it also gives me a pang to think that she is growing away from us. As she grows older, I fear she will feel that school is really her home."[48]

Departures remained wrenching. "Eddie will soon be home for Christmas," wrote one mother. "I am already dreading the parting that will come after the brief holiday."[49] Another woman confessed, "Some of you speak of having trouble with discipline, and the relief it is to have the children back in school, while I am a regular baby about parting with mine."[50]

The letter writers also displayed a broader range of emotions about the pace of learning at home than the *Volta Review* deemed appropriate. Despite considerable pressure to portray themselves as relentlessly optimistic, some women acknowledged discouragement. "Thank you for your kind remarks about my efforts," one mother wrote to another. "I needed a boost, for, in spite of indications to the contrary, I don't always feel like Pollyanna."[51] A Nebraska woman wrote, "My little deaf son's education sometimes seems to me like a long steep hill that is hard to climb and I wonder if we shall ever reach the top."[52] Although the mother added that "it certainly is a consolation to have someone in our group who has almost reached the top," reports of other children's accomplishments sometimes lowered morale. Responding to a request for more information about her daughter, a North Carolina mother wrote, "Frankly, I am ashamed of her progress compared with other children I have read about."[53] A Kansas woman wrote in a similar vein, "Mrs. C. has made such splendid progress with Freddie I am ashamed of my efforts."[54]

In her classic study of women's deference to modern ideals of female physical beauty, Sandra Lee Bartky writes, "Since the standards . . . are impossible fully to realize, requiring as they do a virtual transcendence of nature, a woman may live much of her life with a pervasive feeling of deficiency."[55] Oralism was based on a similar myth of control over nature. The intense training process prescribed by oralists provided one type of communication skill to many moderately deaf, and some severely deaf, children, but virtually none could converse at the level of hearing counterparts. The language development of profoundly deaf children was seriously stunted.

Assuming that maternal responsibility was virtually unbounded, many women blamed themselves when their children failed to fulfill expectations. "I am always under a nervous strain when I take [Kenneth] to and from school," wrote one mother. "I try to get him to stop and look when we cross streets, but he will dash out quickly. I can see more and more the many mistakes I've made. I see that I haven't been as firm with him as I should have been. I've been over anxious about him, and haven't let him feel any responsibility."[56] A Kansas woman, whose son showed little interest in educational games, wrote, "I know it is my mistake somehow, and I need to learn as much as Billy Lee does."[57] A Pennsylvania mother wrote that her daughter's "lip reading isn't progressing as fast as I'd like, but it will come along, I know, after more effort on my part."[58] The many women who expressed a wish for greater patience similarly implied that the problem lay within themselves, rather than with the methods they struggled to apply. Disappointment engendered redoubled commitment, often leading, we may surmise, to deeper discouragement.

LIKE THEIR OFFSPRING, the mothers of deaf children could gain approval from oralist experts and acceptance from the broader society only by conforming to an ideal. Regardless of circumstances, children's personal traits, or the severity of their hearing loss, all women were expected to display optimism, determination, detachment, and self-control. The *Volta Review* pressured mothers to comply with oralist dictates, but also provided a forum for chronicling the more complicated realities of their lives. Some correspondence club members expressed joy as their children's speech clarified, temper tantrums disappeared, and friendships with hearing children flourished. The tone of the letters, however, was not uniformly triumphant. Even mothers who adhered closely to the views sanctioned by the journal wrestled with frustration, shame, sorrow, and despair.

⌒Conclusion: The Uses of the Past

Changes After 1940: A Brief Outline

Caregiving in America has continued to undergo profound transformation since 1940. One major source of change has been the demographic shift. The elderly, who constituted 6.8 percent of the population in 1940, increased to 12.5 percent in 1998.[1] The rate of increase of Americans eighty-five years old and over has been particularly dramatic;[2] the "old old" are the fastest growing segment of the population.[3] A study published in 1989 concluded that 7 million relatives and friends care for elderly people.[4] Other researchers estimate that more than 60 percent of all women provide elder care at some point in their lives.[5]

Although most people sixty-five and over can tend themselves and their households without assistance, approximately one-quarter require at least occasional help,[6] and the prevalence of disability rises steeply with age.[7] The major causes of death in the elderly—heart disease, cancer, and stroke—are chronic conditions that often inflict years of infirmity.[8] Although physicians can now save the lives of many people who previously would have died quickly from these conditions, the survivors frequently endure severe disabilities over extended periods.[9] Many elderly people suffer from multiple chronic ailments, including cognitive impairments.[10]

We saw that caregiving responsibilities struck nineteenth-century women randomly throughout adolescence and adulthood. Care for the frail elderly, however, tends to be concentrated in middle and old age. The average age among primary caregivers of elderly people is sixty-two.[11] Many must cope simultaneously with their own age-related health problems.[12]

Despite the aging of the population, slightly more than half of all sick and disabled people needing care are under the age of sixty.[13] Medical achievements have changed the nature of responsibilities for younger dependent groups as well as for older ones. As a result of advances in acute care, the mortality rate for severe traumatic brain injuries dropped from 90 percent to less than 50 percent in three decades; many survivors experience permanent impairments, requiring long-term care.[14] The growing sophistication of neonatal intensive care has enabled doctors to save many extremely premature infants who would have died twenty years ago. At least 20 percent of these surviving "preemies" have major, lifelong disabilities, such as cerebral palsy, mental retardation, or deafness.[15] Improvements in health care are also partly responsible for the increasing life expectancy of individuals with developmental disabilities. People with Down's syndrome, for example, could expect to live fifty-five years in 1993, up from nine years in 1929.[16]

The AIDS epidemic has created additional caregiving challenges. Some caregivers have themselves been diagnosed as having HIV or perceive themselves as especially vulnerable to the disease. In addition, caregivers of both children and intravenous drug users with AIDS tend to have extremely limited social and financial resources. The relative youth of many friends and family members tending people with AIDS presents another problem. Unlike most who care for the frail elderly, most AIDS caregivers are under forty. At a time when other people their age are building relationships and work lives rather than dealing with mortality, caregivers may feel jarringly disconnected from their contemporaries.[17]

As caregiving increasingly focuses on chronic diseases and disabilities, it lasts longer. Most nineteenth-century women responded to relatively brief events—births, acute illnesses, and deaths. Today, approximately 44 percent of caregivers have been furnishing assistance for one to five years, 20 percent for five years or more.[18] As disabled children live longer, more and more parents worry about who will provide care after they die.[19]

In addition, caregiving has become a very lonely endeavor, at least among some social groups. We saw that nineteenth-century caregiving frequently was a communal endeavor, but one of the sharpest complaints of many caregivers today is the intense isolation they must endure. A woman who cared for an ill husband later recalled, "We were prisoners in our own home. Who can you talk to? Old friends and even family, they just don't understand."[20]

To be sure, we can explain the solitary nature of caregiving variously as resulting from the attenuation of kinship and community bonds, the belief of many caregivers that they should cope with problems alone, or the stigma surrounding such afflictions as AIDS and Alzheimer's disease.[21] Nevertheless, as Martha Farnsworth discovered when her second husband fell ill, caregiving tends to be particularly lonely when it lingers over an extended period. Neighbors and friends who initially rally around rarely remain involved over the long haul. A woman who began caring for her elderly mother in the early 1990s described caregiving as "a lonely and isolating sort of thing to go through, because it seems endless, it just keeps on going. The supporters go home, and you're stuck with the situation."[22]

Changes in the formal health care delivery system also have profoundly affected informal caregivers. Enrollment in private health insurance rose from 10 percent of the population in 1940 to 24 percent in 1945.[23] By 1962, 70 percent of the population had insurance coverage for hospital care, and 65 percent for physicians' services.[24] In 1965 the federal government established Medicaid, a welfare program for poor people, and Medicare, a social insurance program for the elderly.

The growth of health care financing programs led to a dramatic upsurge in the use of institutions. The nursing home industry emerged after World War II and expanded rapidly after the enactment of Medicaid.[25] Only a small fraction of elderly people reside in such facilities, but they represent an important alternative to family care. Although hospitalization had become routine for many conditions by 1940, the emergence of public and private health insurance coverage greatly improved access. The Hill–Burton Act of 1946 further boosted hospitalization by providing for a vast infusion of federal funds.[26] Within the first six years after its passage, hospital admissions jumped 26 percent.[27]

It is important not to assume that the growth of the formal health care system has lightened the work of informal caregiving. I have argued throughout this book that outside services typically transform, rather than eliminate, family responsibilities. Family members act as go-betweens, locating services, making arrangements for patients to participate, providing transportation, and monitoring the quality of care. Despite the widespread belief that families abandon elderly people in nursing homes, many relatives are intimately involved in residents' care.[28]

Moreover, some groups remain unprotected against health care costs. More than 44 million people (16 percent of the population) lacked any form of insurance for acute care in 1999.[29] Coverage for long-term care is especially meager. Although the number of private long-term care insurance plans is rising, they enroll only a tiny fraction of the population.[30] Medicare is based on an acute-care model and thus provides minimal assistance for chronic diseases and disabilities; it pays less than 10 percent of nursing home expenditures. Almost by default, Medicaid has become a primary funding source for long-term institutional care, providing 83 percent of all public spending for nursing homes and 52 percent of total nursing home revenues.[31] Residents first must exhaust their financial resources in order to qualify. Approximately 40 percent of nursing home users initially pay privately, but many become eligible for Medicaid after "spending down." The annual cost of a nursing home stay exceeds the incomes of 80 percent of all elderly people.[32]

Public funding of any kind for community- and home-based services is paltry. Although Medicare recently has devoted more funds to home health care, the program continues to emphasize medically oriented care, not the social support services that alleviate the work of informal caregivers. Recipients must be homebound, under the care of a physician, and in need of part-time or intermittent skilled nursing care or physical or speech therapy.[33] Medicaid spending on community-based services has grown even more rapidly, as a result of legislation passed in 1981 giving states the option of applying for waivers from existing rules in order to provide some community care.[34] Nevertheless, just 5 percent of Medicaid's budget goes to community- and home-based care, compared to 33 percent to nursing homes.[35] Two other programs that fund community services for elderly people are Title III of the Older Americans Act and the Social Services Block Grant. The level of resources devoted to both programs is low.[36]

The inadequacies of public funding programs have several implications for caregivers. First, long-term care remains an overwhelmingly private responsibility. Studies consistently find, for example, that families and friends deliver 70 to 80 percent of the services disabled elderly people receive.[37]

Second, caregivers searching for long-term care for family members encounter many of the same problems as did the Depression-era mothers who wrote to the federal government for help in finding health care for children. A study published in 1992 of families of chronically ill and disabled children reported that the parents "find themselves in a constant round of begging, cajoling, and appealing to higher authorities, often in an effort to obtain the most modest assistance in getting their child's specialized needs met within the house . . . Again and again families reported being treated as if they were trying to defraud the system rather than attempting to secure services to which they were entitled."[38]

Third, rich and poor families face very different options. Some evidence suggests that many nursing homes discriminate against Medicaid patients. High occupancy rates—averaging 95 percent nationwide—enable facilities to be selective about admissions. Because the Medicaid reimbursement rate is lower than the amount nursing homes charge private-pay residents, facilities prefer clients who can afford to pay out of pocket. Hospital discharge planners in California estimate that Medicaid patients are four to seven times more difficult to place than privately funded patients.[39] Caregiving for low-income disabled people thus may be especially prolonged.

Medicaid beneficiaries who do gain admission to nursing homes tend to be relegated to institutions that, according to some measures, offer the poorest quality of care; even within a facility, residents relying on Medicaid sometimes receive worse care than private-pay residents.[40] Although reports about substandard conditions in nursing homes de-

ter even affluent family members from considering institutional placement, relatives of Medicaid beneficiaries may be especially motivated
to continue providing care at home.

Income level also affects the distribution of home- and community-
based services. Because most people who receive such services pay privately, utilization varies directly with income. Not surprisingly, the affluent spend far more than other segments of the population on care.
Moreover, self-pay clients receive more hours of home health care than
those who rely on public funds.[41] The greatest inequities may lie in services provided by workers unaffiliated with established organizations.
Some evidence suggests that disabled people and their caregivers rely
disproportionately on this type of assistance, especially in cities with
large pools of immigrant workers. The support provided by such help-
ers typically is not included in government statistics; however, it repre-
sents a major source of assistance to the affluent that is not available to
others.[42]

Still another reason we should not overstate the extent to which the
growth of formal services has reduced family caregiving is that the
movement of care between home and medical facilities has not been
unidirectional. Deinstitutionalization occurred first and most dramatically in the mental health field. The population of the nation's mental
hospitals plunged from 559,000 to 193,000 between 1955 and 1975.[43]
One observer notes that "mental health professionals were . . . oblivi-
ous to what it might mean for families to replace the ward staff without
the training and resources ordinarily available in the hospital."[44] President Kennedy was a major advocate of managing mentally ill people
outside hospitals, calling for a "bold new approach" based on the establishment of a vast network of community mental health centers. But
adequate funding was never appropriated. Fewer than half the centers
required to serve deinstitutionalized patients were built; even those
typically fail to provide the full range of services originally envisaged.[45]
Other services remain equally scanty. Relatives often search unsuccessfully for adequate halfway houses and hospital-based day treatment
programs, and for such nonmedical services as rehabilitation, housing,
and employment training.[46]

Since the mid-1970s, states have attempted to curb Medicaid expenditures by keeping people out of nursing homes.[47] Strategies for

limiting the supply of beds include certificate-of-need programs and moratorium policies.[48] Although the number of nursing home beds nationwide increased slightly between 1987 and 1996, the supply dropped relative to the size of the elderly population.[49] Preadmission screening programs seek to limit the use of existing beds. A Tennessee woman who tried to obtain Medicaid coverage of nursing home care for her father stated, "I called to get him in at one of the nursing homes but they said he did not qualify medically. This was an extremely frustrating time for me. As long as you can, you try to take care of him at home, but in the back of your mind, you think you can always put him in a nursing home. But, when you are raw, they tell you that . . . he is not sick enough. He had been bedfast for 75 percent of the time for three years. He is on oxygen all the time, which limits his ability."[50]

Acute care also is leaving the hospital. The establishment of a prospective payment system for hospital care under Medicare in 1983 resulted in a drop in the length of stay, shifting care back to the home.[51] The pace of dehospitalization accelerated during the 1990s as managed care grew.[52] Patients arrive home sicker as well as quicker, increasing the intensity of services family members must deliver.[53]

Whereas early-twentieth-century advocates of institutionalization emphasized the disadvantages of family connection, contemporary proponents of deinstitutionalization stress the need to humanize the health care system. Policymakers assert that by shifting care back to the home they are not just saving money but also strengthening family bonds and responding to the widespread disenchantment with technologized and impersonal health care. Such comments, however, often appear disingenuous. The contradictions in the arguments suggest that most such assertions are politically expedient rationalizations. The rhetoric of family love is not extended to the very wealthy, who can afford to purchase the services denied to the vast majority of Americans. And as we have repeatedly seen, caregiving can fracture, as well as consolidate, family ties.

High-tech equipment often follows patients out of the hospital. Technologies recently adapted for the home include dialysis, ventilators, cardiac and apnea monitors, feeding tubes, and infusion pumps for administering narcotics, antibiotics, and chemotherapy. The father of a severely disabled infant commented that "the price of bringing

[him] home was to fill his parents' house with enough medical equipment to open a small clinic."[54] A woman whose husband was dying of
lung cancer stated that her bedroom had become a "mini-ICU."[55]

High-tech home care transforms caregiving work as well as the
domestic environment. Some technologies must be constantly moni-
tored, and many require family caregivers to perform tasks that are
more complex than those managed by licensed vocational nurses in
hospitals.[56] Nineteenth-century women struggled to retain jurisdiction
over skilled medical care, but caregivers today complain about being
entrusted with responsibilities that far exceed their capabilities. A
mother whose infant daughter had drains in her stomach, chest tubes,
and infusion pumps for food and antibiotics later commented, "It was
very stressful. Was I doing the right thing? I really wasn't an expert.
Was I doing everything that she needed?"[57] A woman responsible for
monitoring her husband's feeding tube said, "You understand, I'm 64
years old. In my time, I've never learned anything about computers.
And all these buttons. I was terrified."[58] Even computer-literate caregivers may receive less help than they deem necessary. Some hospitals
discharge technology-dependent patients without providing more than
a few minutes of instruction to family members. Because physicians
have largely abandoned the house call, caregivers rely heavily on home
visits by nurses, but patients dependent on public funds find such visits
are few and far between.[59] One observer notes that some consumers receive more support with new word processing programs than with the
complex technology that sustains gravely ill patients at home.[60]

Caregivers also have new responsibilities for institutionalized patients. The same fiscal constraints that encouraged shorter hospital
stays led to reductions in the size of nursing staffs. At the same time,
early discharge has contributed to a rise in the average level of patient
acuity. Because patients are sicker and staffing levels lower, nurses have
increased workloads.[61] Some find that they are no longer able to respond to the personal and social needs of patients. Family members increasingly complain that staff fail to answer call bells or provide assistance with meals and getting to the toilet. As nurses withdraw such
services, family participation becomes crucial, just as it was in the early
days of hospitals.[62]

Regardless of whether patients are at home or in hospitals, sophisticated medical technology raises ethical issues that previous generations

of caregivers never faced. Should premature infants receive aggressive neonatal treatment? At what point should treatment be withdrawn from people with incurable conditions? Robert Zussman argues that although physicians retain control of many key decisions, "the culture of patient rights" demands the involvement of the patient and often the patient's family. "It is precisely those patients who are least able to participate for whom general decisions—to intubate or not to intubate, to dialyze or not to dialyze, whether to treat aggressively or unaggressively—are usually most pressing. The result is that the patient's family is typically substituted for the patient himself or herself."[63]

Many caregivers face additional pressures at work. Women's labor force participation rate grew from 28 percent in 1940 to nearly 60 percent in 1996.[64] Several researchers have analyzed the clash between paid employment and care for elderly relatives.[65] Some argue that caregiving often has little impact on employment.[66] One reason may be that women often assume that their primary goal should be to insulate their work lives from intrusions of family responsibilities; as a result, they sacrifice vacations, social activities, and time alone. In my study of adult daughters caring for elderly parents, I asked women whether caregiving interfered more with leisure or work. A respondent who lived with her disabled mother answered this way: "By cutting into the job, it cuts into the leisure, because the things I have to do for her take place Monday through Friday. So I take time off from the job to take care of her needs, and then I have to give up my leisure to take care of the job. It's a round-robin."[67] Researchers also note that paid employment sometimes benefits caregivers, buffering the emotional consequences of tending elderly kin and providing an alternative source of personal identity.[68] Nevertheless, today, as in the past, caregiving often adversely affects paid employment. Significant numbers of caregivers relinquish their jobs, reduce their hours of work, rearrange their schedules, and take time off without pay.[69]

Little assistance is available to caregivers trying to respond to these complex, and often conflicting, demands. The chief concern of policymakers is to prevent caregivers from unloading their responsibilities on the state, astronomically increasing its burdens. As a result, policymakers support social services and financial assistance for caregivers only insofar as they are viewed as postponing or preventing institutionalization. The major demand of many caregivers is respite services, which provide temporary relief from care.[70] Although most states have established respite programs, they tend to be grossly underfunded, able to serve only a small number of families and offering very few hours of care.[71] State programs to reimburse caregivers for their services typically limit payments to those caring for patients deemed most vulnerable to institutionalization. Stringent eligibility criteria often exclude caregivers who are spouses, children over the age of eighteen, relatives who live apart from the care receivers, and relatives with incomes over a certain amount. Reimbursement levels tend to be low.[72]

The policy response to the conflict between paid employment and care has also been limited. The Family and Medical Leave Act, passed with widespread acclaim in 1993, covers leaves of no more than twelve weeks, provides for no remuneration, excludes part-time and contingent workers and those employed in small firms, and defines families very narrowly. Workers who are white, middle class, and married are most likely to be able to take advantage of the act.[73] Most state programs have similar restrictions.[74] Employer-based programs to accommodate family caregivers tend to be narrow in scope and concentrated in large businesses.[75]

Unlike respite services, financial compensation, and workplace reforms, programs to help caregivers adapt to their responsibilities enjoy enthusiastic support among policymakers. The low cost of such programs partly explains their appeal. It is far cheaper to establish a ten-week course of lectures for caregivers than to provide them with the services of homemakers and home health aides over a period of months or even years. In addition, many caregivers attest to the benefits of such programs. Support groups alleviate the intense isolation experienced by caregivers today. Educational programs that dispense information about disease processes or the new equipment dispatched to the home boost competence and confidence. Counseling services help caregivers disentangle unresolved emotional issues from the process of delivering care.[76]

Unfortunately, these programs also reinforce the premise that our goal should be helping caregivers adjust to unavoidable burdens rather than making care for the dependent population more just and humane. Moreover, support group leaders, educators, and counselors may contribute to the devaluation of caregiving by encouraging caregivers to distance themselves emotionally from the people they tend. We saw that early-twentieth-century experts warned that emotional involvement with sick and disabled people frequently led to overindulgence, permitting them to ignore doctors' orders. The emphasis today is on the problems emotional intimacy creates for the caregiver rather than the care recipient. Care of aged parents is especially likely to be portrayed as an infantilizing experience, stemming from neurotic attachment and involving regressive merging with the patient.

A recent British novel illustrates the prevailing view. In *Have the Men Had Enough?* Margaret Forster describes the conflicts among various family members over how best to care for Grandma, who suffers from dementia and lives with her daughter Bridget, around the corner from her son and his family. Bridget delivers care primarily to heal past disappointments. As a young mother, Grandma had been too overburdened to nurture her children's emotional needs, and Bridget was "the one taken for granted." Caregiving thus permits her to receive the love and affection previously withheld. Although an early-twentieth-century observer might have described Bridget's attachment to her mother as undermining the quality of care, Forster portrays Bridget as attending sensitively to her mother's needs. The interactions of other family members with Grandma are forced and stilted, but Bridget responds to her mother with grace and ease. Bridget's own life, however, becomes more and more constricted. Lacking a sense of self, she becomes submerged in caregiving responsibilities, fails to sustain her other relationships, and refuses even to consider institutionalization when all other options are foreclosed.[77]

This portrait cannot be dismissed as a caricature. My study of women tending elderly parents found that caregiving frequently revived powerful elements of the original parent-child relationship. Many women stated that they slipped back into patterns formed in childhood or adolescence. Old resentments suddenly had renewed force just when the daughters had to assume more adult roles. A woman who quit her job when she returned home to care for her mother described her situation this way: "Because I'm sequestered with my mother all the time, I feel that I'm reverting back. I don't feel like an adult. This could be my chance to grow, but in the process I'm regressing."[78]

Other women reported very different responses. Some enjoyed the closeness they achieved with parents from whom they had grown distant. Mastering old conflicts, some successfully restructured the parent-child relationship. And some perceived the ability to render care as a marker of adulthood, promoting further growth and development. The primary problem many women faced was not the emotional intensity of caregiving but rather the enormous personal sacrifice it entailed and the meagerness of the rewards and respect it conferred.[79] Such issues point to the need for a broad agenda for change, which I will outline in the final section of this chapter.

Respecting Care

The discourse surrounding caregiving helps us understand why care for sick and disabled family members and friends commands so little respect. Although the social fabric relies on our collective ability to sustain life, nurture the weak, and respond to the needs of intimates, we routinely disparage those services and the people who deliver them. One common explanation is that caregiving shares the low status accorded all of women's domestic labor. Another is that we create the illusion of independence by disregarding the care on which we depend.

Our historical inquiry adds three other explanations. First, we have seen that the privileged typically depreciate the humanity of subordinate groups and deride the work of caring for them. Just as slave owners in the antebellum South viewed enslaved people solely in terms of their productive power and apportioned medical care according to the likelihood of recovery, so many early-twentieth-century charity workers in New York regarded care for sick people partly as a way to increase the ranks of productive workers in an industrial economy. Clients who could not be restored to "wage earning power" were considered burdens, consuming household resources that could better be devoted to paid employment. Charity workers also treated many people with tuberculosis as disease carriers rather than sufferers and sought to segregate them in institutions that were little better than warehouses. And an array of professionals recommended institutionalizing "feebleminded" people not only as social and sexual menaces but also as indifferent to affective family relationships.

Second, the cultural value of the three major components of caregiving—instrumental, spiritual, and emotional—declined between 1850 and 1940. Instrumental services in the nineteenth century encompassed not just cooking, cleaning, and assisting sick people with feeding and mobility but also delivering skilled medical care. Women dispensed herbal remedies, dressed wounds, bound broken bones, reattached severed fingers, cleaned bed sores, and removed bullets. The display of unusual healing abilities conferred honor and prestige on women in diverse locales and social strata. Because knowledge acquired through practical education was considered as important as that taught in schools or gleaned in the laboratory, some women could translate caregiving skills into paid employment. Both Sarah Gillespie and Martha Shaw used their experiences caring for dying family members as qualifications for working as skilled nurses in the homes of neighbors. Other women forged careers as midwives.

Struggling to establish themselves as professionals, nineteenth-century doctors often denigrated women's healing knowledge, banned friends and family from the sickroom, and tried to restrict the medical information available to the public through popular media. Nevertheless, many doctors were well aware of their own educational deficiencies, and some later acknowledged their debts to older women caregivers.

Because sickness and death were regarded as religious, as well as medical, events, caregiving had an important spiritual dimension. Enslaved healers in the antebellum South sought to address both the metaphysical and natural causes of disease and to reconnect patients to their ancestors. White women read the Bible to the sick, prayed with them, and urged them to accept death openly and peacefully. It was equally important for caregivers facing the loss of loved ones to resist both denial and despair. Many looked to religion for succor.

Mid-nineteenth-century medicine dignified the emotional dimension of care. Believing that disease arose from the interaction of specific individuals with their environments, doctors recognized the value of understanding both. Moreover, despite doctors' attempts to limit the number of family and friends around the bed, most agreed that attention, sympathy, and reassurance alleviated emotional stress and facilitated healing. Popular literature further affirmed the emotional work of care, encouraging women to find meaning in their closeness to the sufferings of others.

The broad cultural support for these three components of caregiving eroded during the late nineteenth and early twentieth centuries. Caregivers' knowledge increasingly was dismissed as superstition, acceptance of God's will disparaged as resignation, and tender solicitude condemned as indulgence. The balance of power at the bedside shifted from family caregivers to physicians. Although few effective treatments were available, physicians acquired great prestige by allying themselves with the dazzling new discoveries in bacteriology. In addition, physicians escaped the critical scrutiny of neighbors and kin by moving care into offices and hospitals. As the reputation of doctors rose, they could more persuasively portray family caregivers as ignorant and women's healing knowledge as superstition.

Scientific optimism also undermined the spiritual component of care. Rather than looking to religion for the strength to accept the worst, caregivers were expected to mobilize all available medical resources in the fight for recovery. Doctors helped to foster the illusion that the body no longer was subject to uncontrolled forces. Until death was imminent, Dr. Lawrence Flick, a prominent tuberculosis specialist, continually promised cures to family members who adhered to his advice. Spiritual preparation for the next life and acceptance of mortality had no place in his regime.

Simultaneously, the emotional dimension of care was devalued. The ideal was now the purely rational being freed from any disturbing passions or selfish interests. Both doctors and nurses prided themselves on the self-control that shielded them from the pain and suffering they witnessed. New therapeutic approaches emphasized the importance of monitoring patients' behavior. Rather than producing important knowledge about disease, personal intimacy was believed to distort the understanding of patients' needs, leading to dangerous indulgence.

The third way to understand the eclipse of caregiving is to explore how women's involvement increased their dependence. Nancy Fraser and Linda Gordon argue that throughout the nineteenth and early twentieth centuries, the word "dependence" increasingly attached to women and acquired pejorative connotations. According to their typology, the term has four "registers of meaning":

> The first is an economic register, in which one depends on some other person(s) or institution for subsistence. In a second register, the term denotes a socio-legal status, the lack of a separate legal or public identity . . . The third register is political: dependency

means subjection to an external ruling power . . . The fourth register we call the moral/psychological; dependency in this sense is an individual character trait similar to lack of will power or excessive emotional neediness.[80]

In a book on caregiving, it is especially necessary to add a fifth register—physical weakness, or frailty, which undermines the ability to live independently and thus creates the need for care. Fraser and Gordon contrast the "socially necessary dependence" of the ill with the "dependence that is rooted in unjust and potentially remediable social institutions."[81] But disease often is associated with social inequality. We saw that infectious illnesses ravaged slaves weakened by hard physical labor and inadequate rest, diet, and clothing, and confined to overcrowded, insanitary, poorly ventilated quarters. Rates of tuberculosis among disadvantaged groups in the early twentieth century also were elevated by poor living and working conditions. Moreover, changes in disease patterns and health beliefs transformed attitudes toward both caregivers and the kin they nursed.

Caregiving itself sometimes took a heavy physical toll on those who rendered it. Sarah Gillespie constantly complained about exhaustion and back problems when nursing her dying mother between 1886 and 1888; she considered herself an invalid during the year following her mother's death. Ten days after arriving back in Topeka with her dying infant in 1890, Martha Shaw wrote that she was "all worn out with loss of sleep and rest and care and anxiety." While nursing her second husband in February 1916, she wrote that her nerves were "all *unstrung*."

Caregiving also increased economic dependence. Although growing numbers of nineteenth-century and early-twentieth-century women entered the workforce, women at all rungs of the occupational ladder quit their jobs in response to requests for care. Sarah Gillespie repeatedly relinquished her teaching career to return home to tend her dying mother. Martha Shaw had just left her parents' house to work as a hired girl when she was recalled to nurse her stepmother. When Mary Holywell Everett, a successful physician, learned that her sister was ill in 1876, a male colleague wrote to her, "Even at the risk of losing your practice entirely, duty commands you to remain by the side of your old mother and help her to carry the burden."

To be sure, caregiving could also promote economic independence. I have noted that some nurses and midwives plied the skills they had honed as family caregivers. In addition, household sickness pushed some women reluctantly into the workforce. Although Martha abandoned paid employment upon her marriage to Johnny Shaw, she found a job as a waitress in 1893 when he became too sick to farm. She previously had complained about having to "ask Johnny's consent before I buy anything for myself." Now she "bought a *nice Guitar, in a Pawnshop, for $5.00* [with] some of my *tip-money*." But Martha also noted that she could have found a higher-paying job had she not needed to return home in the middle of the day to nurse her husband.

Caregivers also relied disproportionately on charity, a highly stigmatized form of dependence. Doctors, nurses, and hospital social workers referred many families to the New York Charity Organization Society (COS). Sickness and disability, especially if prolonged, were major causes of impoverishment. The "economic injury" inflicted by tuberculosis was of particular concern to the COS. Wives who replaced sick husbands as breadwinners often earned too little to stave off poverty. Some women who quit jobs to nurse the sick told the COS that they no longer could afford the basic necessities of life. And the costs of care often were overwhelming. Family members appealed to the COS for help in paying for new beds, special foods, the clothes required for admission to sanatoriums, and occasionally even moves to larger and drier apartments.

The COS sought to wield legal authority over clients. Although charity workers typically used persuasion to mold client behavior, they occasionally mobilized state power to compel compliance with physicians' advice. The COS solicited the intervention of the Society for the Prevention of Cruelty to Children, which brought parents to court. Charity workers also reported tuberculosis patients to the Department of Health for forcible detention in city sanatoriums.

Because the Social Security Act of 1935 failed to include health insurance, the poor remained dependent on public assistance for medical care. Women appealing to the government for help in paying for children's health care during the Depression had to submit to the same humiliating procedures as turn-of-the-century COS clients. Investigators demanded deference, conducted surprise home visits, and passed judgment on women's personal "deservedness."

Household illness also intensified the subjection of American Indian people to the federal government. David Arnold writes that "imperial powers [used] medicine as a demonstration of their benevolent and paternalistic intentions, as a way of winning support from a newly subject population, of balancing out the coercive features of colonial rule, and of establishing a wider imperial hegemony than could be derived from conquest alone."[82] Although the field nurses sent by the Office of Indian Affairs to reservations in the 1930s provided desperately needed health care services, the nurses also were important weapons in the campaign to convince American Indians of the benefits of white rule.

Like other subordinate social groups, people who depended on either public or private welfare programs were assigned demeaning character traits. Such traits took special prominence in times of household illness. "Emotional neediness" was seen in caregivers' refusal to part with sick family members, "lack of willpower" in their passive capitulation to God's will. Changing disease patterns and health beliefs helped to harden authorities' attitudes. Because the decline of infectious diseases made children's health problems appear preventable, the ill health of offspring was blamed on ignorance and poor mothering. By intensifying fears of contagion, the germ theory of disease amplified the condemnation of caregivers who disregarded professional advice. And the rise of the eugenics movement eroded the sympathy previously extended to mothers of "feebleminded" and epileptic children.

But the actions of many caregivers belied these representations. Despite the association of caregiving with passivity and dependence, many caregivers we examined aligned themselves with strength, not weakness. We saw Samuella Curd, a nineteenth-century white woman, engage in a prolonged struggle to subdue the powerful feelings evoked by her husband's battle with tuberculosis. Harriet Beecher Stowe counseled her friend that accepting God's will after a terrible loss required "constant painful effort." Other nineteenth-century caregivers watched patients face serious illness and death with courage and integrity and strove to prepare themselves to bear those calamities with similar "fortitude." Instead of shielding themselves from life's tragedies, many caregivers openly confronted sickness and death. In such cases, caregiving may have enhanced, as well as demanded, personal strength.

In addition, various groups of caregivers negotiated questions of knowledge and opposed experts in a variety of ways. Enslaved women concealed family illnesses, surrounded sick and disabled people with the community support that gave meaning to their lives, and administered forbidden medicines. Although turn-of-the-century physicians had powerful new grounds for asserting that they alone were entitled to possess, employ, and transmit medical knowledge, caregivers did not simply acquiesce in physicians' authority. Mothers writing to the Children's Bureau in the early twentieth century sought information from various sources before entrusting their children to the operations doctors had recommended. Even after witnessing some of the most dramatic new diagnostic and surgical procedures, Martha Farnsworth drew on a range of therapeutic approaches when nursing her niece and second husband. Field nurses on reservations in the 1930s acted on the expectation that American Indians would follow a linear progression from accepting western medicine to repudiating all traditional practices. American Indian caregivers, however, retained confidence in their own ways of healing and made selective use of the nurses' services.

Despite the growing impersonality of health care, women also continued to employ what I have termed empathic knowledge. We repeatedly saw caregivers strive to affirm the uniqueness and uphold the dignity of sick and disabled kin. Family members writing to Dr. Lawrence Flick violated his dictates by continuing to respond to patients' wishes. Various groups resisted institutional placements that would erode patients' social ties and cultural identities. Despite pressure to speak the language of productivity and self-reliance, COS clients continued to emphasize the importance of preserving patients' affective bonds. Most American Indian parents on reservations during the 1930s refused to send children with tuberculosis to sanatoriums hundreds of miles away. A mother writing to the Volta Bureau in 1939 conceded that deaf children belonged in residential schools but decided to keep her daughter home because "a little girl needs the love and association of her parents." When institutionalization prevailed, caregivers insisted that administrators respect patients' individuality and protect their self-image. Mrs. Germani, an Italian immigrant mother, reminded charity workers of her dying daughter's "special sensitivities," which made New York City's Metropolitan Hospital unbearable to her. And some mothers sought, at great cost, to sustain relationships with children at Craig Colony for Epileptics in upstate New York and influence their care.

Caregiving fostered interdependence as well as independence. As Joan C. Tronto notes, "Caring is by its very nature a challenge to the notion that individuals are entirely autonomous and self-supporting."[83] I used the extensive records of white, middle-class women in the nineteenth century to demonstrate how caregiving helped to solidify female bonds. Caregiving operated like a giant insurance system, spreading the risks of trouble. The absence of formal health care services made mutual assistance essential. Some women who rushed to neighbors' homes in times of crisis were investing in their own uncertain futures. Others responded to neighbors' requests as repayment for services previously rendered. Nevertheless, women did not view each other solely as instrumental resources for discrete tasks. It would be impossible to disentangle altruism from self-interest in women's support networks or to tease sympathy from duty, but evidence suggests that caregiving sometimes reflected a sense of personal connection. In turn, caregiving helped to deepen and strengthen ties of interdependence. Although some women exchanged only domestic services, caregiving often involved a level of physical intimacy that most women found impossible at other times. In addition, women who provided care together or nursed each other through childbirth and illness established a bond based on a common acknowledgement of suffering as integral to life.

Yet white women's sense of sisterhood tended to be sharply circumscribed. White, middle-class mothers of "feebleminded" children in the early twentieth century sought services that insulated their children from the offspring of "inferior" groups. Mothers embraced oralism partly to differentiate their children from the stigmatized deaf community. Competition for scarce resources further narrowed the focus of caregivers in diverse social groups. In the 1930s, many mothers tried to convince the federal government that their children were uniquely deserving of health care. Here, one of the hallmarks of caregiving—intense preoccupation with a single individual—shaded into exclusivity and parochialism. Caregivers' intimate understanding of care recipients can not only promote sensitivity to their needs but also eclipse the problems of more distant individuals. As we struggle to elevate the work of care, we should strive to imbue it with the tenets of social justice.

Framing an Agenda for Change

Health policy researchers and analysts use history in two competing ways. Highlighting the growth of the frail elderly population, some argue that demands for informal care are greater today than in the past. Nadine F. Marks, for example, writes that "demographic changes have now increased the relative risk of becoming a caregiver at some time— or even multiple times—during a lifetime."[84] This statement ignores the history this book has chronicled. If nineteenth-century women had fewer elder care responsibilities, obligations to birthing women and to sick, disabled, and dying people of all ages were constant and unremitting.

Others, clinging to a romantic vision of a vanished world, advocate a return to nineteenth-century methods of care. According to this argument, the nineteenth century was the golden age, not because women lacked responsibilities for sick and disabled people but because they delivered care selflessly and sensitively. We have seen, however, that some women complained bitterly about the burdens imposed on them and that the care they rendered could be inappropriate or inattentive. Moreover, such factors as the rise of the formal health care system, the transportation revolution, the development of domestic technologies, medical discoveries, and changes in women's lives have transformed the nature of informal care. It is critical that policy recommendations be based on an understanding of the reality of contemporary caregiving, rather than on nostalgia for a mythical past.

A more fruitful use of history might be to delineate the specific features of caregiving that have remained constant over time. Judith M. Bennett argues that despite "a strong professional imperative to focus on history as transformation," continuity is often equally, if not more, important.[85] This final section first examines the legacy of the past and then highlights its implications for the future of caregiving in America.

1. *Caregiving work is divided unevenly between the genders.* Although nineteenth-century men fetched doctors, "watched" other men, and helped

to nurse their own wives and children, the primary responsibilities for care of ailing family and neighbors fell to women.

Rannveig Traustadottir asserts that the contemporary "sexual division of caring for people with disabilities is largely an unstudied topic."[86] The gendered allocation of elder care, however, has been well documented. Women represent 72 percent of all caregivers and 77 percent of adult offspring providing care.[87] Daughters are more likely than sons to live with dependent parents and to serve as the primary caregivers.[88] Sons and daughters also assume responsibility for very different tasks. Sons are more likely to assist parents with household maintenance and repairs, while daughters are far more likely to help with housework, cooking, shopping, and personal care.[89]

2. Although caregiving is primarily women's work, it opposes the interests of different groups of women. Privileged nineteenth-century women typically ignored the caregiving needs of the very women who fulfilled their own. Only the rare slave mistress excused enslaved women from work in the big house to care for sick kin at home. Employers of domestic servants expected them to work long and unpredictable hours, subordinating their own caregiving responsibilities.

Evelyn Nakano Glenn demonstrates that poor women and women of color, who previously might have worked as domestic servants, today increasingly enter low-level service occupations such as home health care.[90] Because most people pay privately for home care services, caregivers benefit when agencies save money by keeping the wages of home health aides low. A study conducted in New York City found that 99 percent of such workers are women, 70 percent are African American, 26 percent are Latina, and 46 percent are immigrants. A high proportion are single mothers with three or four children. They typically earn less than $5,000 a year. Eighty percent cannot afford adequate housing, and 35 percent often cannot buy enough food for their families.[91]

I have noted that some caregivers in affluent families turn for assistance to the large pool of marginal workers who cannot secure better employment. Companions and attendants hired through ad hoc, informal arrangements typically receive little pay, and most lack benefits, whether Social Security, Workers' Compensation, Unemployment, or health insurance. In my study of parent care, I interviewed many daughters who watched their parents' savings dwindle away and thus felt unable to pay more. But a fee that seemed high to the daughters did not constitute a living wage for the workers they hired.[92]

3. *Poor women face special difficulties rendering care, even when they are not doing the work of more privileged women.* Throughout the nineteenth century, caregiving was especially problematic for women with the most arduous household and economic responsibilities. Although low-income women continued to shoulder the heaviest burden of domestic labor at the turn of the century, they also had the least access to health care services and were most likely to work for pay.

Caregiving remains especially onerous for poor women today. The low-status jobs they can obtain tend to have little or no flexibility in hours or days worked. Caregivers thus suffer greater penalties if they phone disabled relatives from work or take time off to help them during working hours.[93] Despite the growth of health care financing programs, caregivers in low-income families continue to confront barriers to such assistance. In addition, poor women typically cannot purchase medical equipment or supplies, retrofit their homes to accommodate a sickroom or wheelchair, or "buy out" of their obligations by hiring other women.

4. *Personal relationships, as well as circumstances, mold caregiving experiences.* As Hilary Graham writes, "Caring . . . is experienced as a labour of love in which the labour must continue even when the love falters."[94] By the time Martha nursed her husband Johnny Shaw, she neither liked nor respected him; she adamantly insisted that she cared for him, not out of tenderness or affection, but out of a sense of duty. Despite our sentimental image of several generations living harmoniously under one roof in the nineteenth century, rancor and acrimony marked Hial Hawley's six-month stay at the home of his daughter Emily Gillespie. But the intimacy shared by many nineteenth-century women also exacerbated the stresses of care. Identifying closely with the kin and neighbors they tended and witnessing afflictions that resonated with their own lives, some caregivers felt emotionally overwhelmed.

We hardly need to be reminded that contemporary family relationships can foster tensions and conflicts, as well as warmth and solicitude. Many spouses and adult children deliver care within unloving or even abusive relationships. Strong positive feelings also can complicate caregiving. In a study of informal caregiving in Great Britain, Clare Ungerson found that adult daughters "could care only if they cut themselves off from feeling altogether and simply got on with the tasks at hand. In other words, in order to care *for* their parents, they found it easier to forget about caring *about* them."[95]

5. *Caregiving responsibilities are not confined to immediate family members.* In the nineteenth century, both white and African American women nursed extensive networks of kin, friends, and neighbors. Although urbanization and social mobility loosened the bonds of kinship and community among white, middle-class Americans in the early twentieth century, many low-income people and people of color continue to feel responsible for the well-being of members of a broad circle.[96] Gay white men have crafted a variety of innovative arrangements, including buddy systems and care teams, to support AIDS sufferers.

6. *External forces shape the amount and nature of caregiving responsibilities.* The intense emotional involvement of many women in caring work suggests that they are not simply responding to those forces. Nevertheless, we saw that the absence of formal services, the gender division of domestic labor, notions of feminine virtue, and economic dependence helped to push many nineteenth-century women into caregiving roles. Today, as then, the decisions women make about care are not simply private choices. Both because men still do not share caregiving responsibilities equally and because high-quality, publicly funded services are not universally accessible, many women lack the power to determine whether and when they will begin to care for sick or disabled people, to control the intrusions of caregiving in their lives, and to delegate responsibilities that have become overwhelming.

7. *Although caregiving imposes serious, often calamitous, costs, it is also a profound human experience and thus cannot be neatly subsumed under the terms "stress" and "burden."* The onerous caregiving responsibilities of nineteenth-century women restricted their entry into the public sphere and added to domestic labor that was grueling even in the best of times. But caregiving also provided women with a sense of mastery, bound them to a broad network of friends and kin, and brought them

into sustained contact with fundamental life experiences. Some used the wisdom they had attained to counsel others facing major losses.

Numerous studies find that caregivers today report a range of physical, emotional, social, and financial problems. Researchers repeatedly observe that caregivers experience stress from responsibilities they find overwhelming. As a result, caregiving increases the incidence of depression and other psychiatric disorders. Although evidence about the impact of caregiving on physical health is far more fragmentary, a few studies suggest that the stress of care can manifest itself in physical problems as well.[97]

Nevertheless, caregiving provides important gratifications. Traustadottir found that emotional closeness offered rewards to mothers of disabled children.[98] Caregiving also continues to provide a sense of worth and accomplishment. According to a recent study of a caregivers' support group, members described their responsibilities not only as "personal tribulation" but also as "a challenge" and even a "triumph." As the researchers observed, "Caregiving was something to behold, to be proud of, a sign of effective human stewardship."[99] Andrea Sankar reported that the great majority of people she interviewed about caring for the dying at home stated that "this was one of the most—if not *the* most—significant accomplishments of their lives."[100] Just as Louisa May Alcott "had the great pleasure of supplying all [her mother's] needs and fancies," so a husband interviewed by Sankar stated, "I think I did a hell of a lot better job than they did in the hospital because I was with her. Whatever she wanted, if it was possible to do for her, I did it."[101] Although most adult daughters I interviewed initially lacked confidence in their caregiving abilities, some stated that caregiving eventually provided an opportunity to gain and display competence. And some asserted that their confrontation with pain, vulnerability, and mortality had enriched their lives. One woman said, "You gain a lot of wisdom and insight and compassion for other people's suffering and problems."[102]

⌒ ALTHOUGH THE PATTERNS delineated above have lasted more than 150 years, they are neither inevitable nor immutable. The growth of the population in need of care demands that we pursue broad reforms. If only the most marginal changes seem politically feasible today, few would argue that we need a vision for more generous times, beginning with the following elements:

Eradicating the gender division of domestic labor. When we recognize that caring work is not confined to child rearing but, rather, extends throughout the life course, this central feminist goal assumes greater urgency.

Spreading the work of care more equitably throughout all sectors of society rather than imposing it on the most socially marginalized groups.

Adopting policies that address the needs of all caregivers, not just those with the greatest privilege and political clout.

Recognizing the randomness of love and the peculiarities of individual experiences. Although many policymakers seek to delegate responsibility to caregivers in the interest of economic efficiency, family histories sometimes make this inappropriate. As John D. Arras and Nancy N. Dubler write, "Perhaps a devoted son should not change the soiled diapers of his mother, a formerly abused daughter should not be asked to take her father in her home."[103]

Embracing the diverse family and community arrangements that environ much informal care today.

Establishing high-quality, comprehensive, and universally accessible long-term care services. Although such programs would require an enormous outlay of government funds, the costs are not unlimited. Many elderly people share with most other Americans the belief that dependence demonstrates personal inadequacy; as a result, the frail elderly often reject whatever services are available. A major component of the "servicing work" of adult daughters is overcoming the resistance of their parents to outside assistance.[104]

The belief that publicly funded programs discourage families from providing informal care further inhibits policymakers from considering them. But throughout this book we have repeatedly seen caregivers refuse to relinquish caregiving obligations. Women who view caregiving as a way to achieve greater intimacy with care recipients, to demonstrate competence, and even to attain "hearts of wisdom" want to be relieved of intolerable burdens, not to unload all their responsibilities on the state.

Notes

Introduction

1. Laurel Thatcher Ulrich, *A Midwife's Tale: The Life of Martha Ballard, Based on Her Diary, 1785–1812* (New York: Alfred A. Knopf, 1990).

2. Evelyn Fox Keller, *Reflections on Gender and Science* (New Haven: Yale University Press, 1985), p. 117. For an analysis of empathic knowledge, see Emily K. Abel and C. H. Browner, "Selective Compliance with Biomedical Authority and the Uses of Experiential Knowledge," in *Pragmatic Women and Body Politics*, ed. Margaret Lock and Patricia A. Kaufert (Cambridge, U.K.: Cambridge University Press, 1998), pp. 310–326.

3. Willard Gaylin, "In the Beginning: Helpless and Dependent," in *Doing Good: The Limits of Benevolence*, ed. Willard Gaylin et al. (New York: Pantheon, 1978), p. 35.

4. Sue E. Estroff, "Identity, Disability, and Schizophrenia: The Problem of Chronicity," in *Knowledge, Power, and Practice: The Anthropology of Medicine and Everyday Life*, ed. Shirley Lindenbaum and Margaret Lock (Berkeley: University of California Press, 1993), p. 248.

5. See Karen V. Hansen, *A Very Social Time: Crafting Community in Antebellum New England* (Berkeley: University of California Press, 1994); Nancy Grey Osterud, *Bonds of Community: The Lives of Farm Women in Nineteenth-Century New York* (Ithaca: Cornell University Press, 1991).

6. Arthur Kleinman, *The Illness Narratives: Suffering, Healing, and the Human Condition* (New York: Basic Books, 1988).

7. Sheila M. Rothman, *Living in the Shadow of Death: Tuberculosis and the Social Experience of Illness in American History* (New York: Basic Books, 1994).

1. *"Hot Flannels, Hot Teas, and a Great Deal of Care"*

1. The diaries of both Emily Hawley Gillespie and Sarah Gillespie Huftalen are located in the Huftalen Collection, State Historical Society of Iowa, Iowa City. All quotations in this chapter, unless otherwise noted, are taken from these diaries. Although Emily wrote virtually every evening, Sarah was not nearly as conscientious. During periods when she was most intensively involved in providing care, she often did not write at all. Moreover, although each diary provides an important check on the account of the other, they cannot be considered independent productions. Emily bought Sarah a diary in 1877. The two often wrote together at night and presumably discussed some of what they were writing. On at least two occasions, Emily opened Sarah's diary, read the last entry, and appended encouraging remarks. When Emily was very ill, she dictated her comments to Sarah. Nevertheless, these diaries do enable us to examine many events from the perspectives of both mother and daughter. The analysis in this chapter builds on *"A Secret to Be Burried": The Diary and Life of Emily Hawley Gillespie, 1858–1888* by Judy Nolte Lensink (Iowa City: University of Iowa Press, 1989) and *"All Will Yet Be Well": The Diary of Sarah Gillespie Huftalen* by Suzanne L. Bunkers (Iowa City: University of Iowa Press, 1993).

2. It is unclear whether Emily actually witnessed the autopsy. If she did, her presence would have great historical significance. Laurel Thatcher Ulrich notes that in the late eighteenth and early nineteenth centuries, doctors sometimes called midwives to watch dissections. "As guardians of women and children," Ulrich writes, "midwives presumably ensured proper reverence for the bodies. From the doctors' point of view, inviting midwives to observe was perhaps a professional courtesy, a way of including them in an important educational event. At the same time, it helped to validate the activity and perhaps to reassure anxious relatives." Laurel Thatcher Ulrich, *A Midwife's Tale: The Life of Martha Ballard, Based on Her Diary, 1785–1812* (New York: Alfred A. Knopf, 1990), p. 251. Perhaps Emily seemed like an appropriate family representative because she had cared for Mrs. Wiley before her death.

3. Elizabeth Hampsten, *Read This Only to Yourself: The Private Writings of Midwestern Women, 1880–1910* (Bloomington: Indiana University Press, 1982). For an analysis of how graphic descriptions of bodily parts could assuage the fears of early-twentieth-century nurses, see Barbara Melosh, *"The Physician's Hand": Work Culture and Conflict in American Nursing* (Philadelphia: Temple University Press, 1982), pp. 54–60.

4. For an analysis of Emily's aspirations, see Lensink, *"A Secret to Be Burried."*

5. Quoted in ibid., p. 103.

6. See, for example, Glenda Riley, *Frontierswomen: The Iowa Experience* (Ames: Iowa State University Press, 1981); Susan Strasser, *Never Done: A History of American Housework* (New York: Pantheon, 1982).

7. Many other farm women also assumed that the money they earned was theirs to spend alone. See Sarah Elbert, "The Farmer Takes a Wife: Women in America's Farming Families," in *Women, Households, and the Economy,* ed. Lourdes Beneria and Catharine R. Stimpson (New Brunswick, N.J.: Rutgers University Press, 1987), pp. 173–197; Joan M. Jensen, *With These Hands: Women Working on the Land* (Old Westbury, N.Y.: Feminist Press, 1981), pp. 32–33.

8. As Lensink notes, it is impossible to determine whether Harriet had a miscarriage or an intentional abortion. *"A Secret to Be Burried,"* p. 422 n.

9. See ibid., p. 40.

10. See Judith Walzer Leavitt, *Brought to Bed: Child-Bearing in America, 1750–1950* (New York: Oxford University Press, 1986).

11. Historians frequently note that nineteenth-century men experienced a precipitous drop in status when they forfeited their positions as household heads. See Brian Gratton, "The New History of the Aged: A Critique," in *Old Age in a Bureaucratic Society: The Elderly, the Experts, and the State in American Society,* ed. David Van Tassel and Peter N. Stearns (Westport, Conn.: Greenwood Press, 1986), pp. 3–24; Tamara Hareven, "Life-Course Transitions and Kin Assistance," in *Old Age,* ed. Van Tassel and Stearns, pp. 110–125; D. S. Smith, "Life Course, Norms, and the Family Systems of Older Americans in 1900," *Journal of Family History* 4, no. 3 (1979): 285–298.

12. Since the first English colonies in America, care for destitute elderly people had been a local government responsibility.

13. According to Deborah Fink, Nebraska farm women frequently interceded between their husbands' need for farm labor and their children's need for education. *Agrarian Women: Wives and Mothers in Rural Nebraska, 1880–1940* (Chapel Hill: University of North Carolina Press, 1992), p. 15.

14. According to Sally McMurry's study of Oneida County, New York, between 1820 and 1885, "a term or two at an academy or 'select school' became part of the experience of many young people from farming families." *Transforming Rural Life: Dairying Families and Agricultural Change, 1820–1885* (Baltimore: Johns Hopkins University Press, 1995), p. 115.

15. See Polly Kaufman, *Women Teachers on the Frontier* (New Haven: Yale University Press, 1984); Mary Hurlbut Cordier, *Schoolwomen of the Prairies and Plains: Personal Narratives from Iowa, Kansas, and Nebraska, 1860s–1920s* (Albuquerque: University of New Mexico Press, 1992).

16. Nineteenth-century families that could not afford domestic servants frequently recruited neighborhood women to help out in times of trouble. Unlike servants, hired girls occupied the same social status as their employers, and they typically spent their days together. See Faye E. Dudden, *Serving Women: Household Service in Nineteenth-Century America* (Middletown, Conn.: Wesleyan University Press, 1983).

17. "Dropsy" referred to the abnormal accumulation of fluid in any part of the body. *Dorland's Illustrated Medical Dictionary,* 26th ed., s.v. "dropsy."

18. Magnetic doctors believed that the application of mild electrical charges could cure disease. Lensink, *"A Secret to Be Burried,"* p. 426 n.

19. Arthur Kleinman, *The Illness Narratives: Suffering, Healing, and the Human Condition* (New York: Basic Books, 1988), p. 31.

2. An Overview of Nineteenth-Century Caregiving

1. My description of women's support networks relies heavily on Judith Walzer Leavitt's pathbreaking analysis of female ties of interdependence during childbirth in *Brought to Bed: Child-Bearing in America, 1750–1950* (New York: Oxford University Press, 1986).

2. "Letters of John and Sarah Everett, 1854–1864," *Kansas Historical Quarterly* 8, no. 2 (May 1939): 149–166. See also Eliza W. Farnham, *Life in Prairie Land* (New York: Harper and Brothers, 1846), p. 82; Kate Roberts Pelissier, "Reminiscences of a Pioneer Mother," *North Dakota History* 24, no. 3 (July 1957): 136.

3. Quoted in John Mack Faragher, *Women and Men on the Overland Trail* (New Haven: Yale University Press, 1979), p. 140.

4. Quoted in ibid., p. 138.

5. Quoted in Lee Virginia Chambers-Schiller, *Liberty, a Better Husband: Single Women in America, The Generations of 1780–1840* (New Haven: Yale University Press, 1982), p. 114.

6. Nannie Stillwell Jackson, *Vinegar Pie and Chicken Bread: A Woman's Diary of Life in the Rural South, 1890–1891*, ed. Margaret Jones Bolsteri (Fayetteville: University of Arkansas Press, 1982).

7. Ibid., p, 47.

8. Ibid., p. 41.

9. Ibid., p. 76.

10. Ibid., pp. 66–67.

11. Ibid., pp. 88–100.

12. Ibid., p. 53.

13. Emily French, *Emily: The Diary of a Hard-Worked Woman*, ed. Janet Lecompte (Lincoln: University of Nebraska Press, 1987), p. 19.

14. Charles E. Rosenberg, *The Care of Strangers: The Rise of America's Hospital System* (New York: Basic Books, 1987), p. 18.

15. Morris J. Vogel, *The Invention of the Modern Hospital: Boston, 1870–1930* (Chicago: University of Chicago Press, 1980), p. 1.

16. "Civil War Wife: The Letters of Harriet Jane Thompson," ed. Glenda Riley, *Annals of Iowa*, 3d ser., 44, no. 4 (Spring 1978): 312–313.

17. "Rowe Creek, 1890–91: Mary L. Fitzmaurice Diary," part 2, ed. Eileen Hickson Donnell, *Oregon Historical Quarterly* 83, no. 3 (Fall 1982): 290.

18. Anne Ellis, *The Life of an Ordinary Woman*, ed. Lucy Fitch Perkins (Boston: Houghton Mifflin Co., 1929), pp. 166–167.

19. See *Records of a California Family: Journals and Letters of Lewis C. Gunn and Elizabeth LeBreton Gunn*, ed. Anna Lee Marston (San Diego: privately published, 1928), p. 227; "Times Hard but Grit Good: Lydia Moxley's 1877 Diary," ed. James Sanders, *Annals of Iowa*, 3d ser., 47, no. 3 (Winter 1984): 276–277; "Mrs. Caroline Phelps' Diary," *Journal of the Illinois State Historical Society* 23, no. 2 (July 1930): 226.

20. Agnes Just Reid, *Letters of Long Ago* (Caldwell, Idaho: Caxton Printers, 1923), pp. 69–70. These letters were written by the daughter, who based them on her mother's experiences; the letters were edited by the mother.

21. Francis A. Long, *A Prairie Doctor of the Eighties: Some Personal Recollections and Some Early Medical and Social History of a Prairie State* (Norfolk, Nebr.: Huse Publishing Co., 1937), p. 91.

22. Nannie T. Alderson and Helena Huntington Smith, *A Bride Goes West* (New York: Farrar and Rinehart, 1942), pp. 196–197.

23. Ibid., pp. 199–200.

24. Lamar Riley Murphy, *Enter the Physician: The Transformation of Domestic Medicine, 1760–1860* (Tuscaloosa: University of Alabama Press, 1991), pp. 32–69.

25. Alta Harvey Heiser, *Quaker Lady: The Story of Charity Lynch* (Oxford, Ohio: Mississippi Valley Press, 1941), p. 135.

26. Harriet Connor Brown, *Grandmother Brown's Hundred Years, 1827–1927* (New York: Blue Ribbon Books, 1929), pp. 152–153. The author based her book on the many stories Maria D. Brown told her, but did not record Maria's speech verbatim.

27. *Lamps on the Prairie: A History of Nursing in Kansas*, comp. Writers' Program of the Work Projects Administration in Kansas (New York: Garland Publishing, 1984), p. 49.

28. "Private Journal of Mary Ann Owen Sims," ed. Clifford Dale Whitman, in *Lives of American Women: A History with Documents*, ed. Joyce Goodfriend and Claudia M. Christie (Boston: Little, Brown and Co., 1981), p. 203.

29. "Diary of Colonel and Mrs. I. N. Ebey," ed. Victor J. Farrar, *Washington Historical Quarterly* 8, no. 2 (April 1917): 151.

30. *Sam Curd's Diary: The Diary of a True Woman*, ed. Susan S. Arpad (Athens: Ohio University Press, 1984), p. 97.

31. Susan M. Reverby, *Ordered to Care: The Dilemma of American Nursing, 1850–1945* (New York: Cambridge University Press, 1987), pp. 16–21.

32. *The Letters of Ellen Tucker Emerson*, vol. 2, ed. Edith E. W. Gregg (Kent, Ohio: Kent State University Press, 1982), p. 656.

33. Reverby, *Ordered to Care*, pp. 16–21.

34. See ibid., p. 15; Martha Saxton, *Louisa May: A Modern Biography of Louisa May Alcott* (New York: Avon Books, 1978).

35. See Mary P. Ryan, *Cradle of the Middle Class: The Family in Oneida County, New York, 1790–1865* (Cambridge, U.K.: Cambridge University Press, 1981).

36. Lucy Sprague Mitchell, *Two Lives: The Story of Wesley Clair Mitchell and Myself* (New York: Simon and Schuster, 1953), p. 110.

37. Judith C. Breault, *The World of Emily Howland: Odyssey of a Humanitarian* (Millbrae, Calif.: Les Femmes, 1976), p. 121.

38. "Almira Raymond Letters, 1840–1880," ed. Olga Freeman, *Oregon Historical Quarterly* 85, no. 3 (Fall 1984): 300.

39. See Sylvia D. Hoffert, *Private Matters: American Attitudes toward Childbearing and Infant Nurture in the Urban North, 1800–1860* (Urbana: University of Illinois Press, 1989), p. 15; Nancy Grey Osterud, *Bonds of Community: The Lives of Farm Women in Nineteenth-Century New York* (Ithaca: Cornell University Press, 1991), p. 118.

40. Malenda M. Edwards to Sabrina Bennett, Bristol, New Hampshire, August 18, 1845, in *Farm to Factory: Women's Letters, 1830–1860*, ed. Thomas Dublin (New York: Columbia University Press, 1981), pp. 85–86.

41. Quoted in Osterud, *Bonds of Community*, p. 126.

42. Samuel Lilienthal to Mary Holywell Everett, New York, September 8, 1876, in Gerda Lerner, *The Female Experience: An American Documentary* (Indianapolis: Bobbs-Merrill, 1977), p. 179.

43. Quoted in ibid.

44. "'Between Hope and Fear': The Life of Lettie Teeple, 1: 1829–1850," ed. John H. Yzenbaard and John Hoffman, *Michigan History* 58, no. 3 (Fall 1974): 272.

45. Sarah Gillespie Huftalen diary, March 15, 1888, Huftalen Collection, State Historical Society of Iowa, Iowa City.

46. Sarah Gillespie Huftalen diary, May 12, 1886.

47. *The Diaries of Sally and Pamela Brown, 1832–1838, and Hyde Leslie, 1887,* *Plymouth Notch, Vermont,* ed. Blanche Brown Bryant and Gertrude Elaine Baker (Springfield, Vt.: William L. Bryant Foundation, 1970), p. 65.

48. Ibid.

49. Ibid., p. 66.

50. Ibid., p. 64.

51. Ibid.

52. Eleanor Arnold, ed., *Voices of American Homemakers* (Bloomington: Indiana University Press, 1985); Ruth Schwartz Cowan, *More Work for Mother: The Ironies of Household Technology from the Open Hearth to the Microwave* (New York: Basic Books, 1983), pp. 16–68; Susan Strasser, *Never Done: A History of American Housework* (New York: Pantheon, 1982).

53. Faye E. Dudden, *Serving Women: Household Service in Nineteenth-Century America* (Middletown, Conn.: Wesleyan University Press, 1983), p. 106; Strasser, *Never Done,* p. 195.

54. "Mrs. Butler's 1853 Diary of Rogue River Valley," ed. Oscar Osburn Winther and Rose Dodge Galey, *Oregon Historical Quarterly* 41, no. 4 (December 1940): 346.

55. *Caleb and Mary Wilder Foote: Reminiscences and Letters,* ed. Mary Wilder Tileston, (Boston: Houghton Mifflin, 1918), pp. 92–93.

56. "Roughing It on Her Kansas Claim: The Diary of Abbie Bright, 1870–1871—Concluded," ed. Joseph W. Snell, *Kansas Historical Quarterly* 37, no. 4 (Winter 1971): 411–412.

57. Emily Hawley Gillespie diary, October 1, 1872, Huftalen Collection, State Historical Society of Iowa, Iowa City.

58. Jackson, *Vinegar Pie,* p. 29.

59. Ibid., p. 67.

60. Ibid., p. 71.

61. "The Letters of Effie Hanson, 1917–1923: Farm Life in Troubled Times," ed. Frances M. Wold, *North Dakota History* 48, no. 1 (Winter 1981): 30. Although these letters were written after the turn of the century, I draw on them because they illustrate themes that were important in the nineteenth century.

62. Ibid., p. 31.

63. "Journal of Marian L. Moore, 1831–1860," in Lerner, *Female Experience,* pp. 176–177.

64. Mary Ann Webber to Albert and Eliza Webber, January 15, 1865, Parker Family Letters, private collection of Marianne Brown, Los Angeles.

65. Mary Ann Webber to Eliza Webber, June 1, 1865.

66. Sarah Gillespie Huftalen diary, March 26, 1887.

67. Emily Conine Dorsey to Silas and Mary Ann Conine, Scipio, Indiana, March 28, 1854, "The Conine Family Letters, 1849–1851: Employed in Honest Business and Doing the Best We Can," ed. Donald E. Baker, *Indiana Magazine of History* 69, no. 4 (December 1973): 146–147.

68. Mary Ann Webber to Alpha Webber, date lost (June 1871), Parker Family Letters.

69. Mary Ann Webber to Children, June 11, 1871; June 15, 1871; June 21, 1871; June 26, 1871; June 27, 1871; July 23, 1871; August 16, 1871.

70. See "Letters of John and Sarah Everett, 1851–1864: Miami County Pioneers," *Kansas Historical Quarterly* 8, no. 1 (February 1939); "Roughing It," ed. Snell, 414; Reid, *Letters of Long Ago*, pp. 91–92.

71. Reid, *Letters of Long Ago*, pp. 78–79.

72. Louisa May Alcott to Ellen Conway, Concord, Massachusetts, May 1, 1878, *The Selected Letters of Louisa May Alcott*, ed. Joel Myerson and Daniel Shealy (Boston: Little, Brown and Co., 1987), pp. 229–230.

73. "Selections from the Plymouth Diary of Abigail Baldwin, 1853–4," *Vermont History* 40, no. 3 (Summer 1972): 221.

74. *Sam Curd's Diary*, ed. Arpad, p. 65.

75. "Roughing It," ed. Snell, p. 411.

76. *Sam Curd's Diary*, ed. Arpad, p. 111.

77. Ibid., pp. 123–124.

78. Mary Ann Webber to Son, July 23, 1871, Parker Family Letters.

79. See Mary Douglas, *Purity and Danger: An Analysis of Concepts of Pollution and Taboo* (London: Routledge and Kegan Paul, 1966).

80. See Samuel J. Crumbine, *Frontier Doctor: The Autobiography of a Pioneer on the Frontier of Public Health* (Philadelphia: Dorrance and Co., 1948), p. 59.

81. Emily Hawley Gillespie diary, November 7, 1887.

82. Mary Ann Webber to Children, September 12, 1868, Parker Family Letters.

83. Amelia Akehurst Lines, *To Raise Myself a Little: The Diaries and Letters of Jennie, a Georgia Teacher, 1851–1886*, ed. Thomas Dyer (Athens: University of Georgia Press, 1982), p. 66.

84. "Effie Hanson," ed. Wold, 30 n. 41.

85. Ibid., p. 31.

86. Gwendoline Kincaid to Mamie Goodwater, September 11, 1899, in *To All Inquiring Friends: Letters, Diaries, and Essays in North Dakota, 1880–1910*, 2d edition, ed. Elizabeth Hampsten (Grand Forks: Department of English, University of North Dakota, 1980), p. 26.

87. Quoted in Brown, *Grandmother Brown's Hundred Years*, p. 157.

88. Laurel Thatcher Ulrich, *A Midwife's Tale: The Life of Martha Ballard, Based on Her Diary, 1785–1812* (New York: Alfred A. Knopf, 1990), p. 62.

89. Edith White, "Memories of Pioneer Childhood and Youth in French Corral and North San Juan, Nevada County, California. With a brief narrative of later life, told by Edith White, emigrant of 1859, to Linnie Marsh Wolfe, 1936," in *Let Them Speak for Themselves: Women in the American West, 1849–1900*, ed. Christiane Fischer (Hamden, Conn.: Archon Books, 1977), p. 276.

90. Sarah Gillespie Huftalen diary, October 22, 1888.

91. See Charlotte G. Borst, *Catching Babies: The Professionalization of Childbirth, 1870–1920* (Cambridge, Mass.: Harvard University Press, 1995), p. 54; Gertrude Jacinta Fraser, *African American Midwifery in the South: Dialogues of Birth, Race, and Memory* (Cambridge, Mass.: Harvard University Press, 1998).

92. See Lewis O. Saum, "Death in the Popular Mind of Pre–Civil War America," in *Passing the Vision of Death in America*, ed. Charles O. Jackson (Westport, Conn.: Greenwood Press, 1977), pp. 65–90.

93. Eliza Webber to Parents, Champlain, New York, July 22, 1863, Parker Family Letters.

94. *Sam Curd's Diary*, ed. Arpad, p. 114.

95. Ibid., p. 59.

96. Ibid., p. 103.

97. Ibid., p. 112.

98. Ibid., p. 115.

99. Ibid., p. 124.

100. Ibid.

101. Ibid., p. 126.

102. Ibid., p. 122.

103. Katherine Ott, *Fevered Lives: Tuberculosis in American Culture since 1870* (Cambridge, Mass.: Harvard University Press, 1996), p. 14.

104. *Mrs. Longfellow: Selected Letters and Journals of Fanny Appleton Longfellow, 1817–1861*, ed. Edward Wagenknecht (New York: Longmans, Green and Co., 1956), p. 21.

105. "Private Journal of Mary Ann Owen Sims," part 1, ed. Clifford Dale Whitman, *Arkansas Historical Quarterly* 35, no. 4 (Winter 1976): 150.

106. *Louisa May Alcott: Her Life, Letters, and Journals*, ed. Ednah D. Cheney (Boston: Roberts Brothers, 1892), p. 272.

107. Ibid., p. 300.

108. Alcott to Conway, p. 230.

109. Quoted in Leavitt, *Brought to Bed*, p. 92.

110. See Charles E. Rosenberg, "The Therapeutic Revolution: Medicine, Meaning, and Social Change in Nineteenth-Century America," in *Sickness and Health in America: Readings in the History of Medicine and Public Health*, ed. Judith Walzer Leavitt and Ronald L. Numbers (Madison: University of Wisconsin Press, 1985), pp. 39–52.

111. Larry Hirschhorn, "Alternative Services and the Crisis of the Professions," in *Co-ops, Communes, and Collectives: Experiments in Social Change in the 1960s and 1970s*, ed. John Case and Rosemary C. R. Taylor (New York: Pantheon, 1979), p. 170.

112. "The Diary of Calvin Fletcher," vol. 1, 1817–1838, "Including Letters of Calvin Fletcher and Diaries and Letters of His Wife Sarah Hill Fletcher," ed. Gayle Thornbrough, in *Lives of American Women*, ed. Goodfriend and Christie, p. 193.

113. Quoted in Sally G. McMillen, *Motherhood in the Old South: Pregnancy, Childbirth, and Infant Rearing* (Baton Rouge: Louisiana State University Press, 1900), p. 175.

114. Quoted in Arthur W. Frank, *The Wounded Storyteller: Body, Illness, and Ethics* (Chicago: University of Chicago Press, 1995), p. 35.

115. Wendy Simonds and Barbara Katz Rothman, *Centuries of Solace: Expressions of Maternal Grief in Popular Literature* (Philadelphia: Temple University Press, 1992), p. 52.

116. Quoted in ibid.

117. Joan D. Hedrick, *Harriet Beecher Stowe: A Life* (New York: Oxford University Press, 1994), p. 281. See also Hedrick, "'Peaceable Fruits': The Ministry of Harriet Beecher Stowe," *American Quarterly* 40, no. 3 (September 1988): 307–332.

118. Hedrick, *Harriet Beecher Stowe*, p. 199.

119. Hedrick, "Ministry," 316.

120. Hedrick, *Harriet Beecher Stowe*, p. 282.

121. Ibid., p. 278.

122. Quoted in ibid., p. 282.

123. Elizabeth V. Spelman, *Fruits of Sorrow: Framing Our Attention to Suffering* (Boston: Beacon Press, 1997), p. 111.

124. Hedrick, "Ministry," 318.

125. Wilma King, *Stolen Childhood: Slave Youth in Nineteenth-Century America* (Bloomington: Indiana University Press, 1995), p. 11.

126. *Sam Curd's Diary*, ed. Arpad, p. 150.

127. See Dudden, *Serving Women*, pp. 15, 31, 38–39, 49, 57, 170, 193, 205.

128. *The Diary of Ellen Birdseye Wheaton*, ed. Donald Gordon (Boston: privately printed, 1923), p. 171.

129. "Dedication of the Cambridge Hospital, April 29, 1886, Cambridge, Mass.," located at the New York Academy of Medicine, New York.

130. *Caleb and Mary Wilder Foote*, ed. Tileston, p. 62.

131. Lines, *To Raise Myself*, p. 249.

132. This section relies heavily on Sharla Fett, "Body and Soul: African American Healing in Southern Antebellum Plantation Communities, 1800–1860" (Ph.D. diss., Rutgers University, 1995).

133. George P. Rawick, ed., *The American Slave: A Composite Autobiography*, vol. 15, *North Carolina Narratives* (Westport, Conn.: Greenwood Press, 1972), pp. 130–131. In all quotations from this source, the spellings used in the interview transcriptions have been standardized.

134. Quoted in John Michael Vlach, *Back of the Big House: The Architecture of Plantation Slavery* (Chapel Hill: University of North Carolina Press, 1993), p. 163.

135. Deborah Gray White, *Ar'n't I a Woman? Female Slaves in the Plantation South* (New York: W. W. Norton, 1985), p. 83.

136. See George P. Rawick, ed., *The American Slave: A Composite Autobiography*, suppl. series 2 *Texas Narratives*, part 1 (Westport, Conn.: Greenwood Press, 1979), p. 635; Todd Savitt, *Medicine and Slavery: The Diseases and Health Care of Blacks in Antebellum Virginia* (Urbana: University of Illinois Press, 1978), p. 84.

137. See Rawick, ed., *Texas Narratives*, part 2, p. 895; B. A. Botkin, *Lay My Burden Down: A Folk History of Slavery* (Athens: University of Georgia Press, 1945), p. 253; Savitt, *Medicine and Slavery*, p. 85.

138. See Savitt, *Medicine and Slavery*, p. 11.

139. See Fett, "Body and Soul," pp. 70, 219.

140. Botkin, *Lay My Burden Down*, p. 167. Spelling standardized.

141. Richard H. Steckel, "Women, Work, and Health under Plantation Slavery in the United States," in *More than Chattel: Black Women and Slavery in the Americas*, ed. David Barry Gaspar and Darlene Clark Hine (Bloomington: Indiana University Press, 1996), p. 249.

142. Ibid., p. 55.

143. King, *Stolen Childhood*, p. 9.

144. Steckel, "Women, Work, and Health," p. 56.

145. King, *Stolen Childhood*, pp. 13, 24.

146. Nell Irvin Painter, "Soul Murder and Slavery," in *U.S. History as Women's History*, ed. Linda Kerber, Alice Kessler-Harris, and Kathryn Kish Sklar (Chapel Hill: University of North Carolina Press, 1995), pp. 125–146.

147. Quoted in Brenda E. Stevenson, *Life in Black and White: Family and Community in the Slave South* (New York: Oxford University Press, 1995), p. 225.

148. See Fett, "Body and Soul."

149. See Elizabeth Barnaby Keeney, "Unless Powerful Sick: Domestic Medicine in the Old South," in *Science and Medicine in the Old South*, ed. Ronald L. Numbers and Todd L. Savitt (Baton Rouge: Louisiana State University Press, 1989), p. 287; Savitt, *Medicine and Slavery*, p. 155.

150. Rawick, ed., *Texas Narratives*, part 2, p. 636. In all quotations from this source, the spellings used in the interview transcriptions have been standardized.

151. See Fett, "Body and Soul," pp. 271–322.

152. Ibid., pp. 208–270.

153. Rawick, ed., *Texas Narratives*, part 5, p. 2284.

154. James O. Breeden, *Advice among Masters: The Ideal in Slave Management in the Old South* (Westport, Conn.: Greenwood, 1980), p. 191.

155. Ibid.

156. Ibid.

157. Rawick, ed., *Texas Narratives*, part 3, p. 1116.

158. See Fett, "Body and Soul," pp. 149–150, 178–179; Elliott J. Gorn, "Folk Beliefs of the Slave Community," in *Science and Medicine*, ed. Numbers and Savitt, p. 323.

159. Botkin, *Lay My Burden Down*, p. 93.

160. See Fett, "Body and Soul," pp. 287–288.

161. See Vanessa Northington Gamble, "Under the Shadow of Tuskegee: African Americans and Health Care," *American Journal of Public Health* 87, no. 11 (November 1997): 1773–1778.

162. Rawick, ed., *Texas Narratives*, part 2, p. 849.

163. Ibid., part 1, p. 197; ibid., part 3, p. 1138; ibid., part 4, p. 1564.

164. Ibid., part 2, p. 610.

165. See David Barry Gaspar and Darlene Clark Hine, "Preface," in *More than Chattel*, ed. Gaspar and Hine, pp. ix–x.

166. See King, *Stolen Childhood*, pp. 71–80, 119–131; Stephanie J. Shaw, "Mothering under Slavery in the Antebellum South," in *Mothering: Ideology, Experience, and Agency*, ed. Evelyn Nakano Glenn, Grace Chang, and Linda Rennie Forcey (New York: Routledge, 1994), pp. 237–258; Brenda E. Stevenson, "Gender Convention, Ideals, and Identity among Antebellum Virginia Slave Women," in *More than Chattel*, ed. Gaspar and Hine, pp. 169–192. The term "weapons" comes from James C. Scott, *Weapons of the Weak: Everyday Forms of Resistance* (New Haven: Yale University Press, 1985).

167. Fett, "Body and Soul."

168. Margaret Washington Creel, *"A Peculiar People": Slave Religion and Community-Culture among the Gullahs* (New York: New York University Press, 1988), p. 311.

169. Rawick, ed., *Texas Narratives*, part 5, p. 2265.

170. Herbert G. Gutman, *The Black Family in Slavery and Freedom, 1750–1925* (New York: Vintage Books, 1976).

171. Ann Patton Malone, *Sweet Chariot: Slave Family and Household Structure in Nineteenth-Century Louisiana* (Chapel Hill: University of North Carolina Press, 1992), p. 259.

172. See White, *Ar'n't I a Woman?*, pp. 119–141. On "othermothers," see Patricia Hill Collins, "The Meaning of Motherhood in Black Culture and Black Mother-Daughter Relationships," in *Double Stitch: Black Women Write about Mothers and Daughters*, ed. Patricia Bell-Scott et al. (Boston: Beacon Press, 1991), pp. 42–60.

173. See White, *Ar'n't I a Woman?*, pp. 115–118.

174. Rawick, ed., *Texas Narratives*, part 2, p. 893.

175. See Lawrence W. Levine, *Black Culture and Black Consciousness: Afro-American Folk Thought from Slavery to Freedom* (New York: Oxford University Press, 1977), p. 63.

176. Ibid., p. 80.

177. See Bruce Jackson, "The Other Kind of Doctor: Conjure and Magic in Black American Folk Religion," in *African-American Religion: Interpretive Essays in History and Culture*, ed. Timothy E. Fulop and Albert J. Raboteau (New York: Routledge, 1997), pp. 415–432.

178. Fett, "Body and Soul," p. 81.

179. Ibid., pp. 81–90.

180. Levine, *Black Culture*, p. 63.

181. Quoted in Jacqueline Jones, "Black Women, Work, and the Family under Slavery," in *Families and Work*, ed. Naomi Gerstel and Harriet Engel Gross (Philadelphia: Temple University Press, 1987), p. 100.

182. Quoted in ibid. Spelling standardized.

183. See White, *Ar'n't I a Woman?*, pp. 81–83, 111, 115, 116.

184. Fett, "Body and Soul," pp. 208–270.

185. Quoted in White, *Ar'n't I a Woman?*, p. 117.

186. Rawick, ed., *Texas Narratives*, part 5, p. 2251.

3. *"Tried at the Quilting Bees"*

1. See Eliot Freidson, *The Profession of Medicine: A Study of the Sociology of Applied Knowledge* (New York: Harper and Row, 1970); Magali Sarfatti Larson, *The Rise of Professionalism: A Sociological Analysis* (Berkeley: University of California Press, 1977); William G. Rothstein, *American Physicians in the Nineteenth Century: From Sects to Science* (Baltimore: Johns Hopkins University Press, 1985); George Rosen, *The Structure of American Medical Practice, 1875–1941* (Philadelphia: University of Pennsylvania Press, 1983); Paul Starr, *The Social Transformation of American Medicine: The Rise of a Sovereign Profession and the Making of a Vast Industry* (New York: Basic Books, 1982).

2. For an excellent discussion of these issues in the case of childbirth, see Judith Walzer Leavitt, *Brought to Bed: Child-Bearing in America, 1750–1950* (New York: Oxford University Press, 1986). See also Leavitt, "'A Worrying Profession': The Domestic Environment of Medical Practice in Mid-Nineteenth-Century America," *Bulletin of the History of Medicine* 69, no. 1 (Spring 1995): 1–29.

3. Starr, *Social Transformation*, p. 162.

4. George S. King, *Doctor on a Bicycle* (New York: Rinehart and Co., 1958), p. 62. See also Marcus Bossard, *Eighty-one Years of Living* (Minneapolis: Midwest Printing Co., 1946), p. 54.

5. Agnes Just Reid, *Letters of Long Ago* (Caldwell, Idaho: Caxton Printers, 1923), p. 52.

6. See Bossard, *Eighty-one Years*, p. 21; Samuel J. Crumbine, *Frontier Doctor: The Autobiography of a Pioneer on the Frontier of Public Health* (Philadelphia: Dorrance and Co., 1948), pp. 58–59; Amalie M. Kass, "'Called to Her at Three o'Clock AM': Obstetrical Practice in Physician Case Notes," *Journal of the History of Medicine and Allied Sciences* 50, no. 2 (April 1995): 208–210; William Allen Pusey, *A Doctor of the 1870s and 80s* (Springfield, Ill.: Charles C. Thomas, 1932), pp. 118, 121; Francis A. Long, *A Prairie Doctor of the Eighties: Some Personal Recollections and Some Early Medical and Social History of a Prairie State* (Norfolk, Neb.: Huse Publishing Co., 1937), p. 90; John Brooks Wheeler, *Memoirs of a Small-Town Surgeon* (New York: Frederick A. Stokes, 1935), p. 290.

7. Pusey, *Doctor*, pp. 118–119.

8. Quoted in Rosen, *Structure*, p. 22.

9. Arthur E. Hertzler, *The Horse and Buggy Doctor* (Garden City, N.Y.: Blue Ribbon Books, 1941), p. 112.

10. D. W. Cathell, *The Physician Himself and What He Should Add to His Scientific Acquirements* (New York: Arno Press, 1972), p. 62.

11. Quoted in Leavitt, *Brought to Bed*, p. 105.

12. See Kass, "Obstetrical Practice."

13. Harold Wilensky, "The Professionalism of Everyone," *American Journal of Sociology* 70 (1964): 148.

14. See Rosen, *American Medical Practice*, pp. 2–3, 7–9; Charles E. Rosenberg, "The Therapeutic Revolution: Medicine, Meaning, and Social Change in Nineteenth-Century America," in *Sickness and Health in America: Readings in the History of Medicine and Public Health*, ed. Judith Walzer Leavitt and Ronald L. Numbers (Madison: University of Wisconsin Press, 1985), pp. 39–52.

15. Charles E. Rosenberg, *The Care of Strangers: The Rise of America's Hospital System* (New York: Basic Books, 1987), p. 70.

16. "Diary of Mrs. Joseph Duncan," ed. Elizabeth Duncan Putnam, *Journal of the Illinois State Historical Society* 21, no. 1 (April 1928): 71.

17. "Private Journal of Mary Ann Owen Sims," part 1, ed. Clifford Dale Whitman *Arkansas Historical Quarterly* 35, no. 4 (Winter 1976): 171.

18. See John Harley Warner, *The Therapeutic Perspective: Medical Practice, Knowledge, and Identity in America, 1820–1885* (Cambridge, Mass.: Harvard University Press, 1986), pp. 91–99.

19. See William G. Rothstein, "The Botanical Movements and Orthodox Medicine," in *Other Healers: Unorthodox Medicine in America*, ed. Norman Gevitz (Baltimore: Johns Hopkins University Press, 1988), p. 39.

20. Rothstein, "Botanical Movements."

21. Quoted in Janet L. Allured, "Women's Healing Art: Domestic Medicine in the Turn-of-the-Century Ozarks," *Gateway Heritage* 12 (Spring 1992): 21.

22. *Lamps on the Prairie: A History of Nursing in Kansas*, comp. Writers' Program of the Work Projects Administration in Kansas (New York: Garland Publishing, 1984), pp. 36–37.

23. See "Letters of John and Sarah Everett, 1854–1864: Miami County Pioneers," *Kansas Historical Quarterly* 8, no. 1 (February 1939): 19; Elizabeth Hampsten, ed., *To All Inquiring Friends: Letters, Diaries, and Essays in North Dakota, 1880–1910*, 2d ed. (Grand Forks: Department of English, University of North Dakota, 1980), p. 132.

24. "Roughing It on Her Kansas Claim: The Diary of Abbie Bright, 1870–1871," ed. Joseph W. Snell, *Kansas Historical Quarterly* 37, no. 3 (Autumn 1971): 247.

25. Harriet Connor Brown, *Grandmother Brown's Hundred Years, 1827–1927* (New York: Blue Ribbon Books, 1929), pp. 156–157.

26. Helen Smith Jordan, ed., *Love Lies Bleeding* (privately published, 1979), p. 174.

27. Ibid., p. 220.

28. Ibid., p. 322.

29. Ibid., p. 446.

30. Quoted in Lamar Riley Murphy, *Enter the Physician: The Transformation of Domestic Medicine, 1760–1860* (Tuscaloosa: University of Alabama Press, 1991), pp. 112–113.

31. Brown, *Grandmother Brown's Hundred Years*, p. 155.

32. See Murphy, *Enter the Physician*, pp. 75–80; Charles E. Rosenberg, "John Gunn: Everyman's Physician," in *Explaining Epidemics and Other Studies in the History of Medicine* ed. Charles E. Rosenberg (New York: Cambridge University Press, 1992), pp. 57–74.

33. Nannie T. Alderson and Helena Huntington Smith, *A Bride Goes West* (New York: Farrar and Rinehart, 1942), pp. 207–208.

34. James L. Thane, Jr., *A Governor's Wife on the Mining Frontier: The Letters of Mary Edgerton from Montana, 1863–1865* (Salt Lake City: University of Utah Library, 1976), pp. 109–110.

35. See Marilyn Ferris Motz, *True Sisterhood: Michigan Women and Their Kin, 1890–1920* (Albany: State University of New York Press, 1983), p. 100.

36. See Murphy, *Enter the Physician*, pp. 63–69.

37. "Mary Anne Owen Sims," part 1, ed. Whitman, 150–151.

38. Mary S. Paul to Father, June 11, 1855, in *Farm to Factory: Women's Letters, 1830–1860*, ed. Thomas Dublin (New York: Columbia University Press, 1981), p. 122.

39. Hallie F. Nelson, *South of the Cottonwood Tree* (Broken Bow, Nebr.: Purcells, 1977), p. 136.

40. Long, *Prairie Doctor*, p. 68.

41. *Lamps on the Prairie*, p. 45. See also Lillie M. Jackson, *Fanning the Embers* (Boston: Christopher Publishing, 1966), p. 60.

42. Mary Ann Webber to Eliza and Albert Webber, Summer 1865, Parker Family Letters, private collection of Marianne Brown, Los Angeles.

43. "The Letters of Effie Hanson, 1917–1923: Farm Life in Troubled Times," ed. Frances M. Wold, *North Dakota History* 48, no. 1 (Winter 1981): 39.

44. *Lamps on the Prairie*, pp. 45–46.

45. Lorraine Code, *What Can She Know? Feminist Theory and the Construction of Knowledge* (Ithaca: Cornell University Press, 1991), p. 222.

46. Mary Smith Webber Adams to Friends, April 29, 1863, Parker Family Letters.

47. Jordan, ed., *Love Lies Bleeding*, p. 435.

48. Quoted in Eleanor Arnold, ed., *Voices of American Homemakers* (Bloomington: Indiana University Press, 1985), p. 96.

49. Freidson, *Profession of Medicine*, p. 169.

50. Quoted in Rosenberg, "Therapeutic Revolution," p. 48.

51. In his study of obstetrics in the mid-nineteenth-century South, Steven Stowe writes, "A physician must come to *know* his patient, and engage himself with her and her family, in order to learn not only the signs of pregnancy but also methods of eliciting and interpreting them in individuals." Stowe, "Obstetrics and the Work of Doctoring in the Mid-Nineteenth-Century American South," *Bulletin of the History of Medicine* 64, no. 3 (Fall 1990): 543.

52. Rothstein, *American Physicians*, p. 288–289; Starr, *Social Transformation*, pp. 118–119.

53. Cited in Starr, *Social Transformation*, p. 118.

54. Long, *Prairie Doctor*, p. 76.

55. Ibid., p. 29.

56. Helen Doyle, "A Child Went Forth: The Autobiography of Dr. Helen MacKnight," in *Let Them Speak for Themselves: Women in the American West, 1849–1900*, ed. Christiane Fischer (Hamden, Conn.: Archon Books, 1977), p. 196.

57. Charles Beneulyn Johnson, *Sixty Years in Medical Harness; or, The Story of a Long Medical Life, 1865–1925* (New York: Medical Life Press, 1926), p. 95. See also William L. Crosthwait and Ernest G. Fischer, *The Last Stitch* (Philadelphia: J. B. Lippincott Co., 1956), pp. 72–75.

58. J. Marion Sims, *The Story of My Life* (1884; reprint, New York: Da Capo Press, 1968), p. 139.

59. Ibid., pp. 140–141.

60. Ibid., p. 141.

61. Ibid., p. 142.

62. Ibid.

63. Ibid., p. 143.

64. Ibid., pp. 145–146.

65. Ibid., p. 146.

66. Crumbine, *Frontier Doctor*, p. 153.

67. Willene Hendrick and George Hendrick, *On the Illinois Frontier: Dr. Hiram Rutherford, 1840–1848* (Carbondale: Southern Illinois University Press, 1981), p. 16.

68. Quoted in Leavitt, *Brought to Bed*, p. 102.

69. Pusey, *Doctor*, p. 94.

70. Quoted in Murphy, *Enter the Physician*, p. 201.

71. Pusey, *Doctor*, p. 94.

72. See Rosen, *American Medical Practice*, p. 28.

73. Hertzler, *Horse and Buggy Doctor*, pp. 112–113. See also Nathan Elliott Wood, *Dollars to Doctors; or, Diplomacy and Prosperity in Medical Practice* (Chicago: Lion Publishing Co., 1903).

74. Long, *Prairie Doctor*, p. 29.

75. See ibid., pp. 67–68; Murphy, *Enter the Physician*, pp. 59, 112.

76. See Murphy, *Enter the Physician*.

4. A "Terrible and Exhausting" Struggle

1. James H. Cassedy, *Medicine in America: A Short History* (Baltimore: Johns Hopkins University Press, 1991), p. 93.

2. Ruth Schwartz Cowan, *More Work for Mother: The Ironies of Household Technology from the Open Hearth to the Microwave* (New York: Basic Books, 1983), p. 73.

3. See, for example, M. L. Berger, "The Influence of the Automobile on Rural Health Care, 1900–1929," *Journal of the History of Medicine and Allied Sciences* 28 (1973): 319–335; Helen Clapesattle, *The Doctors Mayo* (Minneapolis: University of Minnesota Press, 1941), pp. 348–353; Guenter B. Risse, "From Horse and Buggy to Automobile and Telephone: Medical Practice in Wisconsin, 1848–1930," in *Wisconsin Medicine: Historical Perspectives*, ed. Ronald L. Numbers and Judith Walzer Leavitt (Madison: University of Wisconsin Press, 1981), pp. 25–45. For a contemporary discussion of the impact of automobiles on medical practice, see "Satisfaction in Automobiling: A Symposium by Physicians on Their Experiences with Motor-Cars—How to Secure the Most in Comfort and Help at the Least Expense," *Journal of the American Medical Association* 58 (1912): 1049–1080.

4. See Cowan, *More Work for Mother*; Susan Strasser, *Never Done: A History of American Housework* (New York: Pantheon, 1982).

5. The complete diary of Martha Shaw Farnsworth is located in the Martha Farnsworth Collection, no. 28, Kansas State Historical Society, Topeka, Kansas. All quotations in this chapter, unless otherwise noted, are taken from this diary. For an excellent annotated and abbreviated version, see *Plains Woman: The Diary of Martha Farnsworth, 1882–1922*, ed. Marlene Springer and Haskell Springer (Bloomington: Indiana University Press, 1988).

6. See Arthur E. Hertzler, *The Horse and Buggy Doctor* (Garden City, N.Y.: Blue Ribbon Books, 1941), pp. 110–115.

7. On Kansas women and temperance, see Glenda Riley, *The Female Frontier: A Comparative View of Women on the Prairie and the Plains* (Lawrence: University of Kansas Press, 1988), pp. 178–179.

8. Walker Winslow, *The Menninger Story* (Garden City, N.Y.: Doubleday, 1956), p. 47.

9. See Lucy Freeman, ed., *Karl Menninger, M.D., SPARKS* (New York: Thomas Y. Crowell Co., 1973), p. 2.

10. See Riley, *Female Frontier*, p. 94.

11. Winslow, *Menninger Story*, p. 47.

12. See Charles E. Rosenberg, "The Therapeutic Revolution: Medicine, Meaning, and Social Change in Nineteenth-Century America," in *The Therapeutic Revolution: Essays in the Social History of American Medicine*, ed. Morris J. Vogel and Charles E. Rosenberg (Philadelphia: University of Pennsylvania Press, 1979), pp. 3–25.

13. Winslow, *Menninger Story*, pp. 59–60.

14. Flo V. Menninger, *Days of My Life: Memories of a Kansas Mother and Teacher* (New York: Richard R. Smith, 1940), p. 238.

15. See Alice Kessler-Harris, *Out to Work: A History of Wage-Earning Women in the United States* (Oxford: Oxford University Press, 1982), pp. 124–125.

16. According to Joan E. Lynaugh, tuberculosis was the major cause of death in nineteenth-century Kansas City. *The Community Hospitals of Kansas City, Missouri, 1870–1915* (New York: Garland Publishing, 1989), p. 86.

17. See Barbara Bates, *Bargaining for Life: A Social History of Tuberculosis, 1876–1938* (Philadelphia: University of Pennsylvania Press, 1992), p. 17.

18. Information from Liana Overley, Public Relations Coordinator, Grant Hospital, Chicago.

19. Thomas Neville Bonner, *Kansas Doctor: A Century of Pioneering* (Lawrence: University of Kansas Press, 1959), p. 91.

20. Winslow, *Menninger Story*, p. 90.

21. Ibid., pp. 30–35.

22. Ibid., p. 45.

23. Paul Starr, *The Social Transformation of American Medicine: The Rise of a Sovereign Profession and the Making of a Vast Industry* (New York: Basic Books, 1982), pp. 96–97.

24. Lynaugh, *Community Hospitals*, p. 22.

25. Billy M. Jones, *Health-Seekers in the Southwest, 1817–1900* (Norman: University of Oklahoma Press, 1967), p. 146. See also Sheila M. Rothman, *Living in the Shadow of Death: Tuberculosis and the Social Experience of Illness in American History* (New York: Basic Books, 1994), pp. 131–175.

26. Quoted in Jones, *Health-Seekers*, p. 96.

27. See Rothman, *Living in the Shadow*, pp. 161–167.

28. Martha's use of the language of rights reminds us that as reliance on doctors increased, the experience of childbirth changed, even when objective conditions remained the same. From Martha's perspective, dependence on a midwife now represented a serious "deprivation."

29. Richard Sennett and Jonathan Cobb, *The Hidden Injuries of Class* (New York: Vintage, 1972), p. 140.

30. Samuel H. Preston and Michael R. Haines, *Fatal Years: Child Mortality in Late-Nineteenth-Century America* (Princeton: Princeton University Press, 1991).

31. Charles R. King, "Childhood Death: The Health Care of Children on the Kansas Frontier," *Kansas History* 14, no. 1 (Spring 1991), p. 26.

32. See L. Emmett Holt, *The Diseases of Infancy and Childhood* (New York: D. Appleton and Co., 1898), pp. 243–245; Eustace Smith, *A Practical Treatise on Disease in Children* (New York: William Wood and Co., 1894), pp. 555–562.

33. Bonner, *Kansas Doctor*, pp. 71–82.

34. Winslow, *Menninger Story*, p. 70.

35. Menninger, *Days of My Life*, p. 242.

36. John E. Baur, *The Health Seekers of Southern California, 1870–1900* (San Marino, Calif.: Huntington Library, 1959); Jones, *Health-Seekers*, p. 141; Rothman, *Living in the Shadow*, pp. 245–247.

37. Rothman, *Living in the Shadow*, p. 182.

38. See Samuel J. Crumbine, *Frontier Doctor: The Autobiography of a Pioneer on the Frontier of Public Health* (Philadelphia: Dorrance and Co., 1948), pp. 142–165.

39. Lucy S. Mitchell, *Two Lives: The Story of Wesley Clair Mitchell and Myself* (New York: Simon and Schuster, 1953), p. 105.

40. According to Flo Menninger, the heat that summer was unusually oppressive; *Days of My Life*, p. 87.

41. Susan M. Reverby, *Ordered to Care: The Dilemma of American Nursing, 1850–1945* (Cambridge, U.K.: Cambridge University Press, 1987), pp. 15–16.

42. See Eleanor Arnold, ed., *Voices of American Homemakers* (Bloomington: Indiana University Press, 1985). On the diffusion of these goods and services throughout the country, see Joann Vanek, "Household Technology and Social Sta-

tus: Rising Living Standards and Status and Residence Differences in Housework," *Technology and Culture* 19 (July 1978): 361–375.

43. Winslow, *Menninger Story*, p. 104.

44. See Stanley Joel Reiser, *Medicine and the Reign of Technology* (Cambridge, U.K.: Cambridge University Press, 1967), p. 146; Rosemary Stevens, *American Medicine and the Public Interest* (New Haven: Yale University Press, 1971), pp. 80, 147.

45. Bonner, *Kansas Doctor*, pp. 69–70.

46. Starr, *Social Transformation*, p. 259.

47. Reiser, *Reign of Technology*, p. 68.

48. Starr, *Social Transformation*, p. 135.

49. Bonner, *Kansas Doctor*, p. 203.

50. See Cassedy, *Medicine in America*, p. 99.

51. Starr, *Social Transformation*, p. 127.

52. See Ray Fitzpatrick, "Lay Concepts of Illness," in *Perspectives in Medical Sociology*, ed. Phil Brown (Belmont, Calif.: Wadsworth, 1989), pp. 254–267; Raymond H. Murray and Arthur J. Rubel, "Physicians and Healers—Unwitting Partners in Health Care," *New England Journal of Medicine*, 326, no. 1 (Jan. 2, 1992), pp. 61–64.

53. Jane B. Brody, "Alternative Medicine Makes Inroads, but Watch Out for Curves," *New York Times* April 28, 1998, sec. B, p. 10.

54. Bonner, *Kansas Doctor*, p. 70; Reiser, *Reign of Technology*, p. 67.

55. Starr, *Social Transformation*, p. 70.

56. See Roy Porter, *The Greatest Benefit to Mankind: A Medical History of Humanity* (New York: W. W. Norton, 1997), pp. 597–627.

57. David Rosner, *A Once Charitable Enterprise: Hospitals and Health Care in Brooklyn and New York, 1885–1915* (Princeton: Princeton University Press, 1982), p. 4.

58. Judith Walzer Leavitt, *Brought to Bed: Child-Bearing in America, 1750–1950* (New York: Oxford University Press, 1986), p. 189.

59. Lynaugh's study of Kansas City hospitals reveals that the presence of family members in operating theaters was not unusual. See Lynaugh, *Community Hospitals*, p. 82.

60. Permission was not always granted. According to Marilyn Ferris Motz, when Winnie Parker entered a Michigan hospital in 1897, her sister believed that she had a "right and duty" to accompany the patient into the operating room and was shocked to discover that the physicians would not allow this. *True Sisterhood: Michigan Women and Their Kin, 1890–1920* (Albany: State University of New York Press, 1983), p. 102. For an argument against admitting family and friends to operating rooms in 1913, see "The Laity in the Operating Room," *Southern California Practitioner* 28, no. 12 (December 1913): 391.

61. See Rosemary Stevens, *In Sickness and in Wealth: American Hospitals in the Twentieth Century* (New York: Basic Books, 1989), p. 21.

62. Starr, *Social Transformation*, pp. 157–158.

63. *Lamps on the Prairie: A History of Nursing in Kansas*, comp. Writers' Program of the Work Projects Administration in Kansas (New York: Garland Publishing, 1984), p. 94.

64. Reverby, *Ordered to Care*, p. 95.

65. Ibid., p. 98.

66. Winslow, *Menninger Story*, p. 162.

67. Ibid., pp. 67, 83.

68. Ibid., pp. 90, 104.

69. Ibid., pp. 111, 131.

70. Kenneth F. Kiple, *The Cambridge World History of Human Disease* (New York: Cambridge University Press, 1993), p. 720.

71. Menninger, *Days of My Life*, pp. 245–246, 256.

72. Winslow, *Menninger Story*, p. 134.

73. Charles E. Rosenberg, *The Care of Strangers: The Rise of America's Hospital System* (New York: Basic Books, 1987), p. 316.

74. Winslow, *Menninger Story*, p. 81; Menninger, *Days of My Life*, p. 246.

75. Leavitt, *Brought to Bed*, p. 174.

76. Strasser, *Never Done*, p. 305.

77. Recalling his early years of practice in rural Kansas in the nineteenth century, one physician wrote, "When there was serious illness or accident . . . these rural settlers gave us town people lessons in applied Christianity . . . These people were ready night or day to drive long distances to town to get groceries, fuel and medicines, or the doctor, as well as to do the work on the farm or in the home." Crumbine, *Frontier Doctor*, pp. 49–50.

78. See Riley, *Female Frontier*, pp. 93–94.

79. Strasser, *Never Done*, p. 235.

80. Joel D. Howell and Catherine G. McLaughlin, "Race, Income and the Purchase of Medical Care by Selected 1917 Working-Class Urban Families," *Journal of the History of Medicine and Allied Sciences* 47 (1992): 439–461.

81. Starr, *Social Transformation*, p. 245.

82. *Plains Woman*, ed. Springer and Springer, p. 307.

83. Laura Balbo, "Crazy Quilts: Rethinking the Welfare State Debate from a Woman's Point of View," in *Women and the State: The Shifting Boundaries of Public and Private*, ed. Anne Showstack Sassoon (London: Unwin Hyman, 1987), pp. 45–71.

5. *"Just as You Direct"*

1. Rosemary Stevens, *In Sickness and in Wealth: American Hospitals in the Twentieth Century* (New York: Basic Books, 1989), p. 35.

2. Cited in Charles E. Rosenberg, *The Care of Strangers: The Rise of America's Hospital System* (New York: Basic Books, 1987), p. 5.

3. Paul Starr, *The Social Transformation of American Medicine: The Rise of a Sovereign Profession and the Making of a Vast Industry* (New York: Basic Books, 1982).

4. Magali Sarfatti Larson, *The Rise of Professionalism: A Sociological Analysis* (Berkeley: University of California Press, 1977), p. 162.

5. Ronald L. Numbers, "The Rise and Fall of the American Medical Profession," in *Sickness and Health in America: Readings in the History of Medicine and Public Health*, ed. Judith Walzer Leavitt and Ronald L. Numbers (Madison: University of Wisconsin Press, 1985), p. 192.

6. Starr, *Social Transformation*.

7. Ellen D. Baer, "Nurses," in *Women, Health, and Medicine in America: A Historical Handbook*, ed. Rima D. Apple (New Brunswick, N.J.: Rutgers University Press, 1992), p. 454.

8. Barbara Melosh, *"The Physician's Hand": Work Culture and Conflict in American Nursing* (Philadelphia: Temple University Press, 1982), pp. 101–102; Susan M. Reverby, *Ordered to Care: The Dilemma of American Nursing, 1850–1945* (New York: Cambridge University Press, 1987), pp. 121–142.

9. Joel D. Howell, *Technology in the Hospital: Transforming Patient Care in the Early Twentieth Century* (Baltimore: Johns Hopkins University Press, 1995).

10. Rosenberg, *Care of Strangers*, p. 151; Starr, *Social Transformation*, pp. 134–36.

11. Baer, "Nurses," p. 453; Reverby, *Ordered to Care*, pp. 60–76, 97.

12. Edna L. Foley, "Bedside Care," *Public Health Nurse* 15, no. 5 (May 1923): 235.

13. Quoted in *The Diary of Emily Jane Green Hollister: Her Nursing Experiences, 1888–1911*, ed. Deborah D. Smith (Ann Arbor: University of Michigan Historical Center for the Health Sciences, 1991), p. 26. I am grateful to Karen Buhler-Wilkerson and Joan E. Lynaugh for introducing me to this book.

14. Jan Lewis and Peter N. Stearns, "Introduction," in *An Emotional History of the United States*, ed. Peter N. Stearns and Jan Lewis (New York: New York University Press, 1998), p. 10.

15. Rosenberg, *Care of Strangers*.

16. A 1929 study found that Philadelphia physicians in private practice spent slightly more than 10 percent of their workweek making house calls. Cited in Ruth Schwartz Cowan, *More Work for Mother: The Ironies of Household Technology from the Open Hearth to the Microwave* (New York: Basic Books, 1983), pp. 84–85.

17. Chris Feudtner, "The Want of Control: Ideas, Innovations, and Ideals in the Modern Management of Diabetes Mellitus," *Bulletin of the History of Medicine* 69, no. 1 (Spring 1995): 67.

18. Quoted in Keith Wailoo, *Drawing Blood: Technology and Disease Identity in Twentieth-Century America* (Baltimore: Johns Hopkins University Press, 1997), p. 21.

19. Barbara Bates, *Bargaining for Life: A Social History of Tuberculosis, 1876–1938* (Philadelphia: University of Pennsylvania Press, 1992), p. 204; Wailoo, *Drawing Blood*, p. 21; New York Society for the Relief of the Ruptured and Crippled, *Sixth Annual Report of the Social Service Out-Patient Department, October 1, 1918–September 30, 1919*, p. 15.

20. Quoted in David Rosner, *A Once Charitable Enterprise: Hospitals and Health Care in Brooklyn and New York, 1885–1915* (Princeton: Princeton University Press, 1982), p. 78.

21. Quoted in Wailoo, *Drawing Blood*, p. 21.

22. Quoted in Katherine Ott, *Fevered Lives: Tuberculosis in American Culture since 1870* (Cambridge, Mass.: Harvard University Press, 1996), p. 82.

23. Quoted in Bates, *Bargaining for Life*, p. 201.

24. Melosh, *"Physician's Hand,"* p. 56.

25. Quoted in ibid.

26. John Brooks Wheeler, *Memoirs of a Small-Town Surgeon* (New York: Frederick A. Stokes, 1935), p. 315.

27. *Emily Jane Green Hollister*, ed. Smith, p. 35.

28. Ibid., p. 25.

29. Charlotte G. Borst, *Catching Babies: The Professionalization of Childbirth, 1870–1920* (Cambridge, Mass.: Harvard University Press, 1995), p. 17.

30. See Gertrude Jacinta Fraser, *African American Midwifery in the South: Dialogues of Birth, Race, and Memory* (Cambridge, Mass.: Harvard University Press, 1998), pp. 107–124.

31. Molly Ladd-Taylor, *Mother-Work: Women, Child Welfare, and the State, 1890–1930* (Urbana: University of Illinois Press, 1994), p. 182.

32. Ibid.

33. Frances E. Kobrin, "The American Midwife Controversy: A Crisis of Professionalization," in *Sickness and Health*, ed. Leavitt and Numbers, p. 197; Ladd-Taylor, *Mother-Work*, p. 82; Richard A. Meckel, *Save the Babies: American Public Health Reform and the Prevention of Infant Mortality, 1850–1929* (Baltimore: Johns Hopkins University Press, 1990), 172–174; Robyn Muncy, *Creating a Female Dominion in American Reform, 1890–1935* (New York: Oxford University Press, 1991), pp. 117–118; Sandra Schackel, *Social Housekeepers: Women Shaping Public Policy in New Mexico, 1920–1940* (Albuquerque: University of New Mexico, 1992), pp. 50–51; Susan L. Smith, *Sick and Tired of Being Sick and Tired: Black Women's Health Activism in America, 1890–1950* (Philadelphia: University of Pennsylvania Press, 1995), pp. 123–124.

34. Stevens, *In Sickness*, p. 86.

35. See Darlene Clark Hine, *Black Women in White: Racial Conflict and Cooperation in the Nursing Profession, 1890–1950* (Bloomington: Indiana University Press, 1989), p. 6.

36. Reverby, *Ordered to Care*, p. 97.

37. Melosh, *"Physician's Hand,"* pp. 102–103.

38. Cited in Ladd-Taylor, *Mother-Work*, p. 23.

39. Fran Leeper Buss, *La Partera: Story of a Midwife* (Ann Arbor: University of Michigan Press, 1980), p. 114.

40. Smith, *Sick and Tired*, pp. 119–120. See also Fraser, *African American Midwifery*.

41. Quoted in Children's Bureau, U.S. Department of Labor, *Prenatal Care*, publication no. 4 (Washington, D.C.: Government Printing Office, 1913), p. 2.

42. See Ladd-Taylor, *Mother-Work*; Molly Ladd-Taylor, *Raising a Baby the Government Way: Mothers' Letters to the Children's Bureau, 1915–1932* (New Brunswick, N.J.: Rutgers University Press, 1986); Kriste Lindenmeyer, *"A Right to Childhood": The U.S. Children's Bureau and Child Welfare, 1912–46* (Urbana: University of Illinois Press, 1997); Meckel, *Save the Babies*; Muncy, *Creating a Female Dominion*; Jacqueline K. Parker and Edward M. Carpenter, "Julia Lathrop and the Children's Bureau: The Emergence of an Institution," *Social Service Review* 55 (March 1981): 60–77; Theda Skocpol, *Protecting Soldiers and Mothers: The Political Origins of Social Policy in the United States* (Cambridge, Mass.: Harvard University Press, 1992), pp. 480–524; Nancy Pottishman Weiss, "Save the Children: A History of the Children's Bureau, 1903–1918" (Ph.D. diss., University of California, Los Angeles, 1974).

43. Ladd-Taylor, *Raising a Baby*, p. 9.

44. Ibid., p. 2.

45. Children's Bureau, U.S. Department of Labor, *Infant Care*, publication no. 8 (Washington, D.C.: Government Printing Office, 1914); Children's Bureau, *Prenatal Care*.

46. Weiss, "Save the Children," p. 199.

47. Ladd-Taylor, *Raising a Baby*, p. 2.

48. Ibid.

49. Julia Grant, *Raising Baby by the Book: The Education of American Mothers* (New Haven: Yale University Press, 1998), pp. 39–69.

50. Ibid., pp. 21–32; Lamar Riley Murphy, *Enter the Physician: The Transformation of Domestic Medicine, 1760–1860* (Tuscaloosa: University of Alabama Press, 1991).

51. See Sydney A. Halpern, *American Pediatrics: The Social Dynamics of Professionalism, 1880–1980* (Berkeley: University of California Press, 1988), pp. 80–109; Jacquelyn Litt, "Pediatrics and the Development of Middle-Class Motherhood," *Research in the Sociology of Health Care* 10 (1993): 161–173; Meckel, *Save the Babies*, pp. 46–50.

52. Julia Wrigley, "Do Young Children Need Intellectual Stimulation? Experts' Advice to Parents, 1900–1985," *History of Education Quarterly* 29, no. 1 (Spring 1989): 41–75.

53. Andrew Abbott, *The System of Professions: An Essay on the Division of Expert Labor* (Chicago: University of Chicago Press, 1988), p. 60.

54. Halpern, *American Pediatrics*, pp. 80–109.

55. Rima Apple, *Mothers and Medicine: A Social History of Infant Feeding, 1890–1950* (Madison: University of Wisconsin Press, 1987); Celia B. Stendler, "Psychologic Aspects of Pediatrics: Sixty Years of Child Training Practices," *Journal of Pediatrics* 36, no. 1 (January 1950): 128.

56. On the clock as a symbol of science, see Ann V. Millard, "The Place of the Clock in Pediatric Advice: Rationales, Cultural Themes, and Impediments to Breastfeeding," *Social Science and Medicine* 31, no. 2 (1990): 211–221.

57. These examples are cited in Susan Strasser, *Never Done: A History of American Housework* (New York: Pantheon, 1982), p. 237.

58. See Elizabeth M. R. Lomax with Jerome Kagan and Barbara G. Rosenkrantz, *Science and Patterns of Child Care* (San Francisco: W. H. Freeman and Co., 1978), pp. 14. 114.

59. Cited in Grant, *By the Book*, p. 45.

60. Litt, "Pediatrics," 163, 166, 170.

61. Grant, *By the Book*, p. 45.

62. Wrigley, "Young Children," 57.

63. Quoted in Litt, "Pediatrics," 166. See also Grant, *By the Book*, p. 51; Kathleen W. Jones, "'Mother Made Me Do It': Mother-Blaming and the Women of Child Guidance," in *"Bad" Mothers: The Politics of Blame in Twentieth-Century America*, ed. Molly Ladd-Taylor and Lauri Umansky (New York: New York University Press, 1998), pp. 99–126.

64. Grant, *By the Book*, pp. 23–25.

65. Alison M. Jaggar, *Feminist Politics and Human Nature* (Totowa, N.J.: Rowman and Allanheld, 1983), p. 311.

66. Lomax, *Science and Patterns*, pp. 63, 73, 96, 133.

67. These letters are located in the Records of the Children's Bureau, RG 102, National Archives, Washington, D.C. For an excellent collection of selected letters, see Ladd-Taylor, *Raising a Baby*.

68. See Muncy, *Creating a Female Dominion*, pp. 114–115.

69. Margaret Jarman Hagood, *Mothers of the South* (New York: W. W. Norton, 1977), p. 138.

70. Ibid.

71. Mrs. H. C. G., September 11, 1926, file 4-5-7-2-1, Children's Bureau Records.

72. Mrs. B. W., Maine, May 21, 1915, file 4-5-3-2x.

73. Mrs. F. H., Nebraska, July 5, 1915, file 4-4.

74. Mrs. F. S., New York, May 3, 1921, file 4-5-3-3.

75. Mrs. P. K., Illinois, July 28, 1920, file 4-4-4.

76. Mrs. A. L. B., Ohio, April 9, 1916, file 4-4-3-3.

77. On the use of language as an indicator of medicalization, see Penny Van Esterik, *Beyond the Breast-Bottle Controversy* (New Brunswick, N.J.: Rutgers University Press, 1989).

78. Rosemary Stevens, *American Medicine and the Public Interest* (New Haven: Yale University Press, 1971), p. 179.

79. John Harley Warner, *The Therapeutic Perspective: Medical Practice, Knowledge, and Identity in America, 1820–1885* (Cambridge, Mass.: Harvard University Press, 1986).

80. Mrs. D. P., Ohio, November 5, 1930, file 4-5-5-1, Children's Bureau Records.

81. Mrs. Z. C. W., Washington, February 6, 1931, file 4-8-6-2.

82. See Jane Lewis, *The Politics of Motherhood: Child and Maternal Welfare in England, 1900–1939* (London: Croom Helm, 1980).

83. National Center for Health Statistics, U.S. Department of Health and Human Services, *Vital Statistics of the United States, 1985*, vol. 2, *Mortality* (Washington, D.C.: Government Printing Office, 1988), part A, sect. 2, p. 1. See also Grant, *By the Book*, p. 116.

84. Mrs. R. C. M., California, June 18, 1915, file 4-4-3-1x, Children's Bureau Records.

85. Mrs. H. A. S., Virginia, December 4, 1917, file 4-5-3-1-3.

86. Grant, *By the Book*, p. 137.

87. See Barbara Ehrenreich and Deirdre English, *For Her Own Good: 150 Years of the Experts' Advice to Women* (Garden City, N.Y.: Anchor Books, 1979); Sheila Rothman, *Woman's Proper Place: A History of Changing Ideals and Practices, 1870 to the Present* (New York: Basic Books, 1978).

88. Robert S. Lynd and Helen Merrell Lynd, *Middletown: A Study in Contemporary American Culture* (New York: Harcourt, Brace and Co., 1929), p. 151.

89. Mrs. H. M. G., Saskatchewan, Canada, October 5, 1914, file 4-5-3-1x.

90. Mrs. L. J. R., Montana, January 7, 1924, file 4-5-3-3, Children's Bureau Records.

91. Mrs. C. S., New Jersey, April 6, 1927, file 4-5-3-2.

92. Mrs. E. I., Iowa, March 24, 1920, file 4-4-3-3.

93. See, for example, Mrs. E. C., Kentucky, September 23, 1915, file 4-4-3-1-3.

94. Mrs. C. S., Michigan, September 20, 1935, file 4-9-1-1.

95. Mrs. J. C. M., Tennessee, January 1, 1930, file 4-5-2-1-1.

96. Stevens, *American Medicine*.

97. Mrs. J. M. K., Texas, September 8, 1933, file 4-5-15.

98. Mrs. W. H. E., California, May 18, 1918, file 4-4-3-1.

99. Mrs. R. B. H., Texas, March 1, 1920, file 4-4-3-1.

100. Mrs. E. D., New York, March 9, 1927, file 4-5-8-3-1.

101. Mrs. E. D., New York, November 11, 1927, file 4-5-3-3.

102. Mrs. L. R., Montana, November 4, 1923, file 4-5-3-0.

103. Mrs. G. F. H., New York, May 9, 1929, file 4-5-15.

104. Mrs. F. D., Quebec, December 18, 1921, file 4-5-8-1.

105. Mrs. F. H., California, February 5, 1929, file 4-5-11-5-1.

106. Stevens, *In Sickness*, p. 106.

107. Ibid., p. 107.

108. See, for example, Mrs. J. J. C., Texas, March 8, 1929, file 4-5-10-4.

109. Mrs. A. G. L., Missouri, October 16, 1920, file 4-6-4-4.

110. Mrs. C. H. S., Alabama, August 5, 1926, file 4-6-8-1.

111. Mrs. W. D., Massachusetts, June 22, 1928, file 4-4-0-3.

112. Mrs. G. E. S., Wisconsin, January 1, 1931, file 4-5-9-3.

113. Mrs. P. N. O., Iowa, July 23, 1928, file 4-5-6-3. Such letters suggest that some of the factors fueling the current malpractice crisis were operative as early as the first decades of the century.

114. Mrs. C. M., California, September 11, 1935, file 4-5-15.

115. Mr. M. S., New York, October 3, 1921, file 4-6-8-1.

116. Between 1918 and 1929, revenues in the advertising industry increased threefold, reaching $200 million by the eve of the Depression. Strasser, *Never Done*, p. 253.

117. Stevens, *In Sickness*, p. 109.

118. Larson, *Rise of Professionalism*.

119. Quoted in Sheila M. Rothman, *Living in the Shadow of Death: Tuberculosis and the Social Experience of Illness in American History* (New York: Basic Books, 1994), pp. 196–197.

120. The letters were selected randomly from those located in the Papers of Lawrence F. Flick, Archives of the Catholic University of America, Washington, D.C. Forty percent of the letters in this sample were from men. Flick's responses to forty-eight of the letters also are available.

121. See Barbara Bates, *Bargaining for Life: A Social History of Tuberculosis, 1876–1938* (Philadelphia: University of Pennsylvania Press, 1992). I rely heavily on this work throughout this section.

122. Ibid., p. 30.

123. For information about these various remedies, see ibid., p. 31.

124. Ibid., pp. 16, 29.

125. Ibid., pp. 320–321.

126. Pat Jalland, *Death in the Victorian Family* (New York: Oxford University Press, 1996), p. 41.

127. See Ott, *Fevered Lives*, p. 82.

128. Quoted in Bates, *Bargaining for Life*, pp. 227–228.

129. Quoted in ibid., p. 205.

130. Quoted in ibid.

131. J. L. B. to Lawrence F. Flick (hereafter abbreviated as LF), Pennsylvania, August 1906, Flick Papers.

132. J. S. to LF, February 4, 1909.

133. J. U. to LF, February 15, 1925.

134. Theodore M. Porter, "Making Things Quantitative," *Science in Context* 7, no. 3 (1994): 389.

135. C. B. K. to LF, Pennsylvania, October 20, 1907.

136. S. H. L., to LF, Ohio, January 29, 1909.

137. Bates, *Bargaining for Life*, p. 214.

138. W. S. to LF, West Virginia, October 21, 1907.

139. R. L. S. to LF, September 11, 1909.

140. E. R. L. to LF, Pennsylvania, May 8, 1915. Most middle-class homes did not have scales before the mid-1920s. See Joan Jacobs Brumberg, *The Body Project: An Intimate History of American Girls* (New York: Random House, 1997), fig. 25. Although companies advertised scales (along with other paraphernalia) to tuberculosis patients at the turn of the century, many must have been unable to purchase them. See Ott, *Fevered Lives*, pp. 87–99.

141. F. R. L. P. to LF Pennsylvania, November 4, 1909.

142. H. W. F. to LF, Connecticut, August 19, 1906.

143. H. W. F. to LF, Connecticut, August 23, 1906.

144. E. H. to LF, Pennsylvania, May 9, 1909.

145. A. M. W. to LF, March 24, 1910.

146. LF to J. H. H., Pennsylvania, August 23, 1907.

147. LF to S. L. L., Pennsylvania, January 26, 1909.

148. LF to M. W., Pennsylvania, June 26, 1907.

149. LF to H. W. F., Pennsylvania, August 22, 1906.

150. LF to H. D., Pennsylvania, January 11, 1907.

151. LF to G. P., Pennsylvania, July 19, 1916.

152. Brigitte Jordan, "Cosmopolitical Obstetrics: Some Insights from the Training of Traditional Midwives," *Social Science and Medicine* 28, no. 9 (1989): 925.

6. Negotiating Public Health Directives

1. All names in the cases in this chapter are pseudonyms. The case files of the New York Charity Organization Society are located in the Community Service Society Papers, Rare Book and Manuscript Library, Columbia University, New York. The case discussed in this section is case no. R2072, box 286. All quotations in this section, unless otherwise noted, are taken from this case file. For a full discussion of this case, see Emily K. Abel, "Hospitalizing Maria Germani," in *"Bad" Mothers: The Politics of Blame in Twentieth-Century America*, ed. Molly Ladd-Taylor and Lauri Umansky (New York: New York University Press, 1998), pp. 58–65.

2. Committee on the Prevention of Tuberculosis, New York Charity Organization Society, *The Need for Hospitals for New York's Consumptives* (New York: New York Charity Organization Society, 1911), p. 3.

3. Letter from J. F. to H. M. Johnson, n.d., filed with COS case no. R966, box 278, Community Service Society Papers.

4. David Arnold, *Colonizing the Body: State Medicine and Epidemic Disease in Nineteenth-Century India* (Berkeley: University of California Press, 1993), p. 7.

5. Sheila M. Rothman, *Living in the Shadow of Death: Tuberculosis and the Social Experience of Illness in American History* (New York: Basic Books, 1994), pp. 179–193.

6. Quoted in Allan M. Brandt, "AIDS: From Social History to Social Policy," in *AIDS: The Burdens of History*, ed. Elizabeth Fee and Daniel M. Fox (Berkeley: University of California Press, 1988), p. 149.

7. Naomi Rogers, *Dirt and Disease: Polio before FDR* (New Brunswick, N.J.: Rutgers University Press, 1992).

8. Charles E. Rosenberg, "The Bitter Fruit: Heredity, Disease, and Social Thought," in *No Other Gods: On Science and American Social Thought*, ed. Charles E. Rosenberg (Baltimore: Johns Hopkins University Press, 1976), p. 35.

9. See C.-E. A. Winslow, *The Life of Hermann Biggs, M.D., D.Sc., LL.D.: Physician and Statesman of the Public Health* (Philadelphia: Lea and Febiger, 1929), p. 132.

10. "East Side Vendors," *New York Times*, July 30, 1893.

11. Ellen N. LaMotte, "Tuberculosis Work of the Instructive Visiting Nurse Association of Baltimore," 1905 paper located at the New York Academy of Medicine, New York City. For an excellent discussion of white fears about African American household workers in Atlanta, see Tera W. Hunter, *To 'Joy My Freedom: Southern Black Women's Lives and Labors after the Civil War* (Cambridge, Mass.: Harvard University Press, 1997).

12. See Georgina D. Feldberg, *Disease and Class: Tuberculosis and the Shaping of Modern North American Society* (New Brunswick, N.J.: Rutgers University Press, 1995); Hunter, *To 'Joy My Freedom.*

13. *Boston Dispensary Quarterly* 2, no. 2 (Winter 1914): 9.

14. See Alisa Klaus, *Every Child a Lion: The Origins of Maternal and Infant Health Policy in the United States and France, 1890–1920* (Ithaca: Cornell University Press, 1993); Richard A. Meckel, *Save the Babies: American Public Health Reform and the Prevention of Infant Mortality, 1850–1929* (Baltimore: Johns Hopkins University Press, 1990), pp. 124–158.

15. New York Society for the Relief of the Ruptured and Crippled, *Sixth Annual Report of the Social Service Out-Patient Department October 1, 1918–September 30, 1919*, p. 15.

16. Massachusetts Charitable Eye and Ear Infirmary, *First Report of Social Service Work, October 1907–October 1908*, p. 10.

17. Lucy Cornelia Catlin, *The Hospital as a Social Agent in the Community* (Philadelphia: W. B. Saunders Co., 1918), p. 60.

18. COS case no. R2018, box 284, Community Service Society papers.

19. Barnes Hospital, St. Louis Children's Hospital, and Washington University Dispensary, *Annual Report of the Social Service Department*, July 1914, p. 22.

20. Edward F. Brown, Superintendent, Bureau of Welfare of School Children, Department of Social Welfare, New York Association for Improving the Condition of the Poor, "Lecture on Medical Inspection of School Children," 1914, box 50, file 325-2-C, Community Service Society Papers.

21. Josephine Baker, *Fighting for Life* (New York: Macmillan, 1939), p. 58.

22. Luella M. Erion, "Francesco of Arizona," *Public Health Nurse* 13, no. 4 (April 1921): 177.

23. Richard Cabot to Lillian Brandt, July 14, 1909, box 134, Community Service Society Papers.

24. See Linda M. Hunt et al., "Compliance and the Patient's Perspective: Controlling Symptoms in Everyday Life," *Culture, Medicine, and Psychiatry* 13 no. 3 (Spring 1989): 315–334.

25. Charles E. Rosenberg, "Making It in Urban Medicine: A Career in the Age of Scientific Medicine," in *Explaining Epidemics and Other Studies in the History of Medicine*, ed. Charles E. Rosenberg (New York: Cambridge University Press, 1992), p. 227.

26. See Hermann M. Biggs, *The Administrative Control of Tuberculosis* (New

York: New York City Department of Health, 1909); John S. Billings, Jr., *The Registration and Sanitary Supervision of Pulmonary Tuberculosis in New York City* (New York: New York City Department of Health, 1912); John Duffy, *A History of Public Health in New York City, 1866–1966* (New York: Russell Sage, 1974); Elizabeth Fee and Evelynn M. Hammonds, "Science, Politics, and the Art of Persuasion: Promoting the New Scientific Medicine in New York City," in *Hives of Sickness: Public Health and Epidemics in New York City,* ed. David Rosner (New Brunswick, N.J.: Rutgers University Press, 1995); Barron H. Lerner, "New York City's Tuberculosis Control Efforts: The Historical Limitations of the 'War on Consumption,'" *American Journal of Public Health* 83, no. 5 (May 1993): 758–768; Winslow, *Life of Hermann Biggs.*

27. See David S. Barnes, *The Making of a Social Disease: Tuberculosis in Nineteenth-Century France* (Berkeley: University of California Press, 1995); Barbara Bates, *Bargaining for Life: A Social History of Tuberculosis, 1876–1938* (Philadelphia: University of Pennsylvania Press, 1992); Linda Bryder, *Below Magic Mountain: A Social History of Tuberculosis in Twentieth-Century Britain* (New York: Oxford University Press, 1988).

28. On the charity organization movement, see Robert H. Bremner, *From the Depths: The Discovery of Poverty in the United States* (New York: New York University Press, 1964), pp. 51–57; Dawn Marie Greeley, "Beyond Benevolence: Gender, Class, and the Development of Scientific Charity in New York City, 1882–1935" (Ph.D. diss., State University of New York at Stony Brook, 1995); Michael B. Katz, *In the Shadow of the Poorhouse: A Social History of Welfare in America* (New York: Basic Books, 1986), pp. 103–109; James Leiby, *A History of Social Welfare and Social Work in the United States* (New York: Columbia University Press, 1978), pp. 112–127; Roy Lubove, *The Professional Altruist: The Emergence of Social Work as a Career, 1880–1930* (New York: Atheneum, 1980); Walter I. Trattner, *From Poor Law to Welfare State: A History of Social Welfare in America* (New York: Free Press, 1984), pp. 77–107; Joan Waugh, *Unsentimental Reformer: The Life of Josephine Shaw Lowell* (Cambridge, Mass.: Harvard University Press, 1997); Frank Dekker Watson, *The Charity Organization Movement in the United States: A Study in American Philanthropy* (New York: Macmillan, 1992); Kathleen Woodroofe, *From Charity to Social Work in England and the United States* (London: Routledge and Kegan Paul, 1962).

29. Quoted in Katz, *Shadow of the Poorhouse,* p. 69.

30. Lori D. Ginzberg, *Women and the Work of Benevolence: Morality, Politics, and Class in the Nineteenth-Century United States* (New Haven: Yale University Press, 1990), pp. 195–202. See also Elizabeth Lunbeck, *The Psychiatric Persuasion: Knowledge, Gender, and Power in Modern America* (Princeton: Princeton University Press, 1994), pp. 26–45.

31. Bremner, *From the Depths,* pp. 51–54; Katz, *Shadow of the Poorhouse,* p. 83.

32. Linda Gordon, *Heroes of Their Own Lives: The Politics and History of Family Violence* (New York: Penguin Books, 1988), p. 103.

33. Relief Committee, Committee on the Prevention of Tuberculosis, New York Charity Organization Society, *Home Treatment of Tuberculosis in New York City* (New York: New York Charity Organization Society, 1908), p. 1; S. Adolphus Knopf, *A History of the National Tuberculosis Association* (New York: National Tuberculosis Association, 1922).

34. *Charity Organization Society Bulletin,* January 24, 1917.

35. New York Charity Organization Society, *Thirty-fourth Annual Report*, October 1, *1915–September 30, 1916*, p. 5.

36. Cited in Community Service Society, "Educational Nursing Service—Educational Nursing for Family Health," 1948, p. 17, box No. 67, Community Service Society Papers.

37. See David Glassberg, "The Design of Reform: The Public Bath Movement in America," in *Sickness and Health in America: Readings in the History of Medicine and Public Health*, 3d edition, ed. Judith Walzer Leavitt and Ronald L. Numbers (Madison: University of Wisconsin Press, 1997), pp. 485–493.

38. New York Charity Organization Society, *Thirty-ninth Annual Report*, October 1, *1920–September 30, 1921*, p. 34.

39. Association of Tuberculosis Clinics and the Committee on the Prevention of Tuberculosis, New York Charity Organization Society, *Tuberculosis Families in Their Homes: A Study* (New York: New York Charity Organization Society, 1916), p. 25.

40. A physician employed in the New York City Department of Health noted that some working mothers locked children with whooping cough in the home. A. J. Dickson, "Social Service in Relation to Contagious Disease Hospitals," *Monthly Bulletin of the Department of Health, City of New York* 6, no. 1 (1916): 19–20.

41. COS case no. R630, box 265, Community Service Society Papers.

42. COS case no. R10, box 237.

43. See Eileen Boris, *Home to Work: Motherhood and the Politics of Industrial Homework in the United States* (New York: Cambridge University Press, 1994); Miriam Cohen, *Workshop to Office: Two Generations of Italian Women in New York City, 1900–1950* (Ithaca: Cornell University Press, 1992), p. 105.

44. On noncompliance with medical advice as a form of child neglect, see Gordon, *Heroes of Their Own Lives*, pp. 127–130.

45. Billings, *Registration and Sanitary Supervision*, pp. 7–8, 24.

46. In 1921 just eight people were removed from their homes to Riverside Hospital. Louis I. Harris, "Tuberculosis in New York City during 1921," *Monthly Bulletin of the Department of Health, City of New York* 11, no. 10 (October 1922): 235.

47. See Gordon, *Heroes of Their Own Lives*, p. 218.

48. See Susan A. Glenn, *Daughters of the Shtetl: Life and Labor in the Immigrant Generation* (Ithaca: Cornell University Press, 1990), pp. 57–58; David Nasaw, *Children of the City: At Work and at Play* (New York: Oxford University Press, 1985), pp. 10–11.

49. Rothman, *Living in the Shadow*, p. 185; Katz, *Shadow of the Poorhouse*, p. 83.

50. John S. Billings, Jr., *The Tuberculosis Clinics and Day Camps of the Department of Health*, Monograph Series, no. 2, New York City Department of Health (July 1912), pp. 42–45.

51. Relief Committee, *Home Treatment*, pp. 13–19.

52. COS, case no. R704, box 268, Community Service Society Papers.

53. COS, case no. R602, box 263.

54. See Bates, *Bargaining for Life*, p. 110.

55. *Monthly Bulletin of the Department of Health, City of New York* 11, no. 10 (October 1922): 251–252.

56. COS case no. R941, box 278, Community Service Society Papers.

57. Committee on the Prevention of Tuberculosis, New York Charity Organi-

zation Society, *Tuberculosis Hospital Situation, New York City, 1911* (New York: New York Charity Organization Society, 1911), p. 6.

58. Duffy, *Public Health in New York City*, pp. 184–185, 253.

59. Billings, *Registration and Sanitary Supervision*, p. 16.

60. Committee on the Prevention of Tuberculosis, *Need for Hospitals* p. 3.

61. COS case no. R367, box 254, Community Service Society Papers.

62. COS case no. R941, box 278.

63. COS case no. R974, box 279.

64. New York Charity Organization Society, *Twenty-fourth Annual Report, October 1, 1905–September 30, 1906*, p. 102.

65. COS case no. R901, box 276.

66. Board of Health of the New York City Department of Health, *Annual Report for the Year Ending December 31, 1906* (New York: Martin B. Brown, 1907), p. 465.

67. COS case no. R52, box 260.

68. COS case no. R693, box 268.

69. COS case no. R52, box 240.

70. See COS case no. R728, box 270; Case no. R213, box 248.

71. COS case no. R142, box 245.

72. COS case no. R728, box 270.

73. COS case no. R299, box 252.

74. COS case no. R144, box 245.

75. COS case no. R719, box 269.

76. COS case no. R602, box 263.

77. COS case no. R806, box 273.

78. COS case no. R909, box 277.

79. Alfred F. Hess, "The Tuberculosis Preventorium," *Survey* 30, no. 22 (August 30, 1913): 666–668; Alfred F. Hess, "The Significance of Tuberculosis in Infants and Children," *Journal of the American Medical Association* 72, no. 2 (January 11, 1919): 83–88. See also Bates, *Bargaining for Life*, p. 275; Winslow, *Life of Hermann Biggs*, p. 224.

80. Hess, "Tuberculosis Preventorium," 667.

81. Ibid.

82. Ibid.

83. Hess, "Significance of Tuberculosis," 87.

84. Ibid.

85. COS case no. R733, box 270, Community Service Society Papers.

86. COS case no. R213, box 248.

87. COS case no. R840, box 274.

88. COS case no. R974, box 279.

89. COS case no. R728, box 270.

7. Caregiving during the Great Depression

1. Rosemary Stevens, *American Medicine and the Public Interest* (New Haven: Yale University Press, 1971).

2. Technical Committee on Medical Care, *The Need for a National Health Pro-*

gram (Washington, D.C.: Interdepartmental Committee to Coordinate Health and Welfare Activities, 1938), p. 27.

3. See Henry F. Dowling, *City Hospitals: The Undercare of the Underprivileged* (Cambridge, Mass.: Harvard University Press, 1982).

4. Paul Starr, *The Social Transformation of American Medicine: The Rise of a Sovereign Profession and the Making of a Vast Industry* (New York: Basic Books, 1982), p. 271.

5. Michael R. Grey, *New Deal Medicine: The Rural Health Programs of the Farm Security Administration* (Baltimore: Johns Hopkins University Press, 1998).

6. Starr, *Social Transformation*, pp. 134–140.

7. See Allan M. Brandt, "Racism and Research: The Case of the Tuskegee Syphilis Study," in *Sickness and Health in America: Readings in the History of Medicine and Public Health*, 3d edition, ed. Judith Walzer Leavitt and Ronald L. Numbers (Madison: University of Wisconsin Press, 1997), pp. 392–404.

8. Rosemary Stevens, *In Sickness and in Wealth: American Hospitals in the Twentieth Century* (New York: Basic Books, 1989), pp. 137–138.

9. Cited in Edward H. Beardsley, *History of Neglect: Health Care for Blacks and Mill Workers in the Twentieth-Century South* (Knoxville: University of Tennessee Press, 1987), p. 170.

10. See Ruth M. Raup, *The Indian Health Program from 1800 to 1955* (Washington, D.C.: U.S. Department of Health, Education, and Welfare, 1959).

11. Records of the Children's Bureau, 1929–1940, RG 102, central files, National Archives, Washington, D.C. Approximately one-fifth are summaries, not actual letters.

12. See Hilary Graham, "Providers, Negotiators, and Mediators: Women as the Hidden Carers," in *Women, Health, and Healing: Toward a New Perspective*, ed. Ellen Lewin and Virginia Olesen (New York: Tavistock, 1985), pp. 25–52.

13. See Mimi Abramowitz, *Regulating the Lives of Women: Social Welfare Policy from Colonial Times to the Present* (Boston: South End Press, 1988).

14. Mrs. E. K. to Franklin D. Roosevelt (hereafter abbreviated as FDR), Pennsylvania, February 1938, file 4-5-9-2, Children's Bureau Records.

15. Mrs. C. H. B. to FDR, Arkansas, May 1939, file 4-9-1-1.

16. Mrs. L. C. to Eleanor Roosevelt (hereafter abbreviated as ER), Michigan, January 25, 1939, file 4-9-1-1.

17. Mr. J. D. to ER, West Virginia, March 3, 1940, file 4-9-1-1.

18. See Frances Fox Piven and Richard A. Cloward, *Regulating the Poor* (New York: Pantheon, 1971).

19. Mr. A. M. to Children's Bureau, West Virginia, November 20, 1939, file 4-9-1-1.

20. Mrs. R. W. to FDR, Minnesota, January 31, 1940, file 4-9-1-1.

21. Mrs. J. L. to FDR, New York, July 20, 1939, file 4-9-1-1.

22. Mrs. E. D. V. to ER, Louisiana, March 1939, file 4-9-1-1.

23. Mrs. K. G. to FDR, Missouri, May 11, 1939, file 4-9-1-1.

24. Mrs. C. C. to FDR, Washington, February 21, 1938, file 4-5-5-4.

25. Mrs. Z. M. to ER, California, August 1, 1940, file 4-9-1-1.

26. Mrs. L. R. P. to ER, Ohio, February 14, 1940, file 4-9-1-1.

27. Mrs. R. F. to ER, Illinois, August 6, 1939, file 4-9-1-1.

28. Mrs. V. P. to FDR, Texas, February 15, 1939, file 4-9-1-1.

29. See Linda Gordon, "The New Feminist Scholarship on the Welfare State," in *Women, the State, and Welfare,* ed. Linda Gordon (Madison: University of Wisconsin Press, 1990), p. 5; Arnlaug Leira, "Coping with Care: Mothers in a Welfare State," in *Gender and Caring: Work and Welfare in Britain and Scandinavia,* ed. Claire Ungerson (New York: Harvester Wheatsheaf, 1990), p. 155; Frances Fox Piven, "Ideology and the State: Women, Power, and the Welfare State," in *Women, the State, and Welfare,* ed. Gordon pp. 250–265.

30. Mrs. F. H. to ER, Idaho, February 16, 1940, file 4-9-1-1, Children's Bureau Records.

31. Mrs. R. L. H. to Children's Bureau, Tennessee, April 15, 1935, file 7-5-4.

32. Mrs. R. W. D. to ER, Ohio, August 1939, file 7-5-3.

33. Mrs. E. D. to ER, Pennsylvania, November 10, 1939, file 4-9-1-1.

34. Mrs. M. B. K. to Children's Bureau, California, August 16, 1939, file 4-9-1-1.

35. See Joan C. Tronto, *Moral Boundaries: A Political Argument for an Ethic of Care* (New York: Routledge, 1993), p. 142–143.

36. For the changes that occurred in the Children's Bureau during the early 1930s, see Robyn Muncy, *Creating a Female Dominion in American Reform, 1890–1935* (New York: Oxford University Press, 1991); Kriste Lindenmeyer, *"A Right to Childhood": The U.S. Children's Bureau and Child Welfare, 1912–46* (Urbana: University of Illinois Press, 1997).

37. Because of the nature of the records, it is impossible to determine what proportion of the total these cases represented.

38. Mrs. P. B. to State Board of Health, Missouri, May 23, 1938, file 4-9-1-1, Children's Bureau Records.

39. H. R. Perkins to R. W. Ball, August 21, 1940, file 4-9-1-1 (attached to letter of Mrs. J. S. O. to FDR, South Carolina, August 7, 1940).

40. Ball to Perkins, August 22, 1940, file 4-9-1-1.

41. Ball to Jessie M. Bierman, September 23, 1940, file 4-9-1-1.

42. Margery J. Lord to G. M. Cooper, February 6, 1940, file 4-9-1-1 (attached to letter of Miss T. A. to ER, North Carolina, January 22, 1940).

43. R. C. Kash to Clara E. Hayes, March 27, 1940 file 4-9-1-1 (attached to letter of Miss E. D. B. to FDR, Tennessee, March 1940).

44. Mrs. M. B. to ER, West Virginia, November 16, 1938, file 4-9-1-1.

45. J. H. Thornbury to Thomas W. Nale, December 8, 1938, file 4-9-1-1 (attached to letter of Mrs. M. B. to ER, West Virginia, November 16, 1938).

46. For the attitudes of middle-class Americans toward the spending patterns of low-income people during the Depression, see Winifred D. Wandersee, *Women's Work and Family Values, 1920–1940* (Cambridge, Mass.: Harvard University Press, 1981), pp. 27–54.

47. Mrs. R. K. G. to ER, New York, January 27, 1939, file 4-9-1-1.

48. Winifred Bell, *Aid to Dependent Children* (New York: Columbia University Press, 1965).

49. See Robert Stevens and Rosemary Stevens, *Welfare Medicine in America: A Case Study of Medicaid* (New York: Free Press, 1974).

50. Margaret M. Devine to Mary S. Labaree, April 24, 1939, file 4-9-1-1 (attached to letter of Mrs. R. L. to FDR, Kentucky, April 7, 1939), Children's Bureau Records.

51. Mayme Penn to Edwin H. Schorer, May 25, 1939, file 4-9-1-1 (attached to letter of Mrs. K. G. to FDR, Missouri, May 11, 1939).

52. Rosalind Whittemore to Mary E. Milburn, January 7, 1938, file 4-9-1-1 (attached to letter of Mr. A. M. to Children's Bureau, South Dakota, December 27, 1937).

53. Ellen C. Potter to Agnes K. Hanna, August 27, 1938, file 7-6-1-2 (attached to letter of Mrs. A. W. O. to ER, New Jersey, August 16, 1938).

54. L. D. Abernathy to Maude M. Gerdes, September 27, 1940, file 4-9-1-1 (attached to letter of Mrs. S. H. D. to ER, Mississippi, August 29, 1940).

55. See Gordon, "New Feminist Scholarship."

56. See Thomas Biolsi, *Organizing the Lakota: The Political Economy of the New Deal on the Pine Ridge and Rosebud Reservations* (Tucson: University of Arizona Press, 1992); Laurence M. Hauptman, *The Iroquois and the New Deal* (Syracuse: Syracuse University Press, 1981); Donald L. Parman, *The Navajos and the New Deal* (New Haven: Yale University Press, 1976).

57. See Emily K. Abel and Nancy Reifel, "Interactions between Public Health Nurses and Clients on American Indian Reservations during the 1930s," *Social History of Medicine* 9, no. 1 (1996): 89–108; Karen Anderson, *Changing Woman: A History of Racial Ethnic Women in Modern America* (New York: Oxford University Press, 1996), pp. 17–91.

58. See John Adair, Kurt W. Deuschle, and Clifford R. Barnett, *The People's Health: Medicine and Anthropology in a Navajo Community* (Albuquerque: University of New Mexico Press, 1988), pp. 3–11; Catherine L. Albanese, *Nature Religion in America: From the Algonkian Indians to the New Age* (Chicago: University of Chicago Press, 1990), pp. 16–34; Stephen J. Kunitz, *Disease Change and the Role of Medicine: The Navajo Experience* (Berkeley: University of California Press, 1983), pp. 118–145; Virgil J. Vogel, *American Indian Medicine* (Norman: University of Oklahoma Press, 1970), pp. 13–35.

59. See Lynn Gray, "Making the Spirit Whole: An Interview with Clara Sue Kidwell," *East West* no. 16 (November 1986): 46–47; Duane Champagne, ed., *The Chronicle of Native North American History* (Detroit: Gale Research, 1994); L. S. Kemnitzer, "Research in Health and Healing on the Plains," in *Anthropology on the Great Plains*, ed. W. Raymond Wood and Margot P. Liberty (Lincoln: University of Nebraska Press, 1980), pp. 272–283; Kunitz, *Disease Change*, pp. 118–123.

60. For information on federal public health activity on American Indian reservations, see Todd Benson, "Race, Health, and Power: The Federal Government and American Indian Health, 1909–1955" (Ph.D. diss., Stanford University, 1993); D. Putney, "Fighting the Scourge: American Indian Morbidity and Federal Indian Policy, 1897–1928" (Ph.D. diss., Marquette University, 1980); Francis Paul Prucha, *The Great Father: The United States Government and the American Indians*, vol. 11 (Lincoln: University of Nebraska Press, 1984), pp. 841–864; Raup, *Indian Health Program*.

61. "Questionnaire, Nursing Personnel Originals," Brown, Bahl, and Watson Collection, Cline Library, Northern Arizona University. This collection consists of the written responses to interviews conducted during the 1970s with nurses previously employed by the Office of Indian Affairs. Ida Bahl, herself a former nurse, sent questionnaires to all nurses whose names she was able to obtain. Forty-eight responded. Many not only answered the specific questions she posed but also sent long letters describing their experiences. For further information on the field

nurses, see Emily K. Abel, "'We Are Left So Much Alone to Work Out Our Own Problems': Nurses on American Indian Reservations during the 1930s," *Nursing History Review* no. 4 (1996): 43–64.

62. The monthly and annual reports of the field nurses are located in the Records of the Bureau of Indian Affairs, RG 75, file E779, National Archives, Washington, D.C. Individual reports are identified by the nurse's name, the name of the agency where she was stationed, and the date.

63. The interviews lasted between one and two hours and were tape-recorded and transcribed. The primary interviewer was Nancy Reifel, a dentist employed by the Indian Health Service and a member of the Rosebud Sioux. Reifel was familiar with the population and geographical area and previously had conducted a community-based survey of elderly Sioux reservation residents at these locations. She was accompanied by Phoebe Little Thunder, a Pine Ridge Sioux resident of Rosebud Reservation, who located respondents and transcribed and translated the interviews. Although all but one of the interviews were conducted in English, many respondents used occasional Lakota words. For more information about the results of these interviews, see Abel and Reifel, "Interactions."

64. Eva Harting, "Monthly Report," Tongue River Agency, Montana, August 1933, Records of the Bureau of Indian Affairs.

65. Nettie Johnston Story, "Monthly Report," Carson Agency, Montana, August 1933.

66. M. Gertrude Sturges, "Monthly Report," Say-nos-tee, June 1935.

67. Ruth I. Peffley, "Monthly Report," Browning, Montana, April 1934.

68. Margaret Mary Schorn, "Monthly Report," Tulalip Agency, Washington, April 1933.

69. Brookings Institution, *The Problem of Indian Administration: Report of a Survey* (Baltimore: Johns Hopkins University Press, 1928), p. 204.

70. Ibid., p. 201.

71. Sarah Smith, "Monthly Report," Pine Ridge, South Dakota, August 1932.

72. Raup, *Indian Health Program*, p. 30.

73. Anna A. Perry, "Monthly Report," Lac du Flambeau, Wisconsin, September 1933.

74. Zelma Butcher, "Monthly Report," Pine Ridge, South Dakota, August 1934.

75. Brookings, *Indian Administration*, p. 290.

76. Ibid., pp. 223–224.

77. Ruth Riss Seawright to Virginia Brown and Ida Bahl, January 20, 1978, Brown, Bahl, and Watson Collection.

78. "Annual Report of the Phoenix Indian Sanatorium," July 1, 1935, Records of the Bureau of Indian Affairs, RG 75, National Archives, Pacific-Southwest region, Laguna Niguel, California.

79. Response of Carrie M. Brilstra, "Questionnaire, Nursing Personnel Originals," Brown, Bahl, and Watson Collection.

80. Margaret Mary Schorn, "Monthly Report," Tulalip Agency, Washington, April 1933, Records of the Bureau of Indian Affairs, National Archives, Washington, D.C.

8. *"Very Dear to My Heart"*

1. The letters between Mrs. Carter and Julia Lathrop are located among the Records of the Children's Bureau, 1914–1921, RG 102, central files, file 4-7-0-3, National Archives, Washington, D.C. All names in the cases in this chapter are pseudonyms. I published the full correspondence in the *Journal of Women's History* 5, no. 1 (Spring 1993): 79–88.

2. Carter to Lathrop, January 20, 1915.

3. Carter to Lathrop, July 28, 1914.

4. Carter to Lathrop, July 28, 1914.

5. Carter to Lathrop, July 28, 1914.

6. Carter to Lathrop, July 28, 1914.

7. Carter to Lathrop, July 28, 1914.

8. Ellen Dwyer, "Stories of Epilepsy, 1880–1930," in *Framing Disease: Studies in Cultural History*, ed. Charles E. Rosenberg and Janet Golden (New Brunswick, N.J.: Rutgers University Press, 1992), p. 255; Philip M. Ferguson, *Abandoned to Their Fate: Social Policy and Practice toward Severely Retarded People in America, 1820–1920* (Philadelphia: Temple University Press, 1994), p. 86.

9. Association for the Improvement of the Condition of the Poor, "A Brief for Adequate Appropriations for the Completion of Lechtworth Village," 1912, box 34, folder 274.8, Community Service Society Papers, Rare Book and Manuscript Library, Columbia University, New York.

10. Joan Gittens, *Poor Relations: The Children of the State in Illinois, 1818–1990* (Urbana: University of Illinois Press, 1994), p. 181.

11. Quoted in ibid.

12. James W. Trent, Jr., *Inventing the Feeble Mind: A History of Mental Retardation in the United States* (Berkeley: University of California Press, 1994), p. 175.

13. Cited in Dwyer, "Stories of Epilepsy," p. 257.

14. Association for the Improvement of the Condition of the Poor, "Brief for Adequate Appropriations."

15. K. B. Weeks to Hon. Thaddeus C. Sweet, May 1, 1914, file 274.8, box 43, Community Service Society Papers.

16. Dwyer, "Stories of Epilepsy," pp. 258–259; Ferguson, *Abandoned to Their Fate*, p. 108; Mark Friedberger, "The Decision to Institutionalize Families with Exceptional Children in 1900," *Journal of Family History* (Winter 1981): 408; Stephen Jay Gould, *The Mismeasure of Man* 6 (New York: W. W. Norton, 1981), pp. 158–173.

17. Cited in Trent, *Inventing the Feeble Mind*, p. 168.

18. See Alan M. Kraut, *Silent Travelers: Germs, Genes, and the "Immigrant Menace"* (New York: Basic Books, 1994), pp. 73–75; Trent, *Inventing the Feeble Mind*, pp. 168–169.

19. In a survey of 3,000 client families in 1916, the COS found 110 cases of feeblemindedness and 32 cases of epilepsy. New York Charity Organization Society, *Thirty-fourth Annual Report, October 1, 1915–September 30, 1916*, p. 5. In 1925 the agency reported, "Mental disease or defectiveness, diagnosed or suspected, was a problem in 32 percent of the total number of families." New York Charity Organization Society, *Forty-third Annual Report, October 1, 1924–September 30, 1925*, p. 12.

20. COS case no. R745, box 270, Community Service Society Papers, Rare Book and Manuscript Library, Columbia University, New York.

21. COS case no. R747, box 270.

22. Dwyer, "Stories of Epilepsy," pp. 248–272.

23. Gittens, *Poor Relations*, p. 196.

24. COS case no. R102, box 243, Community Service Society Papers.

25. See Trent, *Inventing the Feeble Mind*, pp. 28, 68. A committee formed to investigate charges of brutality in 1915 failed to substantiate the charges but nevertheless concluded that inmates were "insufficiently housed in old buildings" and "cared for in large part by poorly paid attendants." New York State Board of Charities, *Report of the Special Committee Appointed in Compliance with a Joint Resolution of the Legislature, Adopted April 1, 1915, to Investigate Alleged Conditions at the New York City Children's Hospitals and Schools at Randall's Island*, (Albany: J. B. Lyon, 1915), p. 5.

26. COS case no. R655, box 266, Community Service Society Papers.

27. COS case no. R732, box 270.

28. Social Service Department of the Massachusetts General Hospital, *Thirteenth Annual Report, January 1, 1918–January 1, 1919*, p. 18.

29. Cited in Ferguson, *Abandoned to Their Fate*, pp. 144–45.

30. Ellen Dwyer, *Homes for the Mad: Life Inside Two Nineteenth-Century Asylums* (New Brunswick, N.J.: Rutgers University Press, 1987), pp. 164–165.

31. Gittens, *Poor Relations*, pp. 198–200; Trent, *Inventing the Feeble Mind*, pp. 184–224.

32. See Seymour B. Sarason, *The Making of an American Psychologist: An Autobiography* (San Francisco: Jossey-Bass, 1988), p. 142.

33. Agnes K. Hanna to Mrs. L. J. G., Ohio, December 22, 1939, file 7-6-1-3, Children's Bureau Records.

34. P. L. Dodge to Archer Smith, June 29, 1933, file 7-6-1-2 (attached to letter of Mrs. A. K. to Children's Bureau, Florida, February 11, 1933).

35. Trent, *Inventing the Feeble Mind*, p. 187.

36. Mrs. N. H. to Franklin D. Roosevelt (hereafter abbreviated as FDR), Illinois, February 5, 1935, file 4-12-1-1.

37. Mrs. S. M. B. to Children's Bureau, Pennsylvania, May 18, 1930, file 7-6-1-3.

38. Hanna to N. P., New Jersey, January 26, 1939, file 7-6-1-3.

39. Peter L. Tyor and Leland V. Bell, *Caring for the Retarded in America: A History* (Westport, Conn.: Greenwood Press, 1984), p. 139.

40. No southern state institution admitted African Americans until Virginia opened a segregated facility in 1929. Steven Noll, *Feeble-Minded in Our Midst: Institutions for the Mentally Retarded in the South, 1900–1940* (Chapel Hill: University of North Carolina Press, 1995), pp. 94–95.

41. Florentine Hackbusch to Mrs. A. C., September 8, 1939, file 7-6-1-0 (attached to letter of Mrs. A. C. to FDR, Pennsylvania, September 1939), Children's Bureau Records.

42. Hackbusch to Kathryn Welch, September 8, 1939, file 7-6-1-0.

43. "Report of Superintendent of Public Welfare of Sampson County," quoted in letter from Lily E. Mitchell to Hanna, July 12, 1938, file 7-6-1-0 (attached to

letter of Mrs. P. H. G. to Eleanor Roosevelt (hereafter abbreviated as ER), North Carolina, June 1938).

44. Mrs. E. H. M. to Children's Bureau, Texas, June 14, 1932, file 4-5-9.

45. Mrs. W. T. E. to Children's Bureau, Missouri, January 14, 1931, file 4-12-3-1.

46. Mrs. C. to Children's Bureau, September 4, 1935, file 4-12-3-1.

47. Some letter writers wanted medical care such as hospitalization, surgery, medicine, or physicians' services. I do not discuss this group here because their concerns were similar to those of the mothers examined in Chapter 7.

48. Mrs. G. L. to ER, New York, November 20, 1940, file 7-6-1-2.

49. Mrs. L. G. to Children's Bureau, Missouri, September 6, 1939, file 7-6-1-0.

50. Mrs. W. E. M. to Children's Bureau, North Carolina, April 15, 1932, file 7-6-1-2.

51. N. A. T. to ER, November 1938, file 7-6-1-0-0.

52. L. M. to ER, April 1938, file 7-6-1-3.

53. Mrs. R. W. to FDR, Arizona, May 4, 1939, file 7-6-1-2.

54. See Friedberger, "Decision to Institutionalize," 399.

55. Mrs. M. H. to ER, New Mexico, August 24, 1940, file 7-5-2.

56. Mrs. B. B. M. to ER, New York, October 12, 1939, file 7-16-1-2.

57. Quoted in Noll, *Feeble-Minded*, p. 135.

58. Trent, *Inventing the Feeble Mind*, p. 158.

59. Mrs. K. L. B. to Children's Bureau, Vermont, December 30, 1936, file 4-12-1-1.

60. Mrs. W. L. A. to Children's Bureau, Pennsylvania, January 25, 1934, file 4-12-1-1.

61. Rita Charon, "To Build a Case: Medical Histories as Traditions in Conflict," *Literature and Medicine* 11, no. 1 (Spring 1992): 118.

62. Mrs. H. D. B. to Children's Bureau, Maine, July 27, 1933, file 4-12-1-4.

63. Mrs. E. H. M. to Children's Bureau, Texas, June 14, 1932, file 4-5-9.

64. Mrs. A. W. I. to Children's Bureau, Vermont, January 7, 1936, file 4-12-1-1.

65. Mrs. B. L. M. to ER, New Jersey, February 19, 1940, file 7-6-1-3.

66. Mrs. S. E. M. to Children's Bureau, New York, June 25, 1936, file 4-12-1-1.

67. Lorraine Code, "Taking Subjectivity into Account," in *Feminist Epistemologies*, ed. Linda Alcoff and Elizabeth Potter (New York: Routledge, 1993), p. 17.

68. Paula S. Fass, *Outside In: Minorities and the Transformation of American Education* (New York: Oxford University Press, 1989), p. 47.

69. Mrs. S. M. B. to Grace Abbott, Pennsylvania, May 18, 1930, file 7-6-1-3, Children's Bureau Records.

70. Mrs. W. L. B. to ER, Kentucky, September 9, 1936, file 4-12-2-3.

71. Paul Starr, *The Social Transformation of American Medicine: The Rise of a Sovereign Profession and the Making of a Vast Industry* (New York: Basic Books, 1982), pp. 136–138.

72. Mrs. H. D. B. to Children's Bureau, Maine, July 27, 1933, file 4-12-1-4.

73. Mrs. S. M. B. to Grace Abbott, Pennsylvania, May 18, 1930, file 7-6-1-3.

74. Mrs. V. B. to FDR, California, February 13, 1940, file 7-6-1-3.

75. Mrs. R. E. to FDR, Alabama, April 26, 1938, file 7-6-1-3.

76. Mrs. H. M. to Children's Bureau, Tennessee, April 4, 1939, file 7-6-1-3.

77. Mrs. C. S. to ER, Pennsylvania, March 1937, file 7-6-1-2.

78. Mrs. A. M. to ER, New Jersey, January 7, 1938, file 7-6-1-3.

79. Mrs. A. W. I. to Children's Bureau, Vermont, January 7, 1936, file 4-12-1-1.

80. Mrs. N. R. to ER, New York, December 1939, file 7-6-2.

81. Mrs. I. F. to ER, New York, May 18, 1939, file 7-6-1-2.

82. Mrs. A. Y. to ER, December 28, 1938, file 7-6-1-3.

83. Faye D. Ginsburg and Rayna Rapp, "Introduction : Conceiving the New World Order," in *Conceiving the New World Order: The Global Politics of Reproduction,* ed. Faye D. Ginsburg and Rayna Rapp (Berkeley: University of California Press, 1997), p. 11.

84. Mrs. C. W. H. to FDR, Oklahoma, May 2, 1939, file 4-5-9.

85. Helen Featherstone, *A Difference in the Family: Living with a Disabled Child* (New York: Basic Books, 1980); Josh Greenfield, *A Child Called Noah* (San Diego: Harcourt Brace and Co., 1972); Greenfield, *A Client Called Noah* (New York: Henry Holt and Co., 1986); Greenfield, *A Place for Noah* (San Diego: Harcourt Brace Jovanovich, 1978); Barbara Hillyer, *Feminism and Disability* (Norman: University of Oklahoma Press, 1993).

86. Quoted in Noll, *Feeble-Minded,* p. 108.

87. COS case no. R102, box 243, Community Service Society Papers.

88. Gittens, *Poor Relations,* pp. 189–190.

89. Ibid., p. 190.

90. Sarason, *Making of an American Psychologist,* p. 147.

91. Patient case file no. 1045a, Craig Colony Records, New York State Archives, Albany, New York.

92. Patient case files no. 3132, no. 3189.

93. Benjamin W. Baker to Mary E. Milburn, New Hampshire, April 27, 1940, file 7-6-1-2, Children's Bureau Records.

94. Mrs. F. G. to Children's Bureau, New York, April 12, 1935, file 7-6-1-2.

95. See Ella Oppenheimer, M.D. to C. G. McGaffin, M.D., Washington, D.C., May 29, 1935, file 7-6-1-2.

96. Mrs. F. G. to Oppenheimer, New York, May 21, 1935, file 7-6-1-2.

97. Oppenheimer to Mrs. F. G., June 15, 1935, file 7-6-1-2.

98. Mrs. F. G. to Oppenheimer, New York, October 14, 1935, file 7-6-1-2.

99. Oppenheimer to Mrs. F. G., Washington, D.C., October 22, 1935, file 7-6-1-2.

100. Many of these file, however, are closed.

101. In this section I rely heavily on Ellen Dwyer's excellent essay, "Stories of Epilepsy, 1880–1930." See note 8 above.

102. Patient case file no. 3189, Craig Colony Records.

103. Patient case file no. 3142.

104. Quoted in Trent, *Inventing the Feeble Mind,* p. 134.

105. Patient case file no. 3158a.

106. Patient case file no. 3168.

107. Dwyer, "Stories of Epilepsy," pp. 250–265.

108. Patient case file no. 3217.

109. Patient case file no. 3178.

110. Patient case file no. 3132.

111. Patient case file no. 3218.

112. Patient case file no. 3184.

113. Patient case file no. 3184.

114. See patient case file no. 3189.

115. Patient case file no. 3184.

116. Patient case file no. 1045.

117. Patient case file no. 3127.

118. Patient case file no. 3127.

119. Patient case file no. 3155.

120. Patient case file no. 3132.

121. Patient case file no. 3189.

122. See Virginia Held, ed., *Justice and Care: Essential Readings in Feminist Ethics* (Boulder: Westview, 1995).

123. See Dwyer, "Stories of Epilepsy," p. 254.

124. Patient case file no. 321, Craig Colony Records.

125. Kathryn Montgomery Hunter, "Remaking the Case," *Literature and Medicine* 11, no. 1 (Spring 1992): 164.

126. Trent, *Inventing the Feeble Mind*, p. 114.

127. Patient case file no. 3178, Craig Colony Records.

128. See Gittens, *Poor Relations*, pp. 191–193; Trent, *Inventing the Feeble Mind*, pp. 119–127.

129. See Noll, *Feeble-Minded*, pp. 49–50.

130. See Ferguson, *Abandoned to Their Fate*, p. 148.

131. Patient case file no. 3143b, Craig Colony Records.

132. Quoted in Trent, *Inventing the Feeble Mind*, p. 113.

133. Patient case file no. 3142, Craig Colony Records.

134. During the early twentieth century, mothers' perspectives had little impact on public discourse. During the 1950s and 1960s, however, those attitudes found expression in social movements that dramatically transformed the care of all mentally disabled children.

9. "Like Ordinary Hearing Children"

1. For an excellent historical analysis of the oralist campaign, see Douglas C. Baynton, *Forbidden Signs: American Culture and the Campaign against Sign Language* (Chicago: University of Chicago Press, 1996).

2. Ibid., p. 145.

3. See ibid., p. 5; Oliver Sacks, *Seeing Voices: A Journey into the World of the Deaf* (New York: Harper Perennial, 1990), pp. 28, 142.

4. Sacks, *Seeing Voices*, p. 28.

5. Baynton, *Forbidden Signs*, p. 5.

6. See Harlan Lane, *The Mask of Benevolence: Disabling the Deaf Community* (New York: Alfred A. Knopf, 1992); Carol Padden and Tom Humphries, *Deaf in America: Voices from a Culture* (Cambridge, Mass.: Harvard University Press, 1988); Sacks, *Seeing Voices*.

7. Baynton, *Forbidden Signs*, p. 25.

8. Quoted in ibid., p. 6.

9. Baynton, *Forbidden Signs*, p. 102.

10. *Volta Review* (hereafter cited as *VR*), October 1935, p. 594.

11. *VR*, January 1934, p. 60.

12. John Dutton Wright, *The Little Deaf Child: A Book for Parents* (New York: Wright Oral School, 1928). The Volta Bureau encouraged all mothers of deaf children to read this book.

13. Quoted in Baynton, *Forbidden Signs*, p. 67.

14. Baynton, *Forbidden Signs*, pp. 66–67; Joan Gittens, *Poor Relations: The Children of the State in Illinois, 1818–1990* (Urbana: University of Illinois Press, 1994), p. 201.

15. *VR*, January 1937, p. 18.

16. See Barbara Hillyer, *Feminism and Disability* (Norman: University of Oklahoma Press, 1993), pp. 73–77.

17. Quoted in Daniel J. Wilson, "Covenants of Work and Grace: Themes of Recovery and Redemption in Polio Narratives," *Literature and Medicine* 13, no. 1 (Spring 1994): 29.

18. Cited in Baynton, *Forbidden Signs*, p. 5.

19. See Leah Hager Cohen, *Train Go Sorry: Inside a Deaf World* (Boston: Houghton Mifflin, 1994), p. 118; Padden and Humphries, *Deaf in America*, pp. 51–52.

20. See *VR*, March 1935, p. 143.

21. *VR*, April 1939, p. 217.

22. *VR*, February 1939, p. 88.

23. *VR*, April 1939, p. 215.

24. *VR*, February 1939, p. 84; *VR*, April 1939, p. 215.

25. *VR*, January 1937, p. 22.

26. *VR*, September 1936, p. 515.

27. *VR*, February 1934, p. 93.

28. *VR*, April 1936, p. 209.

29. *VR*, May 1936, p. 280.

30. *VR*, July 1936, p. 402.

31. *VR*, August 1936, p. 519.

32. *VR*, September 1936, pp. 518–519.

33. *VR*, June 1937, p. 345.

34. Ibid., p. 346.

35. *VR*, March 1935, p. 143.

36. *VR*, June 1938, p. 337.

37. *VR*, August 1936, p. 456.

38. *VR*, May 1936, p. 282.

39. *VR*, December 1936, p. 708.

40. *VR*, July 1936, p. 436.

41. *VR*, January 1937, p. 19.

42. *VR*, April 1937, p. 217.

43. *VR*, November 1939, p. 650.

44. *VR*, January 1937, p. 18.

45. *VR*, May 1937, p. 282.

46. *VR*, March 1935, p. 143.

47. *VR*, December 1938, p. 697.

48. *VR*, December 1939, p. 698.

49. *VR*, January 1939, p. 21.

50. *VR*, March 1936, p. 146.

51. *VR*, August 1936, p. 452.

52. *VR*, March 1935, p. 197.

53. *VR*, October 1939, p. 602.

54. Ibid.

55. Sandra Lee Bartky, "Foucault, Femininity, and the Modernization of Patriarchal Power," in *Feminism and Foucault: Reflections on Resistance*, ed. Irene Diamond and Lee Quinby (Boston: Northeastern University Press, 1988), pp. 81–88.

56. *VR*, February 1939, p. 84.

57. *VR*, October 1939, p. 603.

58. *VR*, May 1936, p. 281.

Conclusion

1. U.S. Department of Commerce, *65+ in the United States*, Current Population Reports, P23–190 (Washington, D.C.: Government Printing Office, 1998), pp. 2–3.

2. See Richard M. Suzman, David P. Willis, and Kenneth G. Manton, eds., *The Oldest Old* (New York: Oxford University Press, 1992).

3. Department of Commerce, *65+ in the United States*, pp. 2–8.

4. R. I. Stone and P. Kemper, "Spouses and Children of Disabled Elders: How Large a Constituency for Long-Term Care Reform?" *Milbank Quarterly* 67, no. 2,3 (1989): 485–506.

5. P. Moen, J. Robison, and V. Fields, "Women's Work and Caregiving Roles: A Life Course Approach," *Journal of Gerontology: Social Sciences* 49, no. 4 (July 1994): S176–S187.

6. U.S. General Accounting Office, "Long-Term Care: Baby Boom Generation Presents Financing Challenges," testimony before the U.S. Senate Special Committee on Aging, statement of William J. Scanlon, March 9, 1998, p. 5.

7. Sixteen percent of people 65 to 74 living in the community need some type of practical assistance, compared to 47 percent of those 85 and over. U.S. Senate Special Committee on Aging, *Developments in Aging: 1989* (Washington, D.C.: Government Printing Office, 1989), p. 236.

8. Department of Commerce, *65+ in the United States*, pp. 3–14.

9. Ibid.

10. Ibid.

11. Pamela Doty et al., "Informal Caregiving," in *The Continuum of Long-Term Care: An Integrated Systems Approach*, ed. Connie Evashwick (Albany, N.Y.: Delmar Publishers, 1995), p. 130.

12. See Charlene Harrington et al., "A National Long-Term Care Program for the United States: A Caring Vision," *Journal of the American Medical Association* 266, no. 21 (December 4, 1991): 3024.

13. Cited in Nancy R. Hooyman and Judith Gonyea, *Feminist Perspectives on Family Care: Policies for Gender Justice* (Thousand Oaks, Calif.: SAGE, 1995), p. 1.

14. William J. Winslade, *Confronting Traumatic Brain Injury: Devastation, Hope, and Healing* (New Haven: Yale University Press, 1998), p. 41.

15. John M. Lorenz et al., "A Quantitative Review of Mortality and Developmental Disability in Extremely Premature Newborns," *Archives of Pediatric and Adolescent Medicine* 152 (May 1998): 425.

16. Cited in Hooyman and Gonyea, *Feminist Perspectives*, p. 81.

17. Gail M. Powell-Cope and Marie Annette Brown, "Going Public as an AIDS Family Caregiver," *Social Science and Medicine* 34, no. 5 (1992): 571–580; Victoria H. Raveis and Karolynn Siegel, "The Impact of Care Giving on Informal or Familial Care Givers," *AIDS Patient Care* 5, no. 1 (February 1991): 39–43; Barbara Schable et al., "Who Are the Primary Caretakers of Children Born to HIV-Infected Mothers? Results from a Multi-State Surveillance Project," *Pediatrics* 95, no. 4 (April 1995): 511–515; Heather A. Turner, Joseph A. Catania, and John Gagnon, "The Prevalence of Informal Caregiving to Persons with AIDS in the United States: Caregiver Characteristics and Their Implications," *Social Science and Medicine* 38, no. 11 (1994): 1543–1552.

18. R. I. Stone, L. Cafferata, and J. Sangl, "Caregivers of the Frail Elderly: A National Profile," *Gerontologist* 27, no. 5 (1987): 616–626.

19. See Hooyman and Gonyea, *Feminist Perspectives*, p. 267.

20. Quoted in Linda Crossman, Cecilia London, and Clemmie Barry, "Older Women Caring for Disabled Spouses: A Model for Supportive Services," *Gerontologist* 21, no. 5 (1981): 466. A study of parents of chronically ill and disabled children found that 30 percent received no assistance from relatives living outside the household, and 16 percent had no one to call in an emergency. James Knoll, "Being a Family: The Experience of Raising a Child with a Disability or Chronic Illness," in *Emerging Issues in Family Support*, ed. Valerie J. Bradley, James Knoll, and John M. Agosta (Washington, D.C.: American Association on Mental Retardation, 1992), p. 37.

21. See Powell-Cope and Brown, "Going Public," 571–580.

22. Quoted in Emily K. Abel, *Who Cares for the Elderly? Public Policy and the Experiences of Adult Daughters* (Philadelphia: Temple University Press, 1991), p. 159.

23. E. Richard Brown and Roberta Wyn, "Public Policies to Extend Health Care Coverage," in *Changing the U.S. Health Care System: Key Issues in Health Services, Policy, and Management*, ed. Ronald M. Andersen, Thomas H. Rice, and Gerald F. Kominski (San Francisco: Jossey-Bass, 1996), pp. 43–44.

24. Ibid., p. 44.

25. See B. C. Vladeck, *Unloving Care: The Nursing Home Tragedy* (New York: Basic Books, 1980).

26. Between 1947 and 1971, the program distributed a total of $3.7 billion. Paul Starr, *The Social Transformation of American Medicine: The Rise of a Sovereign Profession and the Making of a Vast Industry* (New York: Basic Books, 1982), p. 350.

27. Rosemary Stevens, *In Sickness and in Wealth: American Hospitals in the Twentieth Century* (New York: Basic Books, 1989), p. 220.

28. See Barbara Bowers, "Family Perceptions of Care in a Nursing Home," in *Circles of Care: Work and Identity in Women's Lives*, ed. Emily K. Abel and Margaret K. Nelson (Albany: State University of New York Press, 1990), pp. 178–189.

29. Amy Goldstein, "Ranks of Uninsured Americans Swelling," *Washington Post*, October 4, 1999, sec. A, p. 1.

30. General Accounting Office, "Long-Term Care," p. 2.

31. Katherine R. Levit et al., "National Health Expenditures, 1993," *Health Care Financing Review* 16 (Fall 1994): 247–294.

32. General Accounting Office, "Long-Term Care," p. 1; Pepper Commission, U.S. Bipartisan Commission on Comprehensive Health Care, *A Call for Action* (Washington, D.C.: Government Printing Office, 1990).

33. General Accounting Office, "Long-Term Care," pp. 9–10.

34. Ibid., p. 8.

35. See Steven P. Wallace, Emily K. Abel, and Pamela Stefanowicz, "Long-Term Care and the Elderly," in *Changing the U.S. Health Care System*, ed. Andersen, Rice, and Kominski, p. 183.

36. Ibid.

37. See Abel, *Who Cares for the Elderly?*, pp. 3–4.

38. Knott, "Being a Family," pp. 17, 51.

39. Lewin and Associates, *An Evaluation of the Medi-Cal Program's System for Establishing Reimbursement Rates for Nursing Homes*, report prepared for the Office of the Auditor General, State of California, 1987.

40. Alice M. Rivlin and Joshua M. Wiener, *Caring for the Disabled Elderly: Who Will Pay?* (Washington, D.C.: Brookings Institution, 1988).

41. Korbin Liu, Kenneth G. Manton, and B. Marzetta Liu, "Home Care Expenses for the Disabled Elderly," *Health Care Financing Review* 7, no. 2 (1985): 51–58; Nancy M. Kane, "The Home Care Crisis of the Nineties," *Gerontologist* 29, no. 1 (1989): 27.

42. See Abel, *Who Cares for the Elderly?*, pp. 131–148.

43. Starr, *Social Transformation*, p. 365.

44. A. B. Hatfield, "Families as Caregivers: A Historical Perspective," in *Families of the Mentally Ill: Coping and Adaptation*, ed. A. B. Hatfield and H. B. Lefley (New York: Guilford Press, 1987), p. 8.

45. Starr, *Social Transformation*, p. 365.

46. See Hooyman and Gonyea, *Feminist Perspectives*.

47. Although only 13 percent of Medicaid recipients are sixty-five or over, nursing homes consume 45 percent of the program's spending. Hooyman and Gonyea, *Feminist Perspectives*, p. 91.

48. Madonna Harrington Meyer and Michelle Kesterke Storbakken, "Shifting the Burden Back to Families? How Medicaid Cost-Containment Re-Shapes Access to Long-Term Care in the United States," in *Care Work: Gender, Labor, and Welfare States*, ed. Madonna Harrington Meyer (New York: Routledge, 2000).

49. J. Rhoades, "Nursing Homes—Structure and Selected Characteristics, 1987–1996," *Statistical Bulletin* (June 1998): 1–9.

50. Quoted in Meyer and Storbakken, "Shifting the Burden."

51. Katherine L. Kahn et al., "Comparing Outcomes of Care before and after Implementation of the DRG-Based Prospective Payment System," *Journal of the American Medical Association* 264, no. 15 (October 17, 1990): 1984–1988.

52. See James C. Robinson, "Decline in Hospital Utilization and Cost Inflation under Managed Care in California," *Journal of the American Medical Association* 276, no. 13 (October 2, 1996): 1060–1064; Eugene C. Nelson et al., "A Longitudinal Study of Hospitalization Rates for Patients with Chronic Disease: Results from the Medical Outcomes Study," *Health Services Research* 32, no. 6 (February 1998): 750–758.

53. John D. Arras and Nancy N. Dubler, "Introduction: Ethical and Social Implications of High-Tech Home Care," in *Bringing the Hospital Home: Ethical and Social Implications of High-Tech Home Care*, ed. John D. Arras (Baltimore: Johns Hopkins University Press, 1995), p. 12.

54. Jerry Adler, "Every Parent's Nightmare," *Newsweek*, March 16, 1987, p. 59.

55. Quoted in Sherry R. Schachter and Jimmie C. Holland, "Psychological,

Social, and Ethical Issues in the Home Care of Terminally Ill Patients: The Impact of Technology," in *Bringing the Hospital Home*, ed. Arras, p. 104.

56. Carroll L. Estes and Terry Arendell, "The Unsettled Future: Women and the Economics of Health and Aging" (paper presented at the conference "Who Cares for the Elderly? Caregiving in Women's Lives," University of California, Los Angeles, April 19, 1986), p. 18.

57. Quoted in Ian Fisher, "Families Provide Medical Care, Tubes and All," *New York Times* June 7, 1998, p. 31.

58. Fisher, "Families Provide Medical Care," p. 31.

59. See Arras and Dubler, "Introduction," pp. 1–31.

60. Cited in ibid., p. 10.

61. Peter T. Kilborn, "Nurses Put on Fast Forward in Rush for Cost Efficiency," *New York Times*, April 9, 1998, pp. 1, 23.

62. See Lucy Rose Fischer and Nancy N. Eustis, "DRGs and Family Care for the Elderly: A Case Study," *Gerontologist* 28, no. 3 (1988): 383–389; Suzanne Gordon, "The Impact of Managed Care on Female Caregivers in the Hospital and Home," *Journal of the American Medical Women's Association* 52, no. 2 (Spring 1997): 75–80.

63. Robert Zussman, *Intensive Care: Medical Ethics and the Medical Profession* (Chicago: University of Chicago Press, 1992), p. 88.

64. Cynthia B. Costello, Shari Miles, and Anne J. Stone, *The American Woman, 1999–2000* (New York: W. W. Norton, 1998), p. 265; Hooyman and Gonyea, *Feminist Perspectives*, p. 62.

65. Various studies report that between 23 and 32 percent of employees care for elderly people. See Margaret B. Neal et al., *Balancing Work and Caregiving for Children, Adults, and Elders* (Newbury Park, Calif.: SAGE, 1993).

66. See Andrew E. Scharlach, "Caregiving and Employment: Competing or Complementary Roles?" *Gerontologist* 34, no. 3 (1994): 378–385.

67. Quoted in Abel, *Who Cares for the Elderly?*, p. 127.

68. See Scharlach, "Caregiving and Employment."

69. Susan A. Stephens and Jon B. Christianson, *Informal Care of the Elderly* (Lexington, Mass.: Lexington Books, 1986); Stone, Cafferata, and Sangl, "Caregivers."

70. R. J. V. Montgomery, "Respite Care: Lessons from a Controlled Design Study," *Health Care Financing Review*, Annual Supplement (1988): 133–138; Steven P. Wallace, "The No-Care Zone: Availability, Accessibility, and Acceptability in Community-Based Long-Term Care," *Gerontologist* 30, no. 2 (1990): 254–261. Respite programs take the form of either homemaker services and health care in the home or adult day care and foster care homes in the community.

71. See Hooyman and Gonyea, *Feminist Perspectives*, pp. 201, 204, 276–278; Fisher, "Families Provide Medical Care," p. 30.

72. B. O. Burwell, *Shared Obligations: Public Policy Influences on Family Care for the Elderly*, Medicaid Program Evaluation Working Paper 2.1 (Washington, D.C.: Health Care Financing Administration, 1986).

73. Quoted in Naomi Gerstel and Katherine McGonagle, "The Limits of the Family and Medical Leave Act" (paper presented at the American Sociological Association Meeting, San Francisco, August 1998), p. 2.

74. See Hooyman and Gonyea, *Feminist Perspectives*, p. 226.

75. See ibid., pp. 70–71, 210–234.

76. See Abel, *Who Cares for the Elderly?*, pp. 165–176.

77. Margaret Forster, *Have the Men Had Enough?* (London: Penguin, 1990).

78. Abel, *Who Cares for the Elderly?*, p. 100.

79. Ibid., pp. 73–164.

80. Nancy Fraser and Linda Gordon, "'Dependency' Demystified: Inscriptions of Power in a Keyword of the Welfare State," *Social Politics* 1, no. 1 (Spring 1994): 6.

81. Ibid., 24.

82. David Arnold, "Introduction: Disease, Medicine, and Empire," in *Imperial Medicine and Indigenous Societies*, ed. David Arnold (Manchester, U.K.: Manchester University Press, 1988), p. 16.

83. Joan C. Tronto, *Moral Boundaries: A Political Argument for an Ethic of Care* (New York: Routledge, 1994), p. 134.

84. Nadine F. Marks, "Caregiving across the Lifespan: National Prevalence and Predictors," *Family Relations* 45 (January 1996): 27.

85. Judith M. Bennett, "Confronting Continuity," *Journal of Women's History* 9, no. 3 (Autumn 1997): 79.

86. Quoted in Hooyman and Gonyea, *Feminist Perspectives*, p. 122.

87. Stone, Cafferata, and Sangl, "Caregivers."

88. Raymond T. Coward and Eleanor Rathbone-McCuan, "Illuminating the Relative Role of Adult Sons and Daughters in the Long-Term Care of Their Parents" (paper presented at the Professional Symposium of the National Association of Social Workers, Chicago, November 1985); Stephens and Christianson, *Informal Care of the Elderly.*

89. Baila Miller, "Gender Differences in Spouse Management of the Caregiver Roles," in *Circles of Care*, ed. Abel and Nelson, pp. 92–104.

90. Evelyn Nakano Glenn, "From Servitude to Service Work: Historical Continuities in the Racial Division of Paid Reproductive Labor," *Signs* 18, no. 1 (Autumn 1992): 1–43.

91. Rebecca Donovan, "'We Care for the Most Important People in Your Life': Home Care Workers in New York City," *Women's Studies Quarterly* 17, no. 1, 2 (1989): 56–65.

92. Abel, *Who Cares for the Elderly?*, pp. 137–148.

93. Data from a government survey show that female caregivers employed as operatives and laborers are more likely than those employed in either professional/managerial positions or clerical/sales positions to take time off without pay. U.S. House Committee on Aging, Subcommittee on Human Services, *Exploding the Myths: Caregiving in America*, 1987, pub. no. 99-611.

94. Hilary Graham, "Caring: A Labour of Love," in *A Labour of Love: Women, Work, and Caring*, ed. Janet Finch and Dulcie Groves (London: Routledge and Kegan Paul, 1983), p. 16.

95. Clare Ungerson, *Policy Is Personal: Sex, Gender, and Informal Care* (London: Tavistock, 1987), p. 116.

96. See Patricia Hill Collins, "Black Women and Motherhood," in *Justice and Care: Essential Readings in Feminist Ethics*, ed. Virginia Held (Boulder: Westview, 1995), pp. 117–138.

97. See Abel, *Who Cares for the Elderly?*, pp. 62–63.

98. Rannveig Traustadottir, "Disability Reform and Women's Caring Work" (paper presented at the "International Conference on Gender, Citizenship, and the Work of Care," University of Illinois at Urbana-Champaign, November 14–16, 1997).

99. J. F. Gubrium and R. J. Lynott, "Measurement and the Interpretation of Burden in the Alzheimer's Disease Experience," *Journal of Aging Studies* 1, no. 3 (1987): 279.

100. Andrea Sankar, *Dying at Home: A Family Guide for Caregiving* (Baltimore: Johns Hopkins University Press, 1991), p. 1.

101. Ibid., p. 147.

102. Abel, *Who Cares for the Elderly?*, pp. 96–97.

103. Arras and Dubler, "Introduction," p. 20.

104. See Abel, *Who Cares for the Elderly?*, p. 172–173.

Index